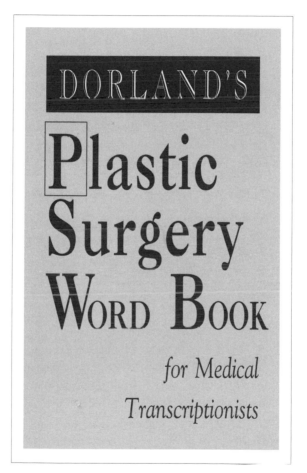

DORLAND'S

Plastic Surgery Word Book

for Medical Transcriptionists

DORLAND'S

Plastic Surgery
Word Book

for Medical Transcriptionists

Series Editor: **SHARON B. RHODES, CMT, RHIT**

Edited & Reviewed by: **Mary E. David, CMT**

W.B. SAUNDERS COMPANY

A Harcourt Health Sciences Company

Philadelphia London New York St. Louis Sydney Toronto

W.B. Saunders Company
A Harcourt Health Sciences Company

The Curtis Center
Independence Square West
Philadelphia, Pennsylvania 19106

Library of Congress Cataloging-in-Publication Data

Dorland's plastic surgery word book for medical transcriptionists / Sharon B. Rhodes, editor; edited & reviewed by Mary E. David.

p. cm.

ISBN 0-7216-9395-4

1. Surgery, Plastic—Terminology.   2. Medical transcription—
   Terminology.   I. Rhodes, Sharon B.   II. David, Mary, CMT.

RD118.D67 2002
617.9′5′014—dc21   2001034186

Dorland's Plastic Surgery Word Book for
Medical Transcriptionists   ISBN 0-7216-9395-4

Printed in the United States of America.

Last digit is the print number: 9 8 7 6 5 4 3 2 1

PREFACE

I am proud to present the *Dorland's Plastic Surgery Word Book for Medical Transcriptionists*—one of the ongoing series of word books being compiled for the professional medical transcriptionist. For over one hundred years, W.B. Saunders has published the *Dorland's Illustrated Medical Dictionary*. With the advent of medical transcription, it became the dictionary of choice for medical transcriptionists.

When I was approached in the fall of 1999 to help develop a new series of word books for W.B. Saunders, I have to admit the thought absolutely overwhelmed me. The *Dorland's Illustrated Medical Dictionary* was one of my first book purchases when I began my transcription career over thirty years ago. To be invited to participate in this project is an honor I could never have imagined for myself!

Transcriptionists need and will continue to need trusted up-to-date resources to help them research difficult terms quickly. In developing the *Dorland's Plastic Surgery Word Book for Medical Transcriptionists*, I had access to the entire Dorland's terminology database for the book's foundation. In addition to this immense database, a context editor, Mary David, CMT, a recognized leader in the field of medical transcription, was selected to review the material from the database, to contribute new and unique terms, and to remove outdated and obsolete ones. With Mary's extensive research and diligent work, I believe this to be the most up-to-date word book for the field of plastic surgery.

In developing the plastic surgery word book, I wanted the size to be manageable so the book would be easy to handle, provide a durable long-lasting binding, and use a type font large enough to read while providing extensive terminology.

Anatomical plates were added as well as identification of anatomical landmarks. Additionally, a list of the most frequently prescribed drugs has been included.

Although I have tried to produce the most thorough word book for plastic surgery available to medical transcriptionists, it is difficult to include every term as the field of medicine is constantly evolving. As you discover new terms, please feel free to share them with me for inclusion in the next edition of the *Dorland's Plastic Surgery Word Book for Medical Transcriptionists.*

I may be reached at the following e-mail address: Sharon@TheRhodes.com

SHARON B. RHODES, CMT, RHIT
Brentwood, Tennessee

Aarskog-Scott syndrome

abacterial

abatement

Abbe
  A. flap
  A. operation
  A. stage I cheiloplasty
  A. stage II cheiloplasty
  A.-Estlander cheiloplasty
  A.-Estlander flap
  A.-Estlander operation

Abbot paste

Abbreviated Injury Scale

ABC
  aneurysmal bone cyst
  avidin-biotin-peroxidase
     complex
  axiobuccocervical

abdomen
  globular a.
  patulous a.
  pendulous a.

abdominal
  a. adipose tissue
  a. apron
  a. axial subcutaneous flap
  a. axial subcutaneous pedi-
     cle flap
  a. binder
  a. contouring
  a. dermolipectomy
  a.-diaphragmatic respira-
     tion
  a. domain
  a. flaccidity
  a. lipectomy
  a. pannus
  a. sculpturing
  a. sequela
  a. wall flap
  a. wall insufficiency
  a. wall zones (1–4)
  a. washout
  a. zipper

abdominoperineal resection

abdominoplasty
  Callia a.
  endoscopically assisted a.
  fleur-de-lis a.
  French-line a.
  Grazer a.
  high lateral tension a.
  male a.
  mini-a.
  mini-tuck a.
  Mladick a.
  modified a.
  modified Weinhold a.
  muscle-access a.
  partial subfascial a.
  Pitanguy a.
  a. procedure
  Regnault a.
  T-excision a.
  W-a.

Abdopatch
  A. Gel Z Adhesive dressing
  A. Gel Z self-adhesive scar
     treatment

ABD pad

abduce

abducent
  a. nerve

abduction
  Gilbert stage shoulder a.
  radial a.

abductor
  a. hallucis flap
  a. hallucis muscle
  a. paralysis
  a. pollicis longus muscle

Abeli tenotomy scissors

Abernethy sarcoma

aberrant
  a. mongolian spot
  a. tissue

ABG
  axiobuccogingival
ABL
  axiobuccolingual
ablate
ablated skin
ablation
  laser a.
  procerus and corrugator a.
  tissue a.
  tumor a.
ablative procedure
ablution
abnormal
  a. frenulum attachment
  a. frenum attachment
  a. occlusion
abnormality
  cutaneous vascular a.
  maxillofacial a.
  tympanomastoid a.
Abocath catheter
abocclusion
aborad
aboral
Aboulker stent
above-elbow (AE) amputation
above-knee (AK) amputation
ABR
  anterior band remover
abradant
abrade
abrasion
  acid a.
  betel nut a.
  bobby pin a.
  cervical a.
  corneal a.

abrasion *(continued)*
  occupational a.
  a. resistance
  superficial a.
abrasive
  aluminum oxide a.
  diatomaceous silicon diox-
    ide a.
  a. disk
  FF a.
  FFF a.
  flint a.
  garnet a.
  iron oxide a.
  a. point
  quartz a.
  recrystallized kaolinite a.
  silicon carbide a.
  silicon dioxide a.
  sodium-potassium alumi-
    num silicate a.
  a. strip
  zirconium silicate a.
abrasiveness
abrasor
abscess
  acute a.
  apical a.
  Bezold a.
  bicameral a.
  buccal space a.
  canalicular a.
  chronic apical a.
  circumscribed a.
  cold a.
  collar-button a.
  dentoalveolar a.
  dorsal hand a.
  follicular a.
  glandular a.
  horseshoe a.
  inferior pole peritonsillar a.
  infraorbital space a.
  interradicular a.
  intramammary a.
  intramastoid a.
  lacrimal a.

abscess *(continued)*
 laryngeal a.
 lateral a.
 lateral alveolar a.
 mammary a.
 masseter a.
 mastoid a.
 metastatic a.
 midpalmar space a.
 milk a.
 Monro a.
 nasal septal a.
 nasopharyngeal a.
 orbital a.
 parapharyngeal space a.
 parotid gland a.
 Pautrier a.
 pericoronal a.
 periprosthetic breast a.
 peritoneal a.
 phlegmonous a.
 premammary a.
 primary a.
 pterygomandibular
  space a.
 radicular a.
 recrudescent a.
 recurrent cutaneous a.
 retrobulbar a.
 retromammary a.
 retroperitoneal a.
 retropharyngeal a.
 run-around a.
 satellite a.
 secondary a.
 stellate a.
 sterile a.
 stitch a.
 subaponeurotic a.
 submammary a.
 submandibular space a.
 submasseteric space a.
 submental space a.
 subperiosteal a.
 subperiosteal a. of frontal
  sinus
 subperiosteal orbital a.
  (SPOA)
 subperitoneal a.

abscess *(continued)*
 temporal fossa a.
 thenar space a.
 Tornwaldt a.
 traumatic a.
 vestibular a.
 von Bezold a.

absolute
 a. construction
 a. pocket
 a. quantity
 a. threshold

absorbable
 a. catgut
 a. gauze
 a. gelatin
 a. gelatin sponge
 a. suture

absorbefacient

absorbent
 a. paper point
 a. point

absorber
 hyCURE hydrolyzed pro-
  tein powder and exu-
  date a.

Absorb-its material

absorption
 a. lacuna
 x-ray a.

abutment
 Dalla Bona ball and
  socket a.
 multiple a.
 multirooted a.

AC
 axiocervical

acacia

acanthesthesia

acanthion

acantholysis

acanthoma
 basal cell a.

acanthoma *(continued)*
    clear cell a.

acanthomatous
    a. ameloblastoma
    a. pattern

acanthosis

acanthotic

accelerator
    Becker a.
    serum thrombotic a.
    a. tip

Accelerator II aspirator

accelerometer

Ac'cents permanent lash liner

access
    cavity a.
    a. flap in osseous surgery
    a. incision
    intraoral a.
    a. opening
    palatal a.
    piriform aperture a.
    a. preparation
    preparotid a.
    submental a.
    translabial a.

Access-Blocker

accessory
    a. cartilage of nose
    a. mammary tissue
    a. maxillary ostium
    a. maxillary sinus ostium
    a. nasal cartilage
    a. node
    a. ostium
    a. palatine canal
    a. sinuses of nose

ACCHN
    adenoid cystic carcinoma
    of head and neck

accident
    cochleovascular a.

accommodation

accordion graft

accretion line

Accu-line Products skin marker

Accu-Measure personal body
    fat tester

accuracy
    submillimetric a.
    a. timer

Accurate Surgical and Scientific
    Instruments (ASSI)

Accusate pulse oximeter

AccuSpan tissue expander

Accu-Spense cavity liner

Accustaple

Accutorr
    A. bedside monitor
    A. monitor

ACE
    autologous-cultured epithe-
    lium

ACE
    A. Autografter
    A. Autografter bone filter
    A. bone screw
    A. bone screw tack
    A. bone screw tacking kit
    A. cortical bone screw

Ace
    A. adherent bandage
    A. bandage
    A. elastic dressing
    A. wrap

ACE/Normed osteodistractor

acentric
    a. glide
    a. relation

acetate
    aluminum a. and acetic
    acid

acetic acid

acetylsalicylic acid (ASA)

Achilles tendon

achondroplasia

acid
    a. abrasion
    acetic a.
    acetylsalicylic a. (ASA)
    alpha-hydroxy a. (AHA)
        (*written also* alphahy-
        droxy acid)
    alpha hydroxy a. gel
    alpha hydroxyl a. (AHA)
    aluminum acetate and ace-
        tic a.
    aminocaproic a.
    arachidonic a.
    ascorbic a.
    azelaic a.
    bicinchoninic a. (BCA)
    boric a.
    carbolic a.
    caustic a.
    cevitamic a.
    citric a.
    glycolic a.
    Gly Derm alpha hydroxy a.
    Gly Derm glycolic a.
    hydrochloric a.
    kojic a.
    lactic a.
    retinoic a.
    salicylic a.
    tannic a.
    trichloroacetic a. (TCA)

acinar
    a. cell
    a. lumen

acinic
    a. cell carcinoma
    a. cell tumor

acinous cell carcinoma

acinus *pl.* acini
    serous a.

Ackerman
    A. bar joint
    A. lingual bar

Ackerman *(continued)*
    A.-Proffitt classification
    A.-Proffitt classification of
        malocclusion

Acland clamp

ACMI light source connector

acne
    a. albida
    a. artificialis
    a. atrophica
    a. cachecticorum
    a. ciliaris
    colloid a.
    comedo a.
    comedonal a.
    a. conglobata
    a. cosmetica
    cystic a.
    a. erythematosa
    a. fulminans
    a. hypertrophica
    a. indurata
    a. keloidalis
    a. keratosa
    a. miliaris
    miliary a.
    a. necrotica
    nodulocystic a.
    papular a.
    a. papulosa
    a. punctata
    pustular a.
    a. rosacea
    a. sebacea
    a. simplex
    a. tarsi
    a. urticata
    a. varioliformis
    a. vulgaris

acneform *(variant of* acneiform)

acnegenic

acneiform
    a. dermatitis
    a. eruption
    a. lesion

acorn carver

acousticofacial
   a. nerve
   a. nerve bundle

acousticopalpebral reflex

ACPS
   acrocephalopolysyndactyly

acquired
   a. cholesteatoma
   a. defect
   a. eccentric jaw relation
   a. nasopharyngeal stenosis

acral lentiginous melanoma

Acrel ganglion

acroangiodermatitis

acrocephalia

acrocephalopolysyndactyly
   (ACPS)

acrocephalosyndactylia (ACS)

acrocephalosyndactyly (ACS)
   type I a.
   type II a.

acrocephaly

acrochordon

acrodermatitis
   papular a.

acrodont

acrodynia

acrofacial
   a. dysostosis
   a. syndrome

acrokeratosis
   paraneoplastic a.
   a. paraneoplastica
   a. verruciformis
   a. verruciformis of Hopf

acrolect

acromegalic face

acromegaly

acromphalus

acropachy
   thyroid a.

acrosclerosis

acrospiroma
   eccrine a.

acrosyndactyly

Acrotorque hand engine

ACS
   acrocephalosyndactylia
   acrocephalosyndactyly

ACTH
   adrenocorticotropic hormone

actinic
   a. cheilitis
   a. damage
   a. keratosis
   a. skin changes

actinomycosis
   cervical a.
   cervicofacial a.

actinophytosis
   staphylococcal a.

action
   bacteriolytic a.
   calorigenic a.
   capillary a.
   centripetal a.
   rasping a.

activated
   a. dermis
   a. resin

active
   a. range of motion (AROM)

activity
   a's of daily living (ADL)
   enzyme a.

ACU-dyne

acuminate wart

acuminatum
   condyloma a.
   giant condyloma a.

Acuspot
   710 A.
   Sharplan Laser 710 A.

acute
   a. disseminated histiocyto-
      sis X
   a. hordeolum
   a. inflammation
   a. phase of burn injury
   a. radiation syndrome

AD
   anterior displacement

Adair
   A. breast clamp
   A. tenaculum

Adamount pocket mounts

Adams
   A. ball
   A. clasp
   A. crushing of nasal sep-
      tum
   A. ectropion operation
   A. otoplasty
   A. saw

Adam's apple

adaptation
   epithelial a.
   marginal a.

adapter (also spelled adaptor)
   a. band
   Luer-Lok a.
   power a.

Adaptic
   A. dressing
   A. gauze
   A. gauze packing

adaptive temporomandibular
   joint remodeling

adaptor (variant of adapter)

ADC
   axiodistocervical

ADD
   angled delivery device

Addison disease

adductor
   a. longus muscle
   a. magnus muscle
   a. paralysis
   a. pollicis

adenoadipose flap

adenocarcinoma
   annular a.
   a. in Barrett esophagus
   mucinous a.
   mucinous cell a.
   papillary a.
   pleomorphic a.

adenoid
   a. cancer
   a. cystic carcinoma
   a. cystic carcinoma of head
      and neck (ACCHN)
   a. face
   a. facies
   a. squamous cell carci-
      noma

adenolipoma

adenolipomatosis

adenoma
   apocrine a.
   basal cell a.
   basaloid monomorphic a.
      (BMA)
   canalicular a.
   Hürthle a.
   malignant a.
   malignant pleomorphic a.
   monomorphic a.
   mucinous a.
   oncocytic a.
   papillary cystic a.
   pleomorphic a.
   recurrent pleomorphic a.

adenoma *(continued)*
  salivary gland pleomor-
    phic a.
  sebaceous a.
  a. sebaceum
  sessile a.
  a. sudoriparum
  thyroid a.

adenomastectomy

adenomatosis
  a. oris

adenomatous

adenopapillary tumor

adenopathy
  scalene a.
  supraclavicular a.

adherence
  immune a.
  a. syndrome

adhesion
  flexor tendon a.
  sublabial a.
  takedown of a's
  tendon a's

adhesive
  Biobrane a.
  biologic fibrogen a.
  cyanoacrylate tissue a.
  hydroxyapatite a.
  Mammopatch gel self a.
  silicone a.
  Tisseel biologic fibrogen a.

adiadochokinesis

Adie syndrome

adipectomy

adipo aspirate

adipocyte

adipodermal graft

adipofascial
  a. axial pattern cross-finger
    flap

adipofascial *(continued)*
  a. flap
  a. sural flap
  a. sural flap procedure
  a. turnover flap

adipose
  a. layers of anterior abdom-
    inal wall
  a. tissue

adiposis
  a. dolorosa
  a. universalis

adipositas
  a. abdominis
  a. ex vacuo

adipositis

adiposity

adjacent
  a. tissue

adjunctive
  a. procedure

adjustable
  a. anterior guide
  a. articulator
  a. axis face-bow
  a. breast implant
  a. external suture
  a. saline breast implant
  a. screw

adjustment
  occlusal a.

adjuvant
  a. chemotherapy
  a. therapy

ADL
  activities of daily living

admaxillary

adnexa
  a. oculi
  ocular a.

adnexal skin tumor

ADNR
  anterior displacement no
    reduction

Adolph Gasser camera system

adrenocorticotropic hormone
  (ACTH)

Adson
  A. bur
  A. forceps
  A. rongeur
  A. rongeur forceps
  A. scalp clip
  A. suction
  A. test
  A.-Brown forceps

adsorbent

adsorption

adult
  a. acquired micrognathia
  a.-type well-differentiated
    liposarcoma

AdultPatch
  Trans-Ver-Sal A.

advancement
  five-flap V-Y a.
  a. flap
  frontal bone a.
  frontal bone a. with strip
    craniectomy
  fronto-orbital a.
  galea frontalis a.
  a. genioplasty
  horizontal maxillary a.
  hyoid a.
  lip border a.
  mandibular a.
  mandibular osteotomy–ge-
    nioglossus a.
  maxillofacial skeletal a.
  monobloc a.
  Tessier type of frontal
    bone a.
  transcranial monobloc
    frontofacial a.

advancement *(continued)*
  volar flap a.
  V-Y a.
  V-Y a. for columellar
    lengthening
  V-Y lip roll mucosal a.
  V-Z a. in buccal sulcus

adventitia
  tunica a.

adventitial

adventitious
  a. breath sounds
  a. membrane

A-E, AE
  above-elbow
    A-E amputation

Aeby
  A. muscle
  A. plane

AED
  aerodynamic equivalent di-
    ameter

aerobic bacteria

aerodynamic equivalent diameter (AED)

aeroembolism

aeroperitoneum

aerotitis media

aerotolerant anaerobe

aesthesioneuroblastoma

aesthetic *(variant of* esthetic)

Aesthetica C topical vitamin C
  skin care product

aesthetician *(variant of* esthetician)

aesthetics *(variant of* esthetics)

afferent
  a.-efferent pathway
  a. loop syndrome

afferent *(continued)*
    a. lymphatic
    a. nerve

affix

afflux

AFH
    anterior facial height

after-glide

afterload

afterperception

aftersensation

age
    mental a. (MA)

Agee
    A. carpal tunnel release
    A. device
    A. fiberoptic carpal tunnel
      operation
    A. sign

agenesis
    corpus callosum a.
    penile a.
    tracheal a.
    vaginal a.

agent
    AGF binding a.
    alkylating a.
    anesthetic a.
    antiinflammatory a.
    antineoplastic a.
    antipruritic a.
    antipyrotic a.
    binding a.
    blocking a.
    chemical a.
    chemotherapeutic a.
    ganglionic blocking a.
    hemostatic a.
    immunosuppressive a.
    keratolytic a.
    lipotropic a.
    myoneural blocking a.
    paralytic a.

agent *(continued)*
    sclerosing a.
    vasoconstrictive a.
    vasodilating a.
    virucidal a.
    wetting a.

AGF
    autologous growth factor
      AGF binding agent
      AGF gel

agger
    a. nasi
    a. perpendicularis

agglutinant

agglutinate
    vasoactive a.

aggregate
    mineral trioxide a. (MTA)

aging
    barnacles of a.
    facial a.

aglossia-adactylia syndrome

agminated blue nevus

agnathia

Agnew
    A. canaliculus knife
    A. canthoplasty
    A. tattooing needle

agranulocytic ulceration

agria

agrius

AHA
    alpha-hydroxy acid
    alphahydroxy acid
    alpha hydroxyl acid

AHI
    apnea-hypopnea index

AHO
    Albright hereditary osteo-
      dystrophy

Aicardi syndrome

air
  a. cyst
  a. embolism
  a. embolus
  a. exchange
  liquid a.
  a. pressure dressing
  a. space

AirFlex carpal tunnel splint

airflow
  a. management

airway
  binasal pharyngeal a.
  laryngeal mask a. (LMA)
  a. management
  nasal a.
  a. obstruction
  upper a.

AJCC
  American Joint Committee
    on Cancer
      AJCC staging

A-K, AK
  above-knee
    A-K amputation

AKA
  above-knee amputation

akinesia
  O'Brien a.
  Van Lint a.

Akros mattress

AL
  axiolingual
    AL reconstruction

ALA
  axiolabial

ala pl. alae
  a. auris
  Burkitt lymphoma of na-
    sal a.

ala (continued)
  a. cristae galli
  a. of the ethmoid
  a.-facial groove
  a. major ossis sphenoidalis
  a. minor ossis sphenoidalis
  nasal a.
  a. nasi
  a. parva ossis sphenoidalis
  a. temporalis ossis sphe-
    noidalis
  thyroid a.

alacrima

alar
  a. area
  a. base
  a. base reduction
  a. batten graft
  a. bone
  a. branch of external maxil-
    lary artery
  a. cartilage
  a.-columella implant
  a.-columella relation
  a. crease
  a. dome and cartilage
  a. facial groove
  a.-facial junction
  a. fascia
  a. flaring
  a. flutter
  a. folds
  a. incision
  a. ligament
  a. muscle
  a. osteotome
  a. reconstruction
  a. retractor
  a. rim
  a. rim collapse
  a. rim excision
  a. suspension stitch
  veiling of the a. rim
  a. wedge excision
  Weir resection of the a.
    base

alarplasty

Albers
  A.-Schönberg disease
  A.-Schönberg marble bones

Albrecht bone

Albright
  A. disease
  disseminated form A. syndrome
  A. hereditary osteodystrophy (AHO)
  A. syndrome
  A.-Hadorn syndrome
  A.-McCune-Sternberg syndrome

Alexander
  A. operation
  A. otoplasty
  A. otoplasty knife
  A.-Ballen orbital retractor

alexandrite
  a. laser
  a. long-pulsed laser

ALEXlazr
  Candela A.
  A. laser

Alezzandrini syndrome

Alfonso eyelid speculum

alganesthesia

algeoscopy

algesia

algesimeter
  Björnström a.

algesimetry (also algesiometry)

algesiometry (variant of algesimetry)

algesthesia

algetic

Algiderm wound packing

alginate
  Hydro-Jel a.

algogenesia

algogenesis

algogenic

algorithm
  bone a.

alignment

alkali caustic

alkylating agent

All Access laser system

Alldress multilayered wound dressing

Allen
  A. test
  A.-Heffernan nasal speculum

alligator forceps

Allis
  A. clamp
  A. hemostat
  A. tissue forceps

Allison forceps

AlloDerm
  A. acellular dermal graft
  A. cellular dermal graft
  A. preserved human dermis

alloderm

allogeneic
  a. bone
  a. bone crib
  a. crib
  a. graft
  a. keratinocyte graft
  a. transplantation

allogenic

allogenically vascularized prefabricated flap

allogotrophia

allograft
  cortical bone a.
  cortical freeze-dried a.
  cancellous freeze-dried a.
  decalcified freeze-dried
    bone a. (DFDBA)
  demineralized freeze-dried
    bone a. (DFDBA)
  freeze-dried a.
  freeze-dried bone a.
  a. joint replacement
  Proplast a.
  a. reaction
  Silastic a.
  a. survival
  a. tissue transplantation
  a. wound covering

alloimplant

AlloMatrix injectable putty
  bone graft substitute

alloplast

alloplastic
  a. AMA
  a. augmentation
  a. chin augmentation
  a. crib
  a. facial implant
  a. graft
  a. graft material
  a. implant
  a. plate
  a. prosthesis
  a. reconstruction
  a. transplant

alloplasty

allotransplantation

allotriodontia

alloy
  Midas a.
  Midigold a.
  Minigold a.

Allport
  A. operation

Allport *(continued)*
  A. ptosis correction proce-
    dure

All-Pro automatic film developer

Allskin marker

aloe

alopecia
  a. adnata
  a. areata
  burn a.
  a. capitis totalis
  cicatricial a.
  a. cicatrisata
  a. circumscripta
  a. follicularis
  a. liminaris
  a. liminaris frontalis
  marginal a.
  a. marginalis
  marginal traumatic a.
  a. orbicularis
  pressure a.
  radiation a.
  scarring a.
  a. seborrheica
  traumatic a.

Alor 5/500

alpha (α)
  a. hydroxy acid (AHA)
  a. hydroxyl acid

alpha-hydroxy acid (AHA) *(written also alphahydroxy acid)*

Alsus-Knapp
  A.-K. eyelid repair
  A.-K. operation

Alter lip retractor

alternating sutures

Altmann classification of congenital aural atresia

Alumafoam nasal splint

aluminum
  a. acetate and acetic acid

Alveoform Biograft

Alveograf binder

alveolar
a. arch
a. arch of mandible
a. arch of maxilla
a. artery
a. atrophy
a. bone
a. bone defect
a. bone density
a. bone graft
a. border
a. border of mandible
a. border of maxilla
a. branch of internal maxillary artery
a. canal
a. canal of maxilla
a. cleft graft
a. dehiscence
a. duct
a. foramina
a. grafting
a. height
a. limbus of mandible
a. limbus of maxilla
a. margin
a. margin of mandible
a. nerve
a. osteitis
a. process
a. process of mandible
a. process of maxilla
a. ridge
a. ridge augmentation
a. soft part sarcoma (ASPS)
a. support
a. supporting bone
a. surface of mandible
a. surface of maxilla

alveolate

alveolobuccal
a. groove
a. sulcus

alveololabial
a. groove
a. sulcus

alveololabialis

alveololingual
a. groove
a. sulcus

alveoloplasty
interradicular a.
intraseptal a.

alveolus *pl.* alveoli
buccal a.
canine a.
cleft a.
cleft lip/a. (CLA)
dental a.
a. dentalis
lingual a.
mandibular a.
maxillary a.
maxillary first molar a.
mesiobuccal a.
mucous a.
salivary gland a.
septum alveoli
serous a.
supramentale mandibu-
  lar a.
tapetum alveoli

Alvis
A. operation
A. ptosis correction proce-
  dure

Alvogyl surgical dressing

AMA
augmentation of the man-
  dibular angle
    alloplastic AMA

Ambil Skin Tone

amelia

ameloblastic
a. carcinoma

ameloblastic *(continued)*
  a. fibroma
  a. fibrosarcoma
  a. sarcoma

ameloblastoma
  acanthomatous a.
  intraosseous a.
  melanotic a.
  mural a.
  peripheral a.
  pigmented a.
  unicystic a.

American Joint Committee on Cancer (AJCC) staging

American Society for Testing and Materials

aminocaproic acid

Ammon
  A. blepharoplasty
  A. canthoplasty
  A. dacryocystotomy
  A. eyelid repair

amnion
  a. graft
  human a.

amniotic
  a. band
  a. membrane dressing

amorphous calcification

amphicrine carcinoma

amplitude
  maximum a.

ampulla
  a. canaliculi lacrimalis
  a. ductus lacrimalis
  a. of lacrimal canaliculus

ampullaris
  crista a.

ampullary
  a. crest
  a. nerve

amputation
  above-knee (AK) a. (AKA)
  above-elbow (AE) a.
  avulsion a.
  below-elbow (B-E) a.
  below-knee (B-K) a.
  Chopart a.
  congenital a.
  degloved a.
  double-flap a.
  fingertip a.
  Hueston finger a.
  labiomaxilloseptocolumellar a.
  labiomental a.
  labiopalatal a.
  linear a.
  Mikulicz-Vladimiroff a.
  modified Chopart a.
  a. neuroma
  nipple-areolar a.
  osteoplastic a.
  synchronous a.
  Tansini breast a.

amyloid
  a. macroglossia
  a. tongue

amyloidosis
  cutaneous a.
  hereditary neuropathic a.
  lichenoid a.
  nodular a.

amyotonia

amyotrophic lateral sclerosis (ALS)

ANA
  antinuclear antibody

anaerobe
  aerotolerant a.

anaerobic
  a. bacteria
  a. culture
  a. streptococcus

anaeroplasty

anakhre

analgesia
  infiltration a.
  local a.
  narcolocal a.
  paretic a.
  permeation a.
  surface a.

analgesic

analysis
  Bolton a.
  cephalometric a.
  Cohen a.
  Cox regression a. of par-
    tially edentulous jaw
  densitometric a.
  dental a.
  facial a.
  immunoradiometric a.
    (IRMA)
  Mantel-Haenszel a.
  Nance a. of arch length
  nasofacial a.
  occlusal a.
  occlusal cephalometric a.
  occlusion a.
  proportional facial a.
  qualitative a.
  quantitative a.
  Tweed a.
  a. of variance (ANOVA)

anaphylactic
  a. crisis
  a. hypersensitivity
  a. reaction
  a. shock

anaphylactogenesis

anaphylactogenic

anaphylactoid
  a. crisis
  a. reaction
  a. shock

anaphylaxis
  acquired a.

anaphylaxis (continued)
  active a.
  aggregate a.
  antiserum a.
  cutaneous a.
  homologous a.
  local a.
  reverse a.

anaplastic

anaplasty

anastomosed graft

anastomosis pl. anastomoses
  arteriovenous a. (AVA)
  Béclard a.
  dog ear of a.
  end-to-end a.
  end-to-end microvascular a.
  end-to-end venous a.
  end-to-side a.
  Galen a.
  Hyrtl a.
  lymphaticovenous a.
  microvascular a.
  nerve a.
  precapillary a.
  small vessel a.
  stirrup a.
  Sucquet a.
  Sucquet-Hoyer a.
  suspension a.
  tension-free a.
  venous-to-venous a.

anatomic
  a. closure
  a. position
  a. repair
  a. ridge
  a. snuff-box

anatomical
  a. Tobin malar prosthetic
    implant

Anbesol
  Maximum Strength A.

anchor
  a. band

anchor *(continued)*
   endosteal implant a.
   fixation a.
   implant a.
   Mitek a.
   Mitek GII suture a.
   Mitek Mini GII a.
   a. splint
   a. suture
   a. with suture ligature
   Zest implant a.

anchorage
   Baker a.
   a. bend
   cervical a.
   a. control
   cranial a.
   dynamic a.
   major a.
   maxillomandibular a.
   multiple a.
   occipital a.
   a. procedure
   reinforced a.
   simple a.

anchoring
   fascial a.
   a. fibril
   a. screw
   a. suture

anconeus muscle

Andermann syndrome

Anders disease

Andersch ganglion

Anderson
   A. columella prosthesis
   A. nasal strut
   A. splint

Andrews six keys to normal occlusion

androgen insensitivity syndrome

Andy Gump
   A. G. deformity

Andy Gump *(continued)*
   A. G. facies

Anel lacrimal duct dilation

anemia
   aplastic a.
   burn wound a.

anesthesia
   axillary a.
   balanced a.
   basal a.
   Bier block a.
   block a.
   caudal a.
   cervical plexus a.
   closed a.
   cocaine a.
   compression a.
   endotracheal a.
   epidural a.
   field block a.
   general a.
   Hunstad system for tumescent a.
   infiltration a.
   infiltrative local a
   inhalation a.
   insufflation a.
   intracavitary a.
   intraligamentary a.
   intranasal a.
   intravenous a.
   laryngeal a.
   ligamental a.
   local a.
   local infiltrative a. (LIA)
   nerve-blocking a.
   palatine block a.
   paraneural a.
   perineural a.
   permeation a.
   plexus a.
   pressure a.
   regional a.
   regional block a.
   selective a.
   stellate block a.
   topical a.
   traumatic a.

anesthesia *(continued)*
   tumescent a.

anesthetic
   a. agent
   eutectic mixture of local a's
      (EMLA)
   general a.
   local a.
   topical a.
   a. tube

anetoderma
   Schweninger-Buzzi a.

aneurysm
   carotid a.

aneurysmal bone cyst (ABC)

ANF
   antinuclear factor

angel's kiss

Angelucci operation

angiitis
   granulomatous a.

angina
   Vincent a.

angiochondroma

angiodermatitis

angioendothelioma

angioendotheliomatosis
   reactive a.

angiofibroma
   juvenile a.
   juvenile nasopharyngeal a.
   nasopharyngeal a.

angiofollicular

angiogenesis
   hyperbaric oxygen–in-
      duced a.

angiogenic

angiography
   magnetic resonance a.
      (MRA)

angiography *(continued)*
   spiral computed tomogra-
      phy a.

angiokeratoma
   a. circumscriptum
   a. corporis diffusum
   a. of Fordyce
   Mibelli a's
   verrucous a.

angiokeratosis

angioleiomyoma
   laryngeal a.

angiolipoleiomyoma

angiolipoma
   subcutaneous a.

angiolupoid

angiolymphangioma

angioma
   a. arteriale racemosum
   capillary a.
   a. cavernosum
   cavernous a.
   cherry a.
   congenital tufted a.
   a. cutis
   hereditary hemorrhagic a.
   hypertrophic a.
   a. pigmentosum atrophi-
      cum
   plexiform a.
   senile a.
   a. serpiginosum
   simple a.
   a. simplex
   spider a.
   strawberry a.
   superficial a.
   telangiectatic a.
   a. venosum racemosum

angiomatoid
   a. fibrous histiocytoma
      (AFH)
   a. myosarcoma

angiomatosis
  cephalotrigeminal a.
  cerebroretinal a.
  encephalotrigeminal a.
  hemorrhagic familial a.
  a. of retina
  retinocerebral a.

angiomatous
  a. lymphoid hamartoma

angiomegaly

angiomyolipoma

angiomyoma
  a. cutis

angiomyoneuroma

angiomyosarcoma

angioneoplasm

angioneurectomy

angioneuroma

angioneuromyoma

angioneuropathy

angioneurotic edema

angio osteohypertrophy syndrome

angiopathy
  giant cell hyaline a.

angiophakomatosis

angioplasty

angioreticuloendothelioma

angiosarcoma

angiosomal flap

angiospasm
  labyrinthine a.

angiospastic

Angle
  A. classification of maloc-
    clusion (Class I, II, III, IV
    malocclusion)

Angle (continued)
  A. splint

angle
  a. of aberration
  acute mandibular plane a.
  alveolar a.
  alveolar profile a.
  antegonial a.
  augmentation of the man-
    dibular a. (AMA)
  auriculocephalic a.
  auriculomastoid a.
  auriculo-occipital a.
  basal mandibular a.
  basilar a.
  Bennett a.
  biorbital a.
  a. bisection technique
  Broca a.
  Broca basilar a.
  Broca facial a.
  buccal a.
  Camper a.
  caudal septal a.
  cephalic a.
  cephalometric a.
  cerebellopontile a.
  cerebellopontine a.
  cervicomental a.
  conchal-mastoid a.
  conchoscaphoid a.
  costophrenic a.
  costovertebral a.
  craniofacial a.
  cricothyroid a.
  Daubenton a.
  distal a.
  distolinguo-occlusal
    point a.
  ethmoid a.
  facial a.
  facial plane a.
  Frankfort mandibular a.
    (FMA)
  Frankfort mandibular inci-
    sor a. (FMIA)
  Frankfort mandibular
    plane a.

angle *(continued)*
    frontal a. of parietal bone
    gonial a.
    incisal a.
    incisal guidance a.
    incisal mandibular plane a.
     (IMPA)
    inferior a. of parietal bone
    intergonial a.
    interincisal a.
    Jacquart a.
    a. of jaw
    labial a.
    labioincisal line a.
    lateral a. of eye
    lateral incisal guide a.
    lingual a.
    linguoincisal line a.
    linguo-occlusal a.
    mandibular a.
    mandibular plane a.
    mastoid a. of parietal bone
    maxillary a.
    medial a. of eye
    mesiobuccal line a.
    mesiobucco-occlusal
     point a.
    mesiolabial line a.
    mesiolabioincisal point a.
    mesiolingual line a.
    mesiolinguoincisal point a.
    mesiolinguo-occlusal
     point a.
    mesio-occlusal line a.
    metafacial a.
    a. of mouth
    a. of Mulder
    nasofrontal a.
    nasolabial a.
    occipital a. of parietal bone
    occlusal plane a.
    occlusal rest a.
    olfactive a.
    olfactory a.
    ophryospinal a.
    orifacial a.
    parietal a.
    parietal a. of the sphenoid
     bone

angle *(continued)*
    piriform a.
    point a.
    prophy a's
    prophylactic a's
    protrusive incisal guide a.
    Quatrefage a.
    radiolunate a.
    Ranke a.
    rest a.
    scaphoconchal a.
    scapholunate a.
    sella-nasion-subspinale a.
     (SNA, S-N-A)
    sella-nasion-supramenta-
     le a. (SNB, S-N-B)
    Serres a.
    sinodural a.
    sphenoid a.
    sphenoidal a.
    sternal a.
    a. sutures
    Topinard a.
    Trautmann a.
    Virchow a.
    Virchow-Holder a.
    visor a.
    Vogt a.
    Weisbach a.
    Welcker a.
    Z a.

angled
    a. cannula
    a. delivery device (ADD)
    a. elevator
    a. scissors
    a. telescope
    a.-vision lens system

angular
    a. artery
    a. cheilitis
    a. elevator
    a. facial vein
    a. gyrus
    a. incision
    a. nasal artery
    a. position of the ramus
    a. stomatitis

angular *(continued)*
a. vein
a. vestibular nucleus

angulate

angulated
ASSI breast dissector a.

angulation
vertical a.

animal graft

animation
facial a.
forehead a.

anisocoria

anisodactylous

anisodactyly

anisognathous

anisomastia

anisomelia

Anita-Busch chondrocutaneous
flap

ankle strategy

ankyloblepharon

ankylocheilia

ankyloglossia
a. superior
a. superior syndrome

ankylosed

ankylosing spondylitis

ankylosis
bony a.
cricoarytenoid a.
extracapsular a.
false a.
fibro-osseous a.
fibrous a.
glossopalatine a.
intracapsular a.
juxta-articular a.
spurious a.

ankylosis *(continued)*
temporomandibular joint a.
TMJ a.
zygomatic-coronoid a.

ankylotic

ankylotomy

annular
a. adenocarcinoma
a. band
a. cartilage
a. ligament
a. stricture

annulare
granuloma a.

annulus
bony a.
a. ciliaris
a. tendineus communis

anodontia
partial a.
total a.
a. vera

anomalous

anomaly *pl.* anomalies
branchial cleft a.
chest wall a.
cleft a.
coloboma, heart a.,
choanal atresia, retarda-
tion, and genital and ear
a's (CHARGE)
congenital a.
congenital hand a.
craniofacial a.
cutaneous vascular a.
dentofacial a.
dysgnathic a.
eugnathic a.
fourth branch a.
hemifacial microsomia a.
kleeblattschädel a.
laryngeal a.
maxillofacial a.
oral a.
pragmatic a.

anomaly *(continued)*
    temporal bone a.
    third branchial a.
    vascular a.
    venous a.

anoplasty

anosmia

anotia

anotus

ANOVA
    analysis of variance

anoxia
    cerebral a.

ANS
    anterior nasal spine

ansa *pl.* ansae
    a. cervicalis
    a. galeni
    Haller a.
    a. hypoglossi

anserinus
    pes a.

antagonist

antecubital fossa

antegonial
    a. angle
    a. notch
    a. notching

antegrade
    a. approach
    a. blood flow
    a. island flap

anterior
    a. active mask rhinoma-
      nometry
    a. auricular muscle
    a. auricular nerve
    a. auricular vein
    a. axillary line
    a. band
    a. band remover (ABR)
    a. chamber hyphema

anterior *(continued)*
    a. chest wall flap
    a. ciliary artery
    a. clinoid process
    a. component
    a. component of force
    a. condylar vein
    a. condyloid foramina
    a. cranial fossa
    a. craniectomy
    a. cricoid split
    a. displacement (AD)
    a. displacement no reduc-
      tion (ADNR)
    a. divergence
    a. ethmoid
    a. ethmoidal air cell
    a. ethmoidal artery
    a. ethmoidal branch of
      ophthalmic artery
    a. ethmoidal foramen
    a. ethmoidal nerve
    a. ethmoid canal
    a. ethmoidectomy
    a. facial height (AFH)
    a. facial vein
    a. force
    a. fracture
    a. hairline incision
    a. helical rim free flap
    a. inferior cerebellar artery
    a. lingual gland
    a. mallear fold
    a. mallear ligament
    a. mandibular posturing
    a. mandibulectomy
    a. meningeal artery
    a. middle meatus
    a. naris
    a. nasal spine (ANS)
    a. nasal spine of maxilla
    a. nasal valve
    a. occlusion
    a. ostium
    a. palatal bar
    a. palatine arch
    a. palatine foramen
    a. palatine groove

anterior *(continued)*
  a. partial laryngectomy
  a. pillar of fauces
  a. pillar tumor
  a. port scalp excision
  a.-posterior discrepancy
  a.-posterior otoplasty
  a. rectus fascia
  a. rhinoscopy
  a. scaler
  a. septum
  serratus a.
  a. sheath
  a. skin flap
  a. skull base
  a. subperiosteal implant
  a. superficialis muscle
  a. superior alveolar artery
  a. superior iliac spine
  a. surface of maxilla
  a. suspension of hyoid
    bone
  a. suspensory ligament
  a. view

anterolateral
  a. thigh flap
  a. thigh free flap

anteroposterior (AP)
  a. dysplasia
  a. facial dysplasia

anterosuperior quadrant

anthelix

Anthony quadrisected minigraft
  dilator

anthropometric measurement

anthropometry

anthroposcopy

antibacterial

antibiotic
  bactericidal a.
  bacteriostatic a.
  broad-spectrum a.
  a. irrigation
  prophylactic a. therapy

antibiotic *(continued)*
  a. prophylaxis
  a.-resistant
  a.-soaked swabs

antibody
  antinuclear a. (ANA)
  collagen a.
  monoclonal a.

antiemetic

antigen
  carcinoembryonic a. (CEA)
  epithelial membrane a.
    (EMA)
  heterogenetic a. (HLA)
  human lymphocyte a's
  organ-specific a.
  tissue-specific a.

antigenic

antigenicity

antihelical fold

antihelix
  superior crus of a.
  unfurling of a.

antihemorrhagic stent

antiinflammatory agent

antineoplastic agent

antinuclear
  a. antibody (ANA)
  a. factor (ANF)

antipruritic agent

antipyretic

antipyrotic agent

antirejection drug therapy

antiretroviral therapy

antiseborrheic

antisepsis

antiserum
  trivalent botulinum a.

antisialagogue

antisialic

antitoxin
  botulinum a.
  botulinus a.
  botulism a.
  bovine a.
  gas gangrene a.
  tetanus a.

antitension line (ATL)

antitragicus
  a. muscle
  musculus a.

antitragohelicina
  fissura a.

antitragus

antitrismus

Antoni classification of schwannoma morphology

antral
  a. carcinoma
  a. mucosal cyst
  a. sarcoma

antrobuccal

antrodynia

antronasal

antroscope

antroscopy

antrostomy
  Caldwell-Luc maxillary a.
  inferior meatal a.
  intraoral a.
  middle meatal a.
  nasal a.

antrotomy

antrum
  a. auris
  ethmoid a.
  a. ethmoidale
  frontal a.
  Highmore a.

antrum *(continued)*
  mastoid a.
  a. mastoideum
  maxillary a.
  Valsalva a.

AO/ASIF titanium craniofacial
  system

AO-Titanium microplate

AP
  anteroposterior

Apert
  A. disease
  A. hirsutism
  A. syndrome
  A.-Crouzon disease

apertognathia
  compound a.
  infantile a.
  a. repair
  simple a.

apertognathism

apertura *pl.* aperturae
  a. externa canaliculi coch-
    leae
  a. piriformis
  a. sinus frontalis
  a. sinus sphenoidalis

aperture
  bony anterior nasal a.
  external a. of canaliculus of
    cochlea
  eye a.
  frontal sinus a.
  orbital a.
  pharyngeal a.
  piriform a.
  a. of sphenoid sinus
  sphenoidal sinus a.
  spurious a. of facial canal

apex *pl.* apices
  a. auriculae
  a. blunderbuss
  a. of the brow
  closed a.
  a. cornea

apex *(continued)*
    darwinian a.
    flaring a.
    a. linguae
    a. locator
    a. nasi
    open a.
    orbital a.
    a. partis petrosae ossis
      temporalis
    a. of petrous part of tempo-
      ral bone
    a. pin
    a. radicis dentis
    radiographic a.
    retropapillary a.
    a. satyri
    a. of tongue

aphalangia

aphasia
    infantile a.
    motor a.

aphtha *pl.* aphthae
    Bednar aphthae
    aphthae major
    Mikulicz aphthae
    aphthae minor

aphthoid

aphthosis

aphthous
    a. stomatitis
    a.-type lesion
    a. ulcer

apical
    a. abscess
    a. cyst
    a. fenestration
    a. radiolucency

apicectomy

API universal foam chin strap

aplasia
    cochlear a.
    condylar a.
    a. cutis congenita

aplasia *(continued)*
    labyrinthine a.
    müllerian duct a.
    salivary gland a.

aplastic
    a. anemia

apnea
    deglutition a.
    a.-hypopnea index (AHI)
    obstructive sleep a.
    peripheral a.
    vagal a.

apneic

aponeurectomy

aponeurosis *pl.* aponeuroses
    abdominal a.
    Denonvilliers a.
    epicranial a.
    a. epicranialis
    extensor a.
    external oblique a.
    fibrovascular a.
    a. of insertion
    internal oblique a.
    levator a.
    a. linguae
    lingual a.
    musculotendinous a.
    a. of musculus transversus
      abdominis
    a. of origin
    palatal a.
    a. palatina
    palatine a.
    palmar a.
    rhomboid a.
    temporal a.
    transversus abdominis a.

aponeurotic
    a. fascia
    a. galea
    a. laxity
    a. musculature

aponeurotica
    galea a.
    lateral galea a.

aponeurositis

aponeurotome

aponeurotomy

apparatus *pl.* apparatus
    attachment a.
    biphase Morris fixation a.
    lacrimal a.
    a. lacrimalis
    a. of Perroncito
    vasomotor a.

appearance
    aesthetic a.
    chamois yellow a.
    cotton-wool a.
    cystlike a.
    esthetic a.
    ground-glass a.
    honeycomb a.
    lamina dura–like a.
    micrognathic a.
    onion peel a.
    "slapped cheek" a.
    "slapped face" a.
    sunken-eye a.
    worm-eaten a.

appendage
    auricular a.
    a's of the eye
    a's of the skin

apple
    Adam's a.

appliance
    arch bar facial fracture a.
    biphasic pin a.
    craniofacial a.
    craniofacial fracture a.
    Denholz a.
    Erich facial fracture a.
    expansion plate a.
    facial fracture a.
    Jackson a.
    Joseph septal fracture a.
    Latham a.
    lip habit a.

appliance *(continued)*
    mandibular advancement a. (MAA)
    Mayne muscle control a.
    monobloc a.
    Muhlmann a.
    multiphase a.
    Nord a.
    obturator a.
    palatal expansion a.
    palate-splitting a.
    prosthetic a.
    Roger Anderson facial fracture a.
    Roger Anderson pin fixation a.
    split plate a.
    surgical a.
    vinyl palatal a.
    Winter facial fracture a.

Appose skin stapler

apposition
    compensatory periosteal bone a.

approach
    antegrade a.
    axillary subpectoral a.
    bicoronal a.
    bicoronal subperiosteal a.
    bilateral a.
    buttonhole a.
    endonasal a.
    extended frontal a.
    external pharyngotomy a.
    extralaryngeal a.
    extraoral a.
    Gillies a.
    infralabyrinthine a.
    infratemporal fossa a.
    intraoral a.
    Kaye minimal-incision anterior a.
    L a.
    lingual a.
    mandibular swing a.
    middle fossa a.
    modified Risdon a.

approach *(continued)*
  retroseptal transconjuncti-
    val a.
  retrosigmoid a.
  Risdon a.
  subciliary a.
  sublabial a.
  sublabial transsphenoi-
    dal a.
  submental a.
  suboccipital a.
  subperiosteal a.
  transblepharoplasty a.
  transconjunctival a.
  transmandibular a.
  transmaxillary a.
  transpalatal a.
  transpalpebral a.
  transsphenoidal a.
  vertical midline a.
approximate
approximated
  skin edges a.
approximation
  direct a.
  a. forceps
  successive a.
  a. sutures
  wound a.
approximator
  a. clamp
  nerve a.
  Neuromeet nerve ending a.
APR
  auropalpebral reflex
apron
  abdominal a.
  a. band
  a. flap
  a. flap procedure
  lingual a.
  redundant abdominal a.
  a. U-shaped incision
Aqua
  A. Glycolic cream

Aqua *(continued)*
  A. Glycolic skin care prod-
    uct
Aquaplast
  A. alloplastic material
  A. dressing
  A. nasal splint
  A. rapid setting splint ma-
    terial
aqueduct
  fallopian a.
arachidonic acid
arborescens
  lipoma a.
arborization
  a. pattern
arc
  auricular a.
  binauricular a.
  longitudinal a. of skull
  nasobregmatic a.
  naso-occipital a.
  reflex a.
  a. of rotation of fasciocuta-
    neous flap
  sensorimotor a.
arcade
  capillary a.
  lumbar a's
  mesenteric a.
arch
  alveolar a.
  alveolar a. of mandible
  alveolar a. of maxilla
  anterior palatine a.
  axillary a.
  branchial a's
  branchial cleft a.
  deep palmar a.
  deep plantar a.
  dentulous dental a.
  faucial a.
  glossopalatine a.
  Gothic a.

arch *(continued)*
    hyoid a.
    hyoid branchial a.
    inferior dental a.
    inferior palpebral a.
    labial a.
    Langer a.
    lingual a.
    lower a.
    malar a.
    mandibular a.
    mandibular branchial a.
    mandibular visceral a.
    maxillary a.
    Mershon a.
    nasal a.
    nasal venous a.
    oral a.
    palatal a.
    palatine a.
    palatoglossal a.
    palatomaxillary a.
    palatopharyngeal a.
    palmar a.
    palmar radial a.
    pharyngeal a's
    pharyngopalatine a.
    plantar a.
    posterior palatine a.
    postoral a's
    premandibular a.
    radiocarpal a.
    saddle a.
    saddle-shaped a.
    superciliary a.
    superficial palmar a.
    superficial plantar a.
    superior palpebral a.
    supraorbital a.
    supraorbital a. of frontal
        bone
    tarsal a.
    upper a.
    utility a.
    W a.
    zygomatic a.

arch bar
    a. b. facial fracture appli-
        ance

arch bar *(continued)*
    a. b. fixation
    a. b's frame
    mandibular a. b.

archwire
    multiple loop a.

Arcon semiadjustable articula-
    tor

arcuata
    eminentia a.
    zona a.

arcuate
    a. eminence
    a. line

arcus *pl.* arcus
    a. adiposus
    a. alveolaris
    a. alveolaris mandibulae
    a. alveolaris maxillae
    a. cornealis
    a. dentalis inferior
    a. dentalis superior
    a. glossopalatinus
    a. juvenilis
    a. marginalis
    a. palatini
    a. palatoglossus
    a. palatopharyngeus
    a. palpebralis inferior
    a. palpebralis superior
    a. pharyngopalatinus
    a. senilis
    a. superciliaris
    a. tarseus inferior
    a. tarseus superior
    a. tendineus
    a. zygomaticus

area *pl.* areae, areas
    alar a.
    alveolar a.
    alisphenoid a.
    articulation a.
    auriculomastoid a.
    bilabial a.
    contact a.
    a. of facial nerve
    glottal a.

area *(continued)*
   hair-bearing a.
   a. hypoglossi
   a's of innervation
   interplacodal a.
   intertriginous a.
   Kiesselbach a.
   labiodental a.
   Laimer-Haeckerman a.
   linguoalveolar a.
   linguodental a.
   Little a.
   mesobranchial a.
   motor a.
   nasal cross-sectional a.
   a. nervi facialis
   olfactory a.
   palatal a.
   parasymphysis a.
   parotid-masseteric a.
   periareolar a.
   postauricular a.
   posterior palatal seal a.
   postpalatal seal a.
   preauricular a.
   prelacrimal a.
   skip a's
   stress-bearing a.
   subglottic a.
   supporting a.
   supra-areolar a.
   surgically denervated a.
   temporal a.
   tissue-bearing a.
   total body surface a.
      (TBSA)
   trigger a.
   velar a.
   Warthin a.

areata

areatus

areflexia

areola *pl.* areolae
   Chaussier a.
   coning of a.
   a. mammae
   a. of mammary gland

areola *(continued)*
   a. of nipple
   a. papillaris
   second a.
   umbilical a.

areolar
   a. demarcation
   a. gland
   a. grafting
   a. incision
   a. reconstruction
   a. tissue

areolomammary complex

Argamaso-Lewis composite flap

argon
   a. beam coagulator
   a. gas
   a. green laser
   a. laser–induced scars
   a. laser photocoagulator
   a. tunable dye laser

Argyle silicone Salem sump

argyria

argyrophilic
   a. collagen fiber
   a. fibril

argyrosis

arhinia *(variant of* arrhinia)

Arie
   A. reductive mammaplasty
   A.-Pitanguy breast reduction
   A.-Pitanguy mammaplasty
   A.-Pitanguy mammary ptosis operation
   A.-Pitanguy operation

Arlt
   A. epicanthus repair
   A. eyelid repair
   A. operation
   A. pterygium excision
   A. recess
   A. sinus
   A.-Jaesche operation

arm
 brawny a.

Army-Navy retractor

Arnold
 A. canal
 foramen of A.
 A. ganglion
 A. nerve
 A.-Chiari malformation

AROSupercut scissors

arrangement
 tongue-in-groove a.

arrhinia (*spelled also* arhinia)

arrow
 a. blade
 a. clasp

ARROWgard central venous
 catheter

arrowhead canthoplasty

arterial
 a. blood gas
 a. flap
 a. forceps
 a. hemorrhage
 a. hypoxemia
 a. insufficiency of lower ex-
  tremities
 a. loop
 a. plexus
 a. pressure
 a. silk suture
 a. spider
 a. ulcer

arterialization

arterialized flap

arteriectasis

arteriectomy

arteriocapillary

arteriogenesis

arteriogram

arteriography

arteriola

arteriole
 capillary a.
 main a. (MA)

arterioplasty

arteriorrhaphy

arteriorrhexis

arteriosclerosis

arteriosclerotic
 a. gangrene
 a. occlusive disease
 a. peripheral vascular disease

arteriospasm

arteriostrepsis

arteriovenous
 a. anastomosis (AVA)
 a. fistula
 a. hemangioma
 a. malformation (AVM)
 a. shunt

arteritis
 cranial a.
 giant cell a.
 Horton a.
 a. nodosa
 temporal a.
 temporal giant cell a.

artery
 aberrant a.
 alar a. of nose
 alveolar a.
 angular a.
 angular nasal a.
 anterior ciliary a.
 anterior ethmoidal a.
 anterior inferior cerebellar a.
 anterior meningeal a.
 anterior superior alveo-
  lar a.

artery *(continued)*
    arcuate a.
    ascending cervical a.
    ascending palatine a.
    ascending pharyngeal a.
    auricular a.
    auriculotemporal a.
    axillary a.
    basilar a.
    bilateral internal mammary
      a. (BIMA)
    buccal a.
    buccinator a.
    a. of bulb of penis
    caroticotympanic a.
    carotid a.
    celiac a.
    chief a. of thumb
    circumflex iliac a.
    circumflex scapular a.
    collateral a.
    collateral digital a.
    common carotid a. (CCA)
    common iliac a.
    common palmar digital a.
    common plantar digital a.
    communicating a.
    cricothyroid a.
    cubital a.
    deep auricular a.
    deep cervical a.
    deep circumflex iliac a.
    deep inferior epigastric a.
    deep a. of the penis
    deep a. of tongue
    descending palatine a.
    digital collateral a.
    dolichoectatic a.
    dorsal a.
    dorsal digital a.
    dorsal a. of foot
    dorsalis pedis a.
    dorsal lingual a.
    dorsal metacarpal a.
    dorsal metatarsal a.
    dorsal a. of nose
    dorsal a. of penis
    a. of Drummond

artery *(continued)*
    ectatic vertebral a.
    end a.
    epigastric a.
    episcleral a.
    esophageal a's
    ethmoidal a.
    external carotid a.
    external mammary a.
    external maxillary a.
    external a. of nose
    external pudendal a.
    facial a.
    first dorsal metatarsal a.
    frontal a.
    gastroepiploic a.
    greater palatine a.
    helicine a.
    inferior alveolar a.
    inferior epigastric a.
    inferior labial a.
    inferior laryngeal a.
    inferior thyroid a.
    inferior tympanic a.
    infrahyoid a.
    infraorbital a.
    innominate a.
    intercostal a.
    internal carotid a. (ICA)
    internal mammary a.
    internal maxillary a.
    internal pudendal a.
    interradicular a.
    ipsilateral common caro-
      tid a.
    labial a.
    labyrinthine a.
    lacrimal a.
    laryngeal a.
    lateral circumflex femoral a.
    lateral circumflex a. of
      thigh
    lateral nasal a.
    lateral plantar a.
    lateral tarsal a.
    lesser palatine a.
    lingual a.
    lowest thyroid a.
    mammary a.

artery *(continued)*
- mandibular a.
- masseteric a.
- maxillary a.
- medial circumflex a. of thigh
- medial plantar a.
- medial tarsal a.
- median a.
- medullary a.
- meningeal a.
- mental a.
- mesenteric a.
- metatarsal a.
- middle meningeal a.
- musculophrenic a.
- nasal a.
- nasal accessory a.
- Neubauer a.
- nutrient a.
- occipital a.
- ophthalmic a.
- palatine a.
- palmar digital a's
- palmar interosseous a's
- palmar metacarpal a's
- palpebral a.
- perforating alveolar a.
- perforating a's of foot
- perforating a's of hand
- perforating a's of internal mammary
- peroneal a.
- petrosal a.
- pharyngeal a.
- pipestem a.
- plantar metatarsal a's
- postauricular a.
- posterior alveolar a.
- posterior auricular a.
- posterior ethmoidal a.
- posterior inferior cerebellar a.
- posterior labial a.
- posterior lateral nasal a's
- posterior palatine a.
- posterior septal a.
- posterior septal a. of nose
- posterior superior alveolar a.

artery *(continued)*
- posterolateral nasal a.
- principal a. of thumb
- profunda femoris a.
- proper palmar digital a.
- proper plantar digital a.
- a. of pterygoid canal
- radial a.
- radial index a.
- ranine a.
- retroauricular a.
- saphenous a.
- septal a.
- septal posterior nasal a.
- small a's
- sphenopalatine a.
- spiral a.
- splayed a's
- stapedial a.
- stylomandibular a.
- stylomastoid a.
- sublingual a.
- submental a.
- subscapular a.
- superficial circumflex iliac a.
- superficial epigastric a.
- superficial palmar a.
- superficial petrosal a.
- superficial temporal a.
- superior alveolar a.
- superior auricular a.
- superior epigastric a.
- superior labial a.
- superior laryngeal a.
- superior pharyngeal a.
- superior superficial epigastric a.
- superior thyroid a.
- supraorbital a.
- supratrochlear a.
- temporal a.
- terminal a.
- thoracoacromial a.
- thoracodorsal a.
- thyroid a.
- thyroid ima a.
- tonsillar a.
- transverse cervical a.
- transverse facial a.

artery *(continued)*
  trigeminal a.
  umbilical a.
  vestibulocochlear a.
  vidian a.
  Zinn a.
  zygomatico-orbital a.

arthralgia
  temporomandibular a.

arthritis
  rheumatoid a. (RA)
  sarcoid a.
  septic a.
  viral a.
  Yersinia a.

arthrochalasis

arthrochondritis

arthroclasia

arthrodentosteodysplasia

arthrodesis
  cricoarytenoid a.
  joint a.
  Moberg a.
  radiolunate a.
  resection-a.
  scaphoid-capitate a.
  small joint a.
  wrist a.

arthrogryposis
  congenital multiple a.
  a. multiplex congenita
  myopathic a. multiplex
    congenita
  neuropathic a. multiplex
    congenita

arthropathy
  acromegalic a.
  Charcot a.
  chondrocalcific a.
  inflammatory a.

arthroplastic implant

arthroplasty
  cemented a.
  gap a.

arthroplasty *(continued)*
  interposition a.
  interpositional gap a.
  intracapsular temporoman-
    dibular joint a.
  metacarpophalangeal (MP)
    joint a.
  metatarsophalangeal (MP)
    joint a.
  perichondral a.
  resection a.
  silicone elastomer a.
  small joint a.

articular
  a. capsule
  a. cartilage
  a. disk
  a. eminence
  a. eminence of temporal
    bone
  a. fossa of mandible
  a. fossa of temporal bone
  a. surface of mandibular
    fossa
  a. tubercle
  a. tubercle of temporal
    bone

articulare

articulate

articulated
  a. chin implant
  a. chin prosthesis

articulating paper forceps

articulatio *pl.* articulationes

articulation
  balanced a.
  capitolunate a.
  carpal a's
  carpometacarpal a's
  Chopart a.
  cranial coronal ring a.
  craniovertebral a.
  cricoarytenoid a.
  cricothyroid a.
  a's of fingers
  a's of foot

articulation *(continued)*
a's of hand
intermetacarpal a's
intermetatarsal a's
interphalangeal a's
mandibular a.
maxillary a.
mediocarpal a.
metacarpophalangeal a's
metatarsophalangeal a's
radiocarpal a.
scaphocapitate a's
scapholunate a.
temporomandibular a.
temporomaxillary a.
transverse tarsal a.
vomerosphenoidal a.

articulator
adjustable a.
Arcon a.
Arcon semiadjustable a.
Denar a.
Denar-Witzig a.
non-Arcon a.
quick-mount face-bow a.
Whip-Mix a.

artifact
skin lesion a.
trigeminal nerve a.

artificial
a. mastoid
a. velum

artiodactylous

aryepiglottic
a. fascia
a. fold
a. fold of Collier
a. muscle

arytenoid
a. cartilage
a. muscle
a. perichondritis

arytenoidectomy

arytenoidopexy

ascending
a. cervical artery

ascending *(continued)*
a. palatine artery
a. pharyngeal artery
a. ramus of the mandible

Asch
A. forceps
A. nasal splint
A. nasal-straightening forceps
A. operation
A. septal forceps
A. septal straightener
A. splint

Ascher syndrome

ascorbic acid

asepsis

aseptic
a. necrosis
a. technique

Asher high-pull face-bow

Ashley breast prosthesis

Asnis 2 guided screw

aspect
buccal a.
inferomedial a.
superolateral a.

Aspiradeps lipodissector

aspirate
adipo a.

aspirating
a. cannula
a. curet
a. dissector
a. needle
a. syringe
a. tube

aspiration
a. biopsy
a. biopsy cytology
a. biopsy needle
a. cannula
cyst a.
fine-needle a. (FNA)
foreign body a.

aspiration *(continued)*
    lipoma a.
    permucosal needle a.
    suction a.

aspirator
    Accelerator II a.
    suction a.
    ultrasonic surgical a.

aspirin
    methocarbamol and a.

ASPS
    alveolar soft part sarcoma

assay
    Maximal Static Response A.
    (MSRA)
    maximal static response a.
    of facial motion

assembly
    malleostapedial a.
    malleus-footplate a.
    malleus-stapes a.

assessment
    functional a. of cancer ther-
    apy—head and neck
    (FACT-HN)

Assézat triangle

ASSI
    Accurate Surgical and Sci-
    entific Instruments
        ASSI bipolar coagulat-
        ing forceps
        ASSI breast dissector
        angulated
        ASSI breast dissector
        spatulated
        ASSI forceps
        ASSI nasal and sinus
        instruments
        ASSI Polar-Mate bipo-
        lar coagulator
        ASSI Super-Cut scis-
        sors

assimilation
    alveolar a.
    labial a.
    velar a.

assisted
    a. respiration

asterion

asternia

asthenopia
    accommodative a.
    muscular a.
    tarsal a.

astomia

Aston
    A. cartilage reduction sys-
    tem
    A. face-lift scissors
    A. nasal retractor
    A. submental retractor

asymmetric
    a. distribution
    a. folds of eyes
    a. maxillomandibular
    growth
    a. reflexes

asymmetry
    facial a.
    forehead a.
    tumofactive a.

Atasoy-Kleinert volar V-Y advancement flap

ataxia
    cerebellar a.
    Friedreich a.
    hereditary a.
    a.-telangiectasia

athelia

Atkins nasal splint

ATL
    antitension line

atonia

atraumatic
    a. bowel clamp
    a. braided silk sutures
    a. chromic sutures
    a. needle

atraumatic *(continued)*
    a. sutures
    a. tissue forceps
    a. visceral forceps

atresia
    aural a.
    bony a.
    choanal a.
    esophageal a.
    laryngeal a.
    meatal a.
    oral a.
    a. plate
    tracheal a.

atretic

atretoblepharia

atretolemia

atretorrhinia

atrophia
    a. cutis
    a. cutis senilis
    a. maculosa varioliformis
      cutis
    a. striata et maculosa

atrophic
    a. acne scar
    a. glossitis
    a. lichen planus
    malignant a. papulosis
    a. pharyngitis
    a. rhinitis
    a. scar

atrophica
    acne a.
    hyperkeratosis figurata
      centrifuga a.
    stria a.

atrophie blanche

atrophied

atrophoderma
    a. albidum
    a. biotripticum
    a. diffusum
    a. maculatum

atrophoderma *(continued)*
    a. neuriticum
    a. of Pasini and Pierini
    a. pigmentosum
    progressive idiopathic a.
    senile a.
    a. senilis
    a. striatum

atrophodermatosis

atrophy
    alveolar a.
    blue a.
    Buchwald a.
    Charcot-Marie-Tooth a.
    dermal a.
    diffuse alveolar a.
    epidermal a.
    fat a.
    a. of fat
    fatty a.
    glandular a.
    hemifacial a.
    hemilingual a.
    horizontal a.
    Hunt a.
    inflammatory a.
    ischemic muscular a.
    linear a.
    macular a.
    myofiber a.
    pathologic a.
    physiologic a.
    pigmentary a.
    primary macular a. of skin
    progressive hemifacial a.
    quadriceps a.
    Romberg hemifacial a.
    skin a.
    striate a. of the skin
    unilateral facial a.
    Wucher a.

attached
    a. cranial section
    a. craniotomy
    a. island

attachment
    abnormal frenulum a.

attachment *(continued)*
    abnormal frenum a.
    Dalbo extracoronal a.
    Dalbo stud a.
    Dalla Bona a.
    epithelial a.
    a. epithelium
    extracoronal a.
    Gottlieb epithelial a.
    high frenum a.
    implant superstructure a.
    lingual a.
    McCollum a.
    multiphase a.

attenuate

atticoantrotomy

atticomastoid

atticotomy

attrition

attritional occlusion

atypia
    epithelial a.
    melanocytic a.

atypical
    a. carcinoid tumor
    a. cleft
    a. erythema multiforme
    a. fibroxanthoma
    a. lipoma
    a. mole
    a. nevus
    a. pityriasis rosea

Auclair operation

Aufrecht sign

Aufricht
    A. elevator
    A. glabellar rasp
    A. nasal rasp
    A. nasal retractor
    A. retractor
    A. scissors
    A. septal speculum
    A.-Lipsett nasal rasp

augmentation
    alloplastic a.
    alloplastic chin a.
    alveolar ridge a.
    autologous a.
    autologous human collagen a.
    breast a.
    calf a.
    camouflage a.
    cheek a.
    chin a.
    connective tissue a.
    Farrior graft a.
    fat a.
    Fomon graft a.
    a. genioplasty
    Gore-Tex lip a.
    a. graft
    Hogan and Converse graft a.
    lip a.
    Longacre graft a.
    malar alloplastic a.
    malar facial a.
    malar shell a.
    a. mammaplasty
    a. of the mandibular angle (AMA)
    mastopexy–breast a.
    midface alloplastic a.
    Millard graft a.
    Musgrave and Dupertuis graft a.
    permanent lip a.
    PermaRidge alveolar ridge a.
    pharyngeal wall a.
    premandible alloplastic a.
    premandibular a.
    preprosthetic a.
    ridge a.
    silicone lip a.
    soft tissue a.
    subantral a.
    submandibular a.
    submuscular breast a.

augmentation *(continued)*
  subpectoral a.
  temporary lip a.
  transaxillary breast a.

augnathus

aural atresia

auricle
  accessory a.'s
  supernumerary a.

auricula *pl.* auriculae
  a. dextra
  a. sinistra

auricular
  a. appendage
  a. artery
  a. cartilage
  a. cartilage graft
  a. composite graft
  a. muscle
  a. nerve
  a. point
  a. prosthesis
  a. reflex
  a. repositioning
  a. tags
  a. trauma
  a. tubercle
  a. tubercle of Darwin
  a. veins

auriculare

auricularis

auriculocephalic angle

auriculocranial

auriculoinfraorbital plane

auriculomastoid

auriculotemporal
  a. artery
  a. nerve
  a. nerve syndrome
  a. neuralgia

auriform

auris *pl.* aures
  a. externa

auris *(continued)*
  a. interna
  a. media
  a. sinister

auropalpebral reflex (APR)

Auspitz sign

Austin
  A. knife
  A. retractor

autoallergic

autoanaphylaxis

autoantibody

autoanticomplement

autoantigen

autoclasia

autoclasis

autoclave

autodermic
  a. graft

autoepidermic graft

autogeneic graft

autogenous
  a. bone graft
  a. cartilage graft
  a. composite tissue
  a. corticocancellous graft
  a. fascia lata sling procedure
  a. fat graft
  a. grafting
  a. transplant

autograft
  bone a.
  cranial a.'s
  cultured a.
  cultured epithelial a.
  a. extender

autografting
  cultured epithelial a.

autographism

autohemotherapy

autoimmune
   a. disorder
   a. hemolysis
   a. phenomenon
   a. reaction

autoimmunity

autologous
   a. augmentation
   a. blood
   a. bone
   a.-cultured epithelium
      (ACE)
   a. fat graft
   a. growth factor (AGF)
   a. iliac crest bone graft
   a. rib bone graft
   a. tissue flaps

autolysis

autonomic

autoplastic graft

autoplasty

autoregulation

autorotation
   backward a. of the mandi-
      ble

autorrhaphy

autosomal
   a. dominant
   a. recessive

autotransfusion

autotransplant

autotransplantation

AVA
   arteriovenous anastomosis

avascular
   a. graft
   a. necrosis (AVN)
   a. tissue

avascularization

Avellis syndrome

aviator's ear

avidin-biotin-peroxidase complex (ABC)

Avitene
   A. fibrillar collagen
   A. microfibrillar collagen
      hemostat

AVM
   arteriovenous malforma-
      tion

AVN
   avascular necrosis

avulsed laceration

avulsion
   a. amputation
   a. of caruncula lacrimalis
   a. of finger
   a. flap injury
   a. fracture
   a. injury
   mechanical a.
   a. of nerve

Axhausen
   A. cleft lip repair
   A. needle holder

axial
   a. advancement flap
   a. anchor screw
   a. dorsal flap
   a. flap
   a. frontonasal flap
   a. pattern vascularized skin
      flap
   a. plane
   a. projection
   a. rotation joint
   a. temporoparietal fascial
      flap

axial-based flap

axilla pl. axillae

axillary
   a. anesthesia
   a. artery
   a. breast tissue

axillary *(continued)*
    a. node
    a. node dissection
    a. subpectoral approach

axiobuccal

axiobuccocervical (ABC)

axiobuccogingival (ABG)

axiobuccolingual (ABL)

axiocervical (AC)

axiodistal

axiodistocervical (ADC)

axiodistogingival

axiodistoincisal

axioincisal

axiolabial (ALA)

axiolabiogingival

axiolabiolingual

axiolingual (AL)

axiolinguocervical

axiolinguogingival

axiolinguo-occlusal

axiomesial

axiomesiocervical

axiomesiodistal

axiomesiogingival

axiomesioincisal

axiomesio-occlusal

axio-occlusal

axis *pl.* axes
    basibregmatic a.
    basicranial a.
    basifacial a.
    binauricular a.
    condylar a.
    craniofacial a.
    external a. of eye
    facial a.
    hinge a.
    mandibular a.
    opening a.
    orbital a.
    radial-ulnar deviation a.
    sagittal a.
    Tessier cleft a.
    a. traction forceps
    transverse horizontal a.
    vertical a.
    vertical a. of eye
    Y a.

axon
    injured a.
    motor a.
    myelinated a.

axonal
    a. continuity
    a. damage
    a. growth

axonotmesis

azelaic acid

Aztec
    A. ear
    A. type

azygous

baby Senn-Miller retractor

bacitracin
 b. dressing
 b. irrigation
 b. ointment
 b. solution
 b. strips

Backhaus
 B. towel clamp
 B. towel clip

back pressure

backward autorotation of the mandible

backward-biting ostrum punch

Bacon
 B. rongeur
 B. rongeur forceps

BacStop check valve

bacteremia
 gram-negative b.
 gram-positive b.

bacteria
 aerobic b.
 anaerobic b.
 vegetative b.

bacterial
 b. barrier
 b. contamination
 b. endocarditis
 b. infection
 b. keratoconjunctivitis
 b. meningitis (BM)
 b. septicemia

bactericidal

bacteriolytic

bacteriostatic

Baek musculocutaneous pedicle technique

Baelz disease

bag
 cheek b.
 malar b.
 trauma induced saddle b.

bag-gel implant

Baghdad
 B. boil
 B. button

bagginess of eyes

Bailey skull bur

Bakamjian
 B. flap
 B. pedicle flap
 B. tubed flap

Baker
 B. anchorage
 B. capsular contracture
 B. classification of capsular contracture (*grades I–IV*)
 B. composite graft
 B. grade
 B. velum

balance
 occlusal b.
 occlusion b.

balanced
 b. anesthesia
 b. articulation
 b. contact between the cusps
 b. force instrumentation technique
 b. occlusion
 b. salt solution (BSS)
 b. suspension
 b. traction

balanic hypospadias

bald tongue

baldness
 Juri II, III degree of male pattern b.
 male pattern b.

ball
    Adams b.
    fatty b. of Bichat
    b. forceps
Ballenger
    B. cartilage knife
    B. ethmoid curet
    B. nose knife
Baller-Gerold syndrome
balloon
    b. cell nevus
    Brighton epistaxis b.
    b. dissection
    epistaxis b.
    esophageal b.
    b. expansion
    nasomaxillary b.
    b. nasostat
    windowed b.
balm
    post laser b.
    protective recovery b.
Baltimore nasal scissors
Balshi packer
Ba-N
    basion-nasion
        Ba-N plane
band
    adapter b.
    amniotic b.
    anchor b.
    annular b.
    anterior b.
    fibrous b.
    iliotibial b.
    lip furrow b.
    mentalis b.
    Muehrcke b.
    palatoglossal b.
    placental b.
    platysmal b.
    Simonart b.
    spiral b. of Gosset
bandage
    abdominal b.

bandage (continued)
    Ace b.
    Ace adherent b.
    adhesive b.
    Band-Aid b.
    Barton b.
    binocular b.
    ClearSite b.
    Coban b.
    compression b.
    Cover-Roll stretch b.
    demigauntlet b.
    elastic b.
    Elasticon b.
    Elastoplast b.
    Esmarch b.
    four-tailed b.
    Galen b.
    Garretson b.
    gauntlet b.
    Gibson b.
    Hamilton b.
    Hammock b.
    Hollister medial adhe-
        sive b.
    Hydron burn b.
    immobilizing b.
    Kerlix gauze b.
    Kiwisch b.
    Kling gauze b.
    many-tailed b.
    oblique b.
    pressure b.
    protective b.
    b. scissors
    Scultetus b.
    Setopress high-compres-
        sion b.
    b. shears
    spica b.
    spiral b.
    Sureseal pressure b.
    Telfa 4×4 b.
    Tricodur compression sup-
        port b.
    Tubigrip elastic support b.
    wet b.
Band-Aid
    B. bandage
    B. dressing

bandeau
　　supraorbital b.

Bane rongeur

banked freeze-dried bone

Banner flap

bar
　　Ackerman lingual b.
　　anterior palatal b.
　　arch b.
　　arch b. facial fracture appliance
　　buccal b.
　　double lingual b.
　　Dynamic Mesh craniomaxillofacial pre-angled connecting b.
　　Erich arch b.
　　facial fracture appliance dental arch b.
　　Goshgarian transpalatal b.
　　Hahnenkratt lingual b.
　　Kazanjian T-b.
　　Kennedy b.
　　labial b.
　　lingual b.
　　mandibular arch b.
　　maxillary arch b.
　　mesostructure b.
　　mesostructure conjunction b.
　　occlusal rest b.
　　palatal b.
　　Passavant b.
　　supraorbital b.
　　T-b. of Kazanjian
　　transpalatal b.

barbula hirci

Bardach
　　B. cleft rhinoplasty
　　B. modification

Bardet-Biedl syndrome

Bard-Parker
　　B.-P. blade
　　B.-P. knife handle
　　B.-P. scalpel

Barkman reflex

Barlow disease

barnacles of aging

Baron palate elevator

barotitis media

Barraquer
　　B. eye shield
　　B. lid retractor

Barrett
　　adenocarcinoma in B. esophagus
　　B. epithelium
　　B. esophagus
　　B. syndrome
　　B. ulcer

barrier
　　antimicrobial b.
　　bacterial b.
　　blood-brain b.
　　b. breach
　　Capset bone graft b.
　　fenestrated sterile field b.
　　b. function
　　b. membrane
　　b. protection
　　b. sheet
　　Nu-Hope Adhesive waterproof skin b.
　　skin b.
　　sterile field b.
　　synthetic b. dressing
　　Vitacuff tissue-interface b.

Barsky
　　B. alar cartilage relocation
　　B. cleft lip repair
　　B. cleft palate raspatory
　　B. elevator
　　B. nasal osteotome
　　B. nasal rasp
　　B. nasal retractor
　　B. nasal scissors
　　B. operation
　　B. pharyngoplasty
　　B. retractor

Bartholin duct

bartholinitis

Barton
    B. bandage
    B. fracture
    reverse B. fracture

basal
    b. bone
    b. cell acanthoma
    b. cell adenoma
    b. cell carcinoma (BCC)
    b. cell epithelioma (BCE)
    b. cell nevus
    b. cell nevus syndrome
    b. cell papilloma
    b. lamina
    b. lamina of ciliary body
    b. mandibular angle
    nodular ulcerative b. cell
      carcinoma
    pigmented b. cell carci-
      noma
    sclerosing b. cell carci-
      noma
    superficial b. cell carci-
      noma

basale
    stratum b.

basalioma

basaloid
    b. cell
    b. carcinoma
    b. monomorphic adenoma
      (BMA)
    b. tumor

basaloma

base
    alar b.
    anterior skull b.
    apical b.
    b. of arytenoid cartilage
    columellar b.
    b. of flap
    mandibular b.
    metal b.
    record b.

base (continued)
    skull b.
    temporary b.
    b. of tongue (BOT)

baseball finger

basedoid

Basedow disease

basedowian

baseline
    b. parameters
    Reid b.
    b. study

basement
    b. membrane
    b. membrane zone
    b. tissue

baseplate
    stabilized b.

basialveolar length

basic fibroblastic growth factor
  (bFGF)

basicranial
    b. flexure

basifacial

basilemma

basilar
    b. artery
    b. kyphosis
    b. plexus
    b. prognathism
    b. projection
    b. segment

basiloma
    b. terebrans

basioglossus

basion
    b.-nasion (Ba-N) plane

basis
    b. cartilaginis arytenoideae
    b. cranii externa

basis *(continued)*
    b. cranii interna
    b. mandibulae
    b. nasi

basisphenoid

basosquamous carcinoma (BSC)

Bass method

basting suture

BAT
    bilateral advancement transposition

bat ear

Bates decision

bathrocephaly

batting
    Dacron b.

Battle sign

Bauer
    B. forceps
    B. retractor
    B.-Tondra-Trusler cleft lip repair
    B.-Tondra-Trusler operation for syndactylism
    B.-Trusler-Tondra cleft lip repair

Bauhin glands

Baumgarten glands

Baumgartner
    B. forceps
    B. needle holder

Baum-Hecht tarsorrhaphy forceps

Baxter V. Mueller laparoscopic instrumentation

Bazex syndrome

Bazin disease

BCA
    bicinchoninic acid

BCC
    basal cell carcinoma

BCE
    basal cell epithelioma

BCI
    blunt carotid injury

BCLP
    bilateral cleft lip and palate

B-E, BE
    below-elbow
        B-E amputation

beak
    cutaneous polly b.
    fibrous polly b.
    parrot b.
    polly b.
    volar b. ligament
    volar b. of the metacarpal

beaklike protrusion of nose

beam
    x-ray b.

beard
    old man's b.

Beard-Cutler operation

bear track pigmentation

beauty mark

Beaver
    B. Mini-Blade
    B. rhinoplasty blade

Bechterew (*variant of* Bekhterev)

Becker
    B. breast prosthesis
    B. dissector cannula
    B. dissector tip
    B. flap
    B. flat dissector tip
    B. Greater Grater dissecting cannula
    B. hair hamartoma
    B. implant

Becker *(continued)*
B. mammary prosthesis
B. nevus
B. operation
B. round tip dissector
B. scissors
B. septal scissors
B. tip
B. tissue expander
B. twist dissector tip
B. vibrating cannula system

Beckman
B. nasal scissors
B. nasal speculum
B.-Colver nasal speculum

Beckwith
B. syndrome
B.-Wiedemann syndrome

Béclard
B. anastomosis
B. triangle

bed
air-fluidized b.
capillary b.
carotid arterial b's
granular b.
monitored b.
nail b.
recipient b.
Skytron operating b.
tissue b.
wound b.

Bednar
B. aphthae
B. tumor

beefy tongue

Beevor sign

Bekhterev *(spelled also* Bechterew)
B. sign
B. spondylitis
B. symptom
B.-Mendel reflex

Bell
B. palsy
B. operation

Bell *(continued)*
B. phenomenon
B. spasm
B. suture

bell
b. flap
b. flap nipple reconstruction

belly
drum b.
frontal b. of the occipitofrontal muscle
muscle b.
b. of the muscle
occipital b. of the occipitofrontal muscle
posterior b.
prune b.

below-elbow (B-E) amputation

below-knee (B-K) amputation

Belz rongeur

Bemis suction canister

bend
anchorage b.

bender
Tessier bone b.

Benelli mastopexy

benign
b. cellular blue nevus
b. cephalic histiocytosis
b. chondroma
b. cystic teratoma
b. dyskeratosis
b. epidermal pigmented lesion
b. epithelial neoplasm
b. familial chronic pemphigus
b. fibrous histiocytoma
b. hemangiopericytoma
b. hyperplasia
b. intraepithelial dyskeratosis
b. juvenile melanoma
b. lipoblastoma

benign *(continued)*
  b. lymphadenosis
  b. lymphocytoma cutis
  b. lymphoepithelial lesion
    (BLL)
  b. mesenchymal neoplasm
  b. mesenchymal tumor
  b. mixed tumor
  b. mucous membrane pem-
    phigoid
  b. necrotizing otitis externa
    (BNOE)
  b. neoplasm
  b. nevus
  b. papular acantholytic
    dermatosis
  b. pemphigus
  b. symmetric lipomatosis
  b. systemic mastocytosis
  b. tumor
Benjamin
  B. binocular slimline laryn-
    goscope
  B. pediatric operating la-
    ryngoscope
  B. syndrome
  B.-Lindholm microsuspen-
    sion laryngoscope
Bennett
  B. angle
  B. epilation forceps
  B. fracture
  B. movement
  reverse B. fracture
Benzac AC Gel
Béraud valve
Berens
  B. mastectomy retractor
  B. mastectomy skin flap re-
    tractor
  B. ptosis forceps
  B. ptosis knife
  B. retractor
Bergman wound retractor
Berke
  B. cilia forceps
  B. double-end lid everter

Berke *(continued)*
  B. operation
  B. ptosis clamp
  B. ptosis correction
  B. ptosis forceps
  B.-Motais ptosis correction
Berkeley Bioengineering ptosis
  forceps
Berlin tulip flap
berlock dermatitis
Bernard
  B. flap
  B. operation
  B.-Burow cheiloplasty
  modified B.-Burow tech-
    nique
  B.-Burow operation
  B.-Burow technique
Bernay sponge
Berndorfer syndrome
Berne
  B. nasal forceps
  B. nasal rasp
Bernstein nasal retractor
Berry ligament
Besnier
  B. rheumatism
  B.-Boeck-Schaumann dis-
    ease
bevel
  marginal b.
beveled septal cartilage
Bezold
  B. abscess
  B. ganglion
  B. mastoiditis
  B. perforation
  B. sign
  B. symptom
bFGF
  basic fibroblastic growth
    factor
Bianchi valve

biauricular

bibulous

bicameral abscess

biceps brachii flap

Bichat
B. fat pad
fatty ball of B.
B. fossa
B. protuberance

bicinchoninic acid (BCA)

Bickel ring

bicoronal
b. approach
b. forehead lift
b. incision
b. ridge
b. scalp flap
b. subperiosteal approach

bicortical
b. iliac bone block
b. superior border screw

bicuspid
mandibular b.
maxillary b.

bidactyly

bidactylous

BIEF
bilateral inferior epigastric artery flap

Bier
B. block
B. block anesthesia

Biermer sign

Biesenberger
B. mammaplasty
B. operation
B. reduction mammaplasty

bifid
b. epiglottis
b. nose

bifid (continued)
b. pinna
b. thumb
b. tongue
b. uvula

bifida
occult spina b.

bifidity of the columella

bifrontal craniotomy

bifurcation
carotid b.
b. of trachea

Biggs mammaplasty retractor

bikini
disposable b.
b. incision
b. wax

bilabial

bilaminar

bilateral
b. abductor paralysis
b. adductor paralysis
b. advancement transposition (BAT)
b. approach
b. balanced occlusion
b. canthopexy
b. cleft lip–associated nose
b. cleft lip and palate (BCLP)
b. coronal synostosis
b. coronoidectomies
b. forehead remodeling
b. fronto-orbital remodeling
b. gluteus maximus transposition
b. hypesthesia
b. inferior epigastric artery flap (BIEF)
b. malposition
b. internal mammary artery (BIMA) reconstruction
b. mandibular sagittal split osteotomy

bilateral *(continued)*
  b. masseteric hypertrophy
  b. mesioclusion
  b. neck dissection
  b. pectoralis major muscle flap
  b. rotational flap
  b. sagittal split osteotomy (BSSO)
  b. sagittal split advancement osteotomy

Bilhaut-Cloquet procedure

biliptysis

bilobed
  b. fasciocutaneous flap
  b. flap
  b. skin flap
  b. skin flap technique
  b. transposition flap

bilumen mammary implant

BIMA
  bilateral internal mammary artery
    BIMA reconstruction

bimaxillary
  b. dentoalveolar protrusion
  b. prognathism
  b. protrusion
  b. protrusive occlusion
  b. relationship

bimeter gnathodynamometer

binasal pharyngeal airway

binaural

binauricular

Binder
  B. implant
  B. submalar implant
  B. syndrome

binder
  abdominal b.
  Alveograf b.
  breast b.
  compression b.

binder *(continued)*
  Dale abdominal b.
  Osteograf b.
  Scultetus b.
  T-b.

binding agent
  AGF b. a.

Bing-Siebenmann malformation

Binne operation

binocular
  b. bandage
  b. dressing
  b. eye dressing
  b. instrument
  b. shield
  b. microscopy

binotic

Bio-Absorbable staple

bioavailability

BioBarrier
  B. membrane
  B. membrane guided tissue regeneration system

Biobrane
  B. adhesive
  B. dressing
  B. experimental skin substitute
  B. glove dressing
  B. graft material
  B. sheet
  B. wound covering
  B. wound dressing

Biobrane/HF

Biocell
  B. anatomical reconstructive mammary implant
  B. RTV implant
  B. smooth surface implant
  B. textured implant
  B. textured shell surface implant
  B. textured silicone
  B. textured surface implant

bioceramic implant material

biocidal

biocompatible
b. bone graft substitute material

BioCurve saline-filled breast implant

biodegradable surgical tack

biodegradation
implant b.

BioDIMENSIONAL
B. saline-filled implant
B. tissue expander

biofeedback
laryngeal image b.

Biogel
B. Diagnostic surgical gloves
B. glove
B. M surgical gloves
B. Neotech surgical gloves
B. Reveal/Indicator surgical gloves
B. Super-Sensitive surgical gloves

Bio-Gide resorbable bilayer barrier membrane

Bioglass
B. bone substitute material
B. bone graft substitute material

biograft
Alveoform B.

BioGran
B. resorbable synthetic bone graft
B. synthetic graft

biologic
b. creep of skin
b. fibrogen adhesive
b. response modifier

biomaterial
Gore-Tex DUALMESH b.
Gore-Tex MYCROMESH b.

biomechanics

BioMedic
B. MicroEncapsulated retinol cream

biomembrane

BioMend periodontal material

Bionix disposable nasal speculum

Bio-Oss
B. collagen
B. corticalis bone graft material
B. freeze-dried demineralized bone
B. maxillofacial bone filler
B. spongiosa bone graft material
B. spongiosa block
B. synthetic bone

Biopatch antimicrobial dressing

biophylaxis

biophysics
dental b.

Bioplant
B. hard tissue replacement synthetic bone
B. HTR synthetic bone

Bioplastique
B. augmentation material
B. polymer

Bioplate screw fixation system

biopsy
aspiration b.
bite b.
core needle b.
b. by curettage
deep-wedge b.
diagnostic excisional b.

biopsy *(continued)*
　directed fine-needle aspira-
　　tion b.
　elliptical b.
　excisional b.
　fine-needle b.
　fine-needle aspiration b.
　　(FNAB)
　b. forceps
　incisional b.
　nasopharyngeal b.
　needle b.
　needle localization
　　breast b.
　open b.
　punch b.
　b. punch
　b. punch forceps
　scalene lymph node b.
　second-look b.
　sentinel lymph node b.
　shave b.
　shave excision b.
　small incisional b.
　b. specimen forceps
　b. suction curet
　surface b.
　ultrasound-guided b.
　vertical lip b.
　wedge b.
　wide resection b.

Bioquant histomorphometry
　system

biorbital angle

bioresorbable
　b. guided tissue membrane
　b. implant

Biospan anatomical tissue ex-
　pander

biosynthetic wound covering

Bio-Vent implant

Biovert implant material

B.I.P.
　Breast Implant Protector
　　B.I.P. biopsy instrument

bipartition
　transcranial facial b.

bipedicle
　b. delay flap
　b. digital visor flap
　b. flap
　b. mucoperiosteal flap
　b. TRAM flap

bipedicled
　b. delay flap
　b. flap

bipennate muscle

bipenniform structure

biphalangeal thumb

biphase
　b. external pin fixation
　b. Morris fixation appa-
　　ratus

biphasic
　b. growth cycle
　b. pin
　b. pin appliance
　b. response

Bi-Phasic exfoliator

biplanar forehead lift

bipolar
　b. cautery
　b. disorder
　b. electrocoagulation
　b. electrosurgery
　b. forceps
　b. transsphenoidal forceps

Birbeck granule

bird-beak
　b.-b. jaw
　b.-b. distal esophagus

bird-face
　b.-f. retrognathism

bird-headed dwarf

Biro dermal nevus scissors

birthmark
  café au lait b.
  hemangioma b.
  macular vascular b.
  port-wine stain b.
  strawberry b.
  telangiectatic facial b.
  vascular malformation b.

Birt-Hogg-Dubé syndrome

bisected
  b. minigraft dilator
  b. mass

bis-GMA
  bisphenol A-glycidyl meth-
    acrylate

bishop collar deformity

Biskra button

bismuth pigmentation

bistoury
  Brophy b.
  Brophy b. knife
  Converse b.
  Converse button-end b.
  b. knife
  nasal b.

bite
  b. biopsy
  deep b.
  b. force
  mature b.
  skeletal open b.
  stork b.
  underhung b.

biteplane

biting
  cheek b.
  b. forceps
  lip b.
  b. punch
  tongue b.

bivalve nasal splint implant

Bivona epistaxis catheter

Björk flap tracheostomy

Björnström algesimeter

B-K, BK
  below-knee
    B-K amputation

Black retractor

black
  b. braided suture
  b. eschar
  b. mole cancer
  b. silk suture
  b. twisted suture

blade
  arrow b.
  Bard-Parker b.
  Beaver chondroplasty b.
  Beaver rhinoplasty b.
  carving b.
  chondroplastic b.
  Davis-Crowe tongue b.
  EDGE coated b.
  b. endosteal implant
  Goulian b.
  jigsaw b.
  lancet b.
  Lite b.
  nasal knife b.
  Padgett b.
  Personna Plus MicroCoat
    surgeon's b.
  ramus b.
  Rubin b.
  scalpel b.
  scapular b.
  Sharpoint b.
  Sharpoint crescent b.
  Sharpoint V-lance b.
  Sharptome crescent b.
  sickle b.
  Super-Cut b.
  Typhoon cutter b.
  Universal nasal saw b.
  X-Acto b.

blade-form
  b.-f. device
  b.-f. implant

Blade-Vent implant system

Blainville ears

Blair
  B. cleft palate clamp
  B. cleft palate elevator
  B. cleft palate knife
  B. knife
  B. operation
  B. nasal chisel
  B. palate hook
  B. ptosis correction operation
  B. serrefine
  B.-Brown graft
  B.-Brown implant
  B.-Brown knife
  B.-Brown operation
  B.-Brown retractor
  B.-Brown skin graft
  B.-Brown skin graft knife

Blaisdell skin pencil

Blake
  B. drain
  B. dressing forceps
  B. silicone drain

Blakesley
  B. ethmoid forceps
  B. forceps
  B. lacrimal trephine
  B. septal bone forceps
  B. septal compression forceps
  B. uvula retractor
  B.-Weil upturned ethmoid forceps
  B.-Wilde nasal forceps

blanch

blanched cutaneous elevation

blanching
  b. of hand
  b. reaction

Blandin
  B. ganglion
  B. glands

Blandin (continued)
  B.-Nuhn cyst
  B. and Nuhn glands

blanket
  Bair Hugger patient warming b.
  cooling b.
  mucous b.
  b. suture

Blasius
  B. duct
  B. lid operation
  B. operation

Blaskovics
  B. eyelid shortening technique
  B. operation
  B. ptosis correction

blastomycetic dermatitis

blastomycosis
  cutaneous b.
  keloidal b.
  laryngeal b.

blastomycosis-like pyoderma

Blauth
  B. classification of hypoplasia of thumb (types I, II, IIIA, IIIB, IV, V)
  B. hypoplastic thumb (Types I, II, IIIA, IIIB, IV, V)

bleach
  walking b.

bleaching cream

bleb

bleed
  silicone b.
  silicone gel b.
  b. of tattoo pigment

bleeder
  superficial b's

Blenderm tape

blennorrhagia

blennorrhagic

blennorrhagica
keratoderma b.
keratosis b.

blennorrhea
Stoerk b.

blepharal

blepharectomy

blepharedema

blepharelosis

blepharism

blepharitis
b. angularis
b. ciliaris
b. oleosa
b. rosacea
seborrheic b.

blepharoadenoma

blepharoatheroma

blepharochalasia

blepharochalasis
b. forceps

blepharoclonus

blepharocoloboma

blepharodermatochalasis

blepharodiastasis

blepharokeratoconjunctivitis

blepharomelasma

blepharopachynsis

blepharophimosis

blepharophyma

blepharopigmentation

blepharoplasty
Ammon b.
Bossalino b.
Budinger b.

blepharoplasty *(continued)*
Burow b.
Castanares bilateral b.
b. clip
CO_2 laser b.
combined upper b.
combined upper lid b.
cosmetic b.
Fox b.
functional b.
laser incisional b.
laser lower lid transconjunctival b.
long-skin flap b.
lower b.
modified Loeb and de la Plaza technique b.
skin/muscle flap b.
transconjunctival b. (TCB)
transconjunctival lower lid b.
upper b.

blepharoplegia

blepharoptosis
acquired b.
b. adiposa
aponeurotic b.
cicatricial b.
congenital b.
dysmyogenic b.
false b.
Fasanella-Servat b. operation
involutional b.
mechanical b.
myogenic b.
neurogenic b.
b. repair
senile b.
structural b.
traumatic b.

blepharoptosis-related blindness

blepharorrhaphy

blepharospasm

blepharosphincterectomy

blepharostat
  b. clamp
  McNeill-Goldmann b.
  b. ring
  Schachar b.

blepharostenosis

blepharosynechia

blepharotomy

blindness
  blepharoptosis-related b.
  cortical b.
  functional b.

BlisterFilm transparent wound
  dressing

BLL
  benign lymphoepithelial le-
    sion

Bloch
  B.-Sulzberger disease
  B.-Sulzberger syndrome

block
  axillary technique of bra-
    chial plexus b.
  bicortical iliac bone b.
  Bier b.
  Bio-Oss spongiosa b.
  b. anesthesia
  brachial plexus b.
  catheter technique for bra-
    chial plexus b.
  caudal b.
  cryogenic b.
  digital b.
  epidural b.
  external nasal nerve b.
  field b.
  ganglion b.
  inferior alveolar nerve b.
  infraorbital b.
  infraorbital nerve b.
  intercostal nerve b.
  interscalene b.
  intranasal b.
  local nerve b.

block (continued)
  mandibular b.
  mandibular nerve b.
  median nerve b.
  mental nerve b.
  metal and rubber b.
  nasopalatine nerve b.
  b. needle
  nerve b.
  paraneural b.
  phrenic nerve b.
  radial nerve b.
  regional b.
  ring b.
  Spaeth facial nerve b.
  stellate ganglion b.
  subclavian perivascular b.
  supraorbital nerve b.
  supratrochlear nerve b.
  Teflon b.
  thoracic nerve b.
  d-tubocurarine b.
  ulnar nerve b.
  Van Lint-Atkinson lid akine-
    tic b.
  wrist b.

Blom
  B.-Singer tracheoesopha-
    geal fistula
  B.-Singer vocal reconstruc-
    tion

blood
  anticoagulated b.
  autologous b.
  b. coagulation factor
  cord b.
  b. expander
  b. perfusion monitor
  b. product
  sludged b.
  whole b.

blood-borne
  b.-b. macrophage
  b.-b. pathogen

bloodless
  b. field
  b. operation

Bloom syndrome

blow-out fracture
    b.-o. f. of orbital floor

blown pupil

blue
    b. atrophy
    Bonney b.
    methylene b.
    b. nevus
    b. rubber bleb nevus syn-
        drome
    b. spot

Blue Peel
    B. P. chemical method
    B. P. chemical peel

Blumberg sign

blunderbuss
    apex b.

blunt
    b. and sharp dissection
    b. bullet-tip cannula
    b. carotid injury (BCI)
    b. dissection
    b. lacrimal probe
    b. suction-assisted lipo-
        plasty
    b. suction lipectomy

BM
    bacterial meningitis
    buccomesial

BMA
    basaloid monomorphic ad-
        enoma

BMD
    bone mineral density

BMI
    body mass index

BMP
    bone morphogenic protein

BMP-2
    bone morphogenic
        protein-2

BMT
    bone marrow transplant

BNOE
    benign necrotizing otitis
        externa

BO
    bucco-occlusal

board
    cartilage cutting b.
    graft b.

Bobath method

Bochdalek
    B. ganglion
    B. muscle
    B. valve

Bodenham
    B. dermabrasion cylinder
    B.-Blair skin graft knife
    B.-Humby skin graft knife

body
    adipose b. of cheek
    alveolar b.
    carotid b.
    b. contouring
    b. dysmorphic disorder
    fat b. of cheek
    fat b. of orbit
    foreign b.
    b. of the hamate
    hypoplastic mandibular b.
    b. image disorder
    b. image dissatisfaction
    loose b.
    mammillary b.
    b. of mandible
    b. mass index (BMI)
    b. of maxilla
    multivesicular b.
    parotid b.
    Schaumann b's
    b. sculpting
    b. sculpture
    b. of sphenoid bone
    thyroid b.
    b. of tongue

body *(continued)*
   Verocay b's

Boeck sarcoid

Boehringer Autovac autotransfusion system

Boerhaave syndrome

Bogorad syndrome

Bohn nodules

Boies
   B. cutting forceps
   B. nasal elevator
   B. nasal fracture elevator
   B. plastic surgery elevator
   B.-Lombard mastoid ron-
     geur

boil
   Baghdad b.

Boiler septal trephine

Boll cells

bolster
   cotton b. dressing
   b. finger
   muscular b.
   b. sutures
   tie-over b.

Bolton
   B. analysis
   B. nasion plane
   B. plane
   B.-Broadbent plane

bolus *pl.* boluses
   b. dressing
   b. injection
   intravenous b.

Bondek absorbable suture

bone
   accessory b.
   alar b.
   Albers-Schönberg marble
     b's
   Albrecht b.
   alisphenoid b.

bone *(continued)*
   allogeneic b.
   alveolar b.
   alveolar supporting b.
   anterior suspension of
     hyoid b.
   articular eminence of tem-
     poral b.
   b. autograft
   autologous b.
   banked freeze-dried b.
   basal b.
   basihyal b.
   basilar b.
   basioccipital b.
   basisphenoid b.
   Bertin b's
   Bio-Oss freeze-dried demi-
     neralized b.
   Bio-Oss synthetic b.
   Bioplant hard tissue re-
     placement synthetic b.
   Bioplant HTR synthetic b.
   bregmatic b.
   calvarial b.
   cancellous b.
   cancellous cellular b.
   capitate b.
   carpal b's
   carpal row b's
   chalky b's
   cheek b.
   b. chisel
   cortical b. allograft
   corticocancellous b.
   cranial b. grafting
   b. cutter
   decalcified freeze-dried b.
   decalcified freeze-dried
     cortical b. (DFDCB)
   b. decay
   Dembone demineralized
     human b.
   Dembone freeze-dried b.
   demineralized b. (DMB)
   demineralized freeze-
     dried b. (DFBD)
   b. deposition
   dermal b.

bone *(continued)*
    ectethmoid b's
    endochondral b.
    epactal b's
    epihyal b.
    epipteric b.
    ethanol-treated freeze-dried
      b. tissue
    ethmoid b.
    facial b.
    b. file
    b. fixation wire
    b. flap
    Flower b.
    b. forceps
    freeze-dried demineralized b. (FDDB)
    frontal b.
    b. grafting
    b. growth chambers
    b. growth stimulator
    hamate b.
    haversian b.
    hemiseptum of interalveolar b.
    horizontal plate of palatine b.
    hyoid b.
    immature b.
    b. implant material
    b.-inductive protein
    inferior maxillary b.
    inferior turbinate b.
    b. ingrowth
    intermaxillary b.
    interproximal b.
    intrajugular process of temporal b.
    invasive fungal infection of temporal b.
    jaw b.
    jugal b.
    lacrimal b.
    Lambone demineralized laminar b.
    Lambone freeze-dried b.
    lamellar b.
    lamellated b.
    laminar b.

bone *(continued)*
    lateral mastoid b.
    lateral surface of zygomatic b.
    lingual b.
    lunate b.
    malar b.
    malar surface of zygomatic b.
    marble b's
    b. margin
    marginal process of malar b.
    marginal tubercle of zygomatic b.
    b. marrow
    b. marrow transplant (BMT)
    masticatory b.
    mastoid b.
    b. matrix
    maxillary b.
    maxillary process of zygomatic b.
    maxillary surface of perpendicular plate of palatine b.
    medial turbinate b.
    meiopragic b.
    metatarsal b.
    b. mineral density (BMD)
    monocortical b.
    b. morphogenic protein (BMP)
    b. morphogenic protein-2 (BMP-2)
    nasal b.
    occipital b.
    orbital b.
    orbitosphenoidal b.
    Osteomin freeze-dried b.
    osteonic b.
    Paget disease of b.
    palatal b.
    palate b.
    palatine b.
    palatomaxillary groove of palatine b.
    parietal b.

bone *(continued)*
    particulate cancellous b.
    and marrow (PCBM)
    petrous b.
    Pirle b.
    postsphenoid b.
    prefrontal b.
    prefrontal b. of von Barde-
    leben
    pterygoid b.
    b. rasp
    b. recession
    b. reconstruction
    regenerated b.
    b. remodeling
    replacement b.
    b. resection
    b. resorption
    Riolan b's
    scroll b's
    semilunar b.
    septal b's
    b. sequestrum
    sesamatic b.
    sieve b.
    sphenoid b.
    sphenoidal turbinate b's
    b. spicule
    spine of sphenoid b.
    spongy b.
    squamous b.
    styloid b.
    superior maxillary b.
    superior surface of hori-
    zontal plate of palatine b.
    superior turbinate b.
    supporting b.
    supraorbital rim of fron-
    tal b.
    supreme turbinate b.
    sutural b's
    synthetic b.
    table b's of skull
    b. tack system
    tarsal b's
    temporal b.
    temporal process of zygo-
    matic b.

bone *(continued)*
    temporal surface of fron-
    tal b.
    temporal surface of zygo-
    matic b.
    thickened b.
    b. threshold
    b. trabecula
    trabecular b.
    turbinate b.
    upper jaw b.
    vaginal process of sphe-
    noid b.
    vascular bundle implanta-
    tion into b.
    Vesalius b.
    b. wax
    b. window
    wormian b's
    woven b.
    xenogeneic b.
    yoke b.
    zygomatic b.
    zygomatic process of fron-
    tal b.
    zygomatic process of tem-
    poral b.

bone graft
    AlloMatrix injectable putty
    b. g. substitute
    alveolar b. g.
    autogenous b. g.
    autologous iliac crest b. g.
    autologous rib b. g.
    biocompatible b. g. substi-
    tute material
    Bioglass b. g. substitute
    material
    BioGran resorbable syn-
    thetic b. g.
    calvarial b. g.
    cancellous b. g.
    cancellous cellular b. g.
    cantilevered b. g.
    Capset b. g. barrier
    Collagraft b. g. matrix
    composite inlay antral and
    nasal b. g.

bone graft *(continued)*
 conchal cartilage–ethmoid
  b. g.
 cortical b. g.
 cranial b. g.
 demineralized b. g.
 double-barreled fibular
  b. g.
 free b. g.
 free autogenous cortico-
  cancellous iliac b. g.
 Grafton DBM b. g.
 heterotrophic b. g.
 iliac crest b. g.
 inlay b. g.
 in situ tricortical iliac crest
  block b. g.
 intercalary b. g.
 nonvascularized b. g.
 onlay b. g.
 orthotopic b. g.
 OsteoGen b. g.
 overlay cantilever b. g.
 PerioGlas synthetic b. g.
 primary b. g.
 revascularized b. g.
 scapula crest pedicled b. g.
 sliding inlay b. g.
 b. g. substitute
 synthetic b. g.
 undemineralized b. g.
 underlayer cantilever b. g.
 vascularized b. g. (VBG)
 vascularized metaphyseal
  b. g.
 vascularized scapular b. g.

bonelet

bone plate
 cortical b. p.
 Jaeger b. p.
 Leibinger 3-D b. p.
 mandibular staple b. p.
  (MSBP)
 Senn b. p.
 Sherman b. p.
 staple b. p.
 Y b. p.

bone powder
 Ultimatics demineralized
  cortical b. p.

BoneSource HA cement

Bonn miniature iris scissors

bonnet
 gluteal b.

Bonnet-Dechaume-Blanc syndrome

Bonney blue

Bonwill triangle

bony
 b. ankylosis
 b. annulus
 b. atresia
 b. atretic plate
 b. bridging
 b. caval opening
 b. chin button
 b. crater
 b. deformity
 b. destruction
 b. erosion
 b. excess
 b. impaction
 b. ingrowth
 b. kyphos
 b. mobilization
 b. orbit of eye
 b. palate
 b. pathologic change
 b. pogonion
 b. prominence
 b. protuberance
 b. rasping
 b. reconstruction
 b. regeneration
 b. repositioning
 b. ridge
 b. septation
 b. septum
 b. union
 b. vault collapse
 b. volume

Boo-Chai craniofacial cleft

Böök syndrome

boomerang
 b.-shaped skin paddle
 b.-shaped rectus abdominis
  musculocutaneous free
  flap

boot
 Gelocast Unna b.

border
 alveolar b.
 alveolar b. of mandible
 alveolar b. of maxilla
 caudal b.
 indurated b.
 inferior b. of mandible
 irregular b.
 lateral upper lip vermi-
  lion b.
 mandibular b.
 mucocutaneous b.
 orbital b. of sphenoid bone
 posterior b. of petrous portion of temporal bone
 raised b.
 sphenoidal b.
 superior b. of petrous portion of temporal bone
 b. tissue
 tragal b.
 vermilion b.
 vermilion b. of lip
 white roll b.

boric acid

Borst-Jadassohn type intraepidermal epithelioma

Bosker
 B. TMI Reconstruction sys-
  tem
 B. TMI surgery
 B. transmandibular recon-
  structive surgical system

boss
 b. of bone

boss (continued)
 carpal b.

Bossalino
 B. blepharoplasty
 B. operation

bosselated
 b. surface

bosselation

bossing
 frontal b.
 tip b.

Bosworth
 B. nasal saw
 B. nasal wire speculum
 B.-Joseph nasal saw

BOT
 base of tongue

Botox

bottom-shaped nose

botryomycosis

botulinum
 b. toxin
 b. toxin type A

botulism
 wound b.

bouche de tapir

bougie
 Jackson steel-stem woven
  filiform b.
 Maloney b.

bougienage

bound
 upper b.

bouquet
 Riolan b.

boutonnière deformity

Bovero muscle

bovine
 b. cartilage

bovine *(continued)*
    b. collagen
    b. face

bovine-derived bone filler

Bowen
    B. disease
    B. precancerous dermato-
        sis

bowenoid
    b. cells
    b. papulosis

bowl
    conchal b.
    ear b.
    b. of ear
    mastoid b.

Bowman
    B. ciliary muscle
    B. glands

box
    anatomic snuff-b.

boxer's ear

boxing of nipple

Boyer
    B. bursa
    B. cyst

Bozzolo sign

brace
    jaw b.
    Rhino Triangle b.
    SOMI (sternal-occipital-
        mandibular immobi-
        lizer) b.

brachial
    closed b. plexus injury
    b. dermolipectomy
    b. fascia
    b. plexus
    b. plexus block

brachialis muscle

brachioradialis
    b. flap

brachioradialis *(continued)*
    b. muscle

brachiocyrtosis

brachybasophalangia

brachycephalic

brachycephalofrontonasal dys-
    plasia

brachycephalism

brachycephalous

brachycephaly
    frontal b.
    occipital b.

brachycheilia

brachychilia

brachycnemic

brachycranic

brachydactylic

brachydactyly
    Haws type b.
    b. type C

brachyesophagus

brachyfacial

brachyglossal

brachygnathia

brachygnathous

brachykerkic

brachyknemic

brachymelia

brachymesophalangia

brachymetacarpalia

brachymetacarpia
    cryptodontic b.

brachymetapody

brachymetatarsia

brachymorphic

brachyphalangia

brachyprosopic

brachyrhinia

brachyrhyncus

brachyskelous

brachystaphyline

brachysyndactyly

brachytelephalangia

brachyturricephaly

brachytypical   •

brachyuranic

bracket
    metal b.
    multiphase b.

Brackmann
    B. facial nerve monitor
    B. grade

braided
    b. sutures
    b. Vicryl suture
    b. wire

branch
    alar b. of external maxillary
        artery
    alveolar b. of internal max-
        illary artery
    anterior ethmoidal b. of
        ophthalmic artery
    auricular b.
    buccal b.
    cervical b. of facial nerve
    external b. of the superior
        laryngeal nerve
    facial nerve b's
    frontal b.
    ganglionic b's
    internal b. of the superior
        laryngeal (IBSL) nerve
    labial b's
    lingual b.
    mammary b's

branch (continued)
    marginal mandibular b.
    mental b's
    nasal b's
    nerve b.
    orbital b's
    perforating b's
    pharyngeal b. of pterygo-
        palatine ganglion
    sphenopalatine b. of inter-
        nal maxillary artery
    stylohyoid b.
    superficial palmar b. of ra-
        dial artery
    zygomatic b.
    zygomaticofacial b.
    zygomaticotemporal b.

branchial
    b. arches
    b. cleft arch
    b. cleft anomaly
    b. cleft cyst
    b. cleft sinus
    b. cleft sinusectomy
    b. cyst
    b. fistula
    hyoid b. arch
    mandibular b. arch
    b. pouch
    b. sinus

branchiogenic
    b. carcinoma
    b. cyst

branchiogenous

branchioma

Brand tendon repair

Brandt brassiere

Brandy
    B. scalp stretcher I, rear
        closure
    B. scalp stretcher II, front
        closure

brandy nose

Brånemark
    B. implant

Brånemark *(continued)*
    B. implant system
    B. osseointegration implant

branny desquamation

brassiere
    Brandt b.
    dermal b. technique
    Foerster surgical sup-
        port b.
    skin b.

Braun
    B. graft
    B. skin graft
    B.-Wangensteen graft

Brawley frontal sinus rasp

brawny
    b. edema
    b. induration

Brazilian leishmaniasis

breach
    barrier b.

breadth
    bizygomatic b.
    b. of mandible
    b. of mandibular ramus
    maxilloalveolar b.
    midfacial b.
    b. of palate
    zygomatic b.

breakdown
    b. of bone
    skin b.

breast
    b. augmentation
    b. binder
    b. cancer
    constricted b.
    b. contour
    contralateral b.
    fibrocystic b. disorder
    b. folds
    b. hypertrophy
    b. hypoplasia

breast *(continued)*
    hypoplastic tuberous b.
    b. implant
    B. Implant Protector
        (B.I.P.)
    b. lift
    b. mobility
    b. mound
    b. mound reconstruction
    b. parenchyma
    pole of the b.
    postmenopausal b's
    b. prosthesis
    b. ptosis
    b. reconstruction
    b. reduction
    shotty b.
    Snoopy b.
    b. symmetry
    b. tenaculum
    b. tissue
    tubular b's
    b. implant valve
    b. volume

breast-conserving surgery

breathing
    frog b.
    glossopharyngeal b.
    mouth b.

Breda disease

bregma

bregmatic
    b. bone
    b. fontanelle

bregmatomastoid suture

Brent
    B. eyebrow reconstruction
    B. pressure earring for ke-
        loid surgery

brephoplastic graft

Breschet
    B. canal
    B. hiatus
    B. sinus

Breschet *(continued)*
  B. veins

Breslow
  B. classification for malignant melanoma
  B. measurements
  B. microstaging system for malignant melanoma
  B. thickness

brevis
  extensor digitorum b. (EDB)
  palmaris b.

Brewerton view radiograph

Brickner sign

bridge
  b. flap
  intercellular b.
  Maryland b.
  b. of nose
  palmar skin b.

Bridgemaster nasal splint

bridging
  bony b.

Brill-Symmers disease

Brinker tissue retractor

Brink PeriPyriform implant

Brissaud-Marie syndrome

Bristow
  B. zygomatic elevator
  B.-Bankart soft tissue retractor

brittle bone disease

Broca
  B. angle
  B. basilar angle
  B. facial angle

Brockman clubfoot procedure

Broders
  B. index *(grades 1–4)*

Broders *(continued)*
  B. tumor classification *(grades 1–4)*

Brooke
  B. Army Hospital splint
  B. disease
  B. epithelioma
  B. tumor

Brophy
  B. bistoury
  B. bistoury knife
  B. cleft palate knife
  B. dressing forceps
  B. knife
  B. operation
  B. plastic surgery scissors
  B. plate
  B. scissors
  B. tenaculum

brow
  apex of the b.
  contour of the b.
  coronal b. lift
  endoscopic b. lift
  endoscopically assisted b. lift
  b. ptosis
  ptotic b.
  b. tape

brow lift
  coronal b. l.
  endoscopic b. l.
  endoscopic b. l. with simultaneous carbon dioxide laser resurfacing
  endoscopically assisted b. l.
  open coronal b. l.
  subperiosteal b. l.

Brown
  B. cleft palate knife
  B. cleft palate needle
  B. dermatome
  B. electric dermatome
  B. lip clamp
  B. nasal splint

Brown *(continued)*
  B. push-back palatoplasty
  B. syndrome
  B.-Adson forceps
  B.-Adson side-grasping forceps
  B.-Blair dermatome
  B.-Blair operation
  B.-Blair skin graft knife
  B.-Brenn stain
  B.-Brenn staining method
  B.-Burr modified Gillies retractor
  B. and McDowell alar cartilage relocation

brown
  b. adipose tissue
  b. fat

browpexy
  endoscopy b.

brow-upper lid complex

Broyle ligament

brucellosis

Bruch glands

Brücke muscle

Bruening nasal-cutting septal forceps

Bruhn method

Brun plastic surgery scissors

Brunn membrane

BSC
  basosquamous carcinoma
  burn scar contracture

BSS
  balanced salt solution

BSSO
  bilateral sagittal split osteotomy

BTR
  buccal triangular ridge

bubas braziliana

buccal
  b. alveolar plate
  b. alveolus
  b. angle
  b. artery
  b. aspect
  b. cervical ridge
  b. crossbite
  b. defect
  b. embrasure
  b. envelope flap
  b. epithelium
  b. fat
  b. fat pad
  b. glands
  b. lymph node
  b. mucosa
  b. mucosa graft
  b. mucosal flap
  b. muscle
  b. mucosal defect
  b. mucosal flap
  b. musculomucosal flap
  b. nerve
  b. neuralgia
  b. occlusion
  b. triangular ridge (BTR)

buccinator
  b. artery
  b. fascia
  b. muscle
  b. myomucosal flap
  b. nerve

buccoaxiogingival

buccocervical

buccodistal

buccogingival

buccolabial

buccolingual

buccomandibular zone

buccomaxillary

buccomesial (BM)

bucco-occlusal (BO)

buccopalatal

buccopharyngeal
  b. fascia

buccoversion

buccula

Buchwald atrophy

Buck
  B. fascia
  B. knife

bucket-handle view of facial
  bones

buckling fracture of the phalanx

bud
  limb b.
  tooth b.

Budinger blepharoplasty

Buerger disease

bulb
  hair b.
  jugular b.
  olfactory b.
  saphenous b.

bulbiform

bulbous
  b. nasal tip
  b. turbinates

bulge
  periocular b.

bulk pack technique

bulky pressure dressing

bulla *pl.* bullae
  ethmoid b.
  ethmoidal b.
  b. ethmoidalis
  b. ethmoidalis cava nasi
  b. ethmoidalis ossis eth-
    moidalis
  hemorrhagic b.
  intraepidermal b.

bulldog
  b. forceps
  b. nasal scissors
  vascular b.

Buller eye shield

bullous
  b. erythema multiforme
  b. hemorrhagic pyoderma
    gangrenosum
  b. lesion
  b. lichen planus
  b. pemphigoid

bull's eye lesion

bumper
  lip b.

bundle
  acousticofacial nerve b.
  extravelar muscle b.
  fiber b.
  inferior alveolar neurovas-
    cular b.
  muscle b.
  nerve b.
  nerve fiber b.
  neurovascular b.
  orbital neurovascular b.
  sensory nerve fiber b.
  transverse b's of palmar
    aponeurosis
  vascular b.

Bunnell
  B. bipedicle digital visor
    flap
  B. bipedicle flap
  B. dressing
  B. flap
  B. sign
  B. suture

bur (*spelled also* burr)
  Adson b.
  Bailey skull b.
  Cavanaugh sphenoid b.
  cranial b.
  Hall mastoid b.
  b. hole

bur *(continued)*
    Hudson cranial b.
    Lindeman b.
    Masseran trepan b.
    rhinoplasty diamond b.
    Sachs skull b.
    sphenoidal b.

buried
    b. de-epithelialized local
      flap
    b. dermal flap
    b. free forearm flap transfer
    b. sutures

Burkitt
    B. lymphoma
    B. lymphoma of nasal ala

burn
    acid b.
    acute phase of b. injury
    alkali b.
    b. alopecia
    cement b.
    chemical b.
    concrete b.
    electrical b.
    first degree b.
    b. eschar
    flash b.
    full-thickness b.
    laryngeal b.
    Lund and Browder chart
      for b. estimation
    Parkland fluid requirement
      formula for b. patients
    partial-thickness b.
    powder b.
    b. process
    radiation b.
    b. reconstruction
    road b.
    b. scar contracture (BSC)
    b. scar treatment
    second degree b.
    b. shock
    slag b.
    thermal b.
    third degree b.

burn *(continued)*
    three zones of a b. wound
    b. wound
    b. wound anemia
    b. wound management
    b. wound regimen
    x-ray b.

Burow
    B. blepharoplasty
    B. cheiloplasty
    B. flap
    B. flap operation
    B. operation
    B. solution
    B. technique
    B. triangle
    B. triangle deformity

bursa *pl.* bursae
    Boyer b.
    Fleischmann b.
    hyoid b.
    Luschka b.
    nasopharyngeal b.
    pharyngeal b.
    retrohyoid b.
    retromammary b.
    Tornwaldt b.

burr *(variant of* bur*)*

Burton
    B. line
    B. sign

Buschke-Ollendorf sign

button
    Aleppo b.
    Baghdad b.
    Biskra b.
    bony chin b.
    Converse fracture-wiring b.
    b. farcy
    implant b.
    lingual b.
    oriental b.

buttonhole approach

buttonholing of skin

buttress
  maxillary b.
  nasomaxillary b.
  pterygomaxillary b.
  zygomatic b.
  zygomatic b. of maxilla
  zygomaticomaxillary b.

buttressing

B-W graft

Byzantine arch palate

C

CA
    carcinoma
    cervicoaxial

cable
    c. graft
    c. tie
    c. wire sutures

cacogenesis

cacomelia

cacomorphosis

cadaveric
    c. donor
    c. graft

CAD/CAM
    computer-assisted design/
      computer-assisted manu-
      facturing

café au lait
    c. au l. birthmark
    c. au l. macule (CALM)
    c. au l. spots

Caffey
    C. disease
    C. syndrome
    C.-Silverman disease

Cagot ear

Cairns
    C. maneuver
    C. retractor

calcific
    c. density
    c. shadow

calcification
    amorphous c.
    c. of breast implant
    capsular c.
    dystrophic c.
    diffuse c.
    soft tissue c.
    spiculated c.
    subcutaneous c.

calcified
    c. lymph node
    c. node
    c. nodule
    c. tissue

calciform papilla

calcifying
    c. cyst
    c. epithelial odontogenic
      tumor
    c. epithelioma of Malherbe
    c. and keratinizing odonto-
      genic cyst
    c. odontogenic cyst

calcinosis circumscripta

calciphylaxis

Calcitek drill system

Calcitite hydroxyapatite coating

calcitonin

calculus *pl.* calculi
    hard c.
    lacrimal c.
    mammary c.
    nasal c.
    pharyngeal c.
    salivary c.

Caldwell
    C. projection
    C. view
    C.-Luc incision
    C.-Luc maxillary antros-
      tomy
    C.-Luc operation
    C.-Luc window operation

calf augmentation

calibrated
    c. clubfoot splint
    c. probe
    c. position
    c. triangle of septal carti-
      lage

calipers
Accu-Measure skinfold c.
bone-measuring c.
breast c.
Castroviejo c.
Cottle c.
digital c.
FatTrack Digital body fat c.
FatTrack skinfold c.
Harpenden skinfold c.
Ladd c.
Lafayette skinfold c.
Lange/Jamar skinfold c.
Lange skinfold c.
McGaw skinfold c.
Mitutoyo Digimatic c.
skinfold c.
Tenzel c.
Vernier c.
x-ray c.

Cali-Press graft press

Callahan
C. fixation forceps
C. flange
C. lacrimal rongeur
C. method
C. modification speculum
C. retractor
C. rongeur
C. scleral fixation forceps

Callaway formula

Callia abdominoplasty

callus distraction

CALM
café au lait macule

caloric
c. nystagmus
c. requirements for burn
patients

calorie-to-nitrogen ratio

calorimetry
indirect c.

Caltagirone skin graft knife

calvarectomy

calvaria *pl.* calvariae

calvarial
c. bone
c. bone graft
c. clamp
c. defect
c. deformity
c. repair

calvarium flap

calvities

CAM
cell adhesion molecule

cambrium layer

camera
Zeiss operating c.

Cameron elevator

camouflage
c. augmentation
cosmetic c.
c. make-up

Campbell
C. nerve rongeur
C. retractor

Campbell De Morgan spots

Camper
C. angle
C. chiasm
C. fascia
fascia of C.
C. line
C. plane

camptodactylia

camptodactylism

camptodactyly
congenital c.

camptomelia

campylodactyly

campylognathia

canal
  accessory palatine c.
  alisphenoid c.
  alveolar c.
  alveolar c. of maxilla
  alveolodental c's
  anterior condyloid c. of oc-
    cipital bone
  anterior vertical c.
  Arnold c.
  basipharyngeal c.
  Breschet c.
  calciferous c's
  carotid c.
  carpal c.
  c's of cartilage
  ciliary c's
  common c.
  condylar c.
  craniopharyngeal c.
  dehiscent mandibular c.
  diploic c's
  Dorello c.
  ear c.
  ethmoid c.
  external auditory c. (EAC)
  facial c.
  fallopian c.
  Ferrein c.
  fibro-osseous flexor ten-
    don c.
  flexor c.
  galactophorous c's
  greater palatine c.
  Guidi c.
  c. of Guidi
  Guyon c.
  Hannover c.
  haversian c's
  hypoglossal c.
  infraorbital c.
  interfacial c's
  irruption c.
  Kürsteiner c's
  lacrimal c.
  lateral c.
  c's for lesser palatine
    nerves

canal (continued)
  mandibular c.
  mandibular neurovascu-
    lar c.
  maxillary c.
  mental c.
  mesiobuccal c.
  nasolacrimal c.
  nasopalatine c.
  nutrient c. of bone
  orbital c.
  palatine c.
  palatomaxillary c.
  palatovaginal c.
  Petit c.
  pharyngeal c.
  pterygoid c.
  pterygopalatine c.
  c's of Recklinghausen
  recurrent c.
  Rivinus c's
  ruffed c.
  Santorini c.
  c's of Scarpa
  serous c.
  sphenopalatine c.
  sphenopharyngeal c.
  Stensen c.
  Sucquet c's
  Sucquet-Hoyer c's
  supraciliary c.
  supraorbital c.
  tarsal c.
  temporal c.
  Tourtual c.
  vidian c.
  Volkmann c's
  vomerine c.
  vomerobasilar c.
  vomerorostral c.
  vomerovaginal c.
  Walther c's
  zygomaticofacial c.
  zygomaticotemporal c.

canalicular

canaliculitis

canaliculus pl. canaliculi
  c. innominatus

canaliculus *(continued)*
    intercellular c.
    lacrimal c.
    c. lacrimalis
    secretory c.
    Thiersch canaliculi

canalis

canalization

canaloplasty

Canals-N root canal filling material

cancellated

cancellous
    c. bone
    c. bone graft
    c. cellular bone (CCB)
    c. freeze-dried allograft

cancellus

cancer
    acinar c.
    acinous c.
    adenoid c.
    black c.
    black mole c.
    boring c.
    breast c.
    claypipe c.
    colloid c.
    cystic c.
    endothelial c.
    epidermal c.
    epithelial c.
    glandular c.
    c. in situ
    laryngeal c.
    melanotic c.
    mule-spinners' c.
    oral c.
    oral cavity c.
    pitch-workers' c.
    skin c.
    smoker's c.
    spindle cell c.
    tar c.
    telangiectatic c.

cancer *(continued)*
    tubular c.
    villous duct c.

cancerous

cancriform

cancrum *pl.* cancra
    c. nasi
    c. oris

Candela
    C. ALEXlazr
    C. GentleLASE
    C. laser
    C. pulsed dye laser
    C. ScleroLaser

candidal
    c. angular cheilitis
    c. infection

candidiasis
    acute atrophic oral c.
    chronic hyperplastic c.
    cutaneous c.
    esophageal c.
    c. in face-lift skin flap
    localized mucocutaneous c.
    mucocutaneous c.
    oral c.
    oropharyngeal c.

Canfield facial plastics garment

canine
    c. alveolus
    c. eminence
    maxillary c.
    c. muscle
    c. prominence
    c. smile

canine-to-canine lingual splint

canister
    Bemis suction c.
    Lipovacutainer c.
    Sorensen reusable c.

canker sore

Cann-Ease moisturizing nasal gel

cannula *pl.* cannulas, cannulae
  angled c.
  aspirating c.
  aspiration c.
  Becker dissector c.
  Becker Greater Grater dissecting c.
  blunt bullet-tip c.
  blunt-tipped c.
  CellFriendly c.
  Cobra c.
  Coleman aspiration c.
  Concorde suction c.
  Cosmetech c.
  extractor/injector c.
  Fasanella lacrimal c.
  flap c.
  flap dissector c.
  four-pronged liposuction c.
  frontal sinus c.
  G-bevel c.
  Goddio disposable c.
  Gonzalez specialized dissecting c.
  Gram c.
  Illouz c.
  infusion/infiltration c.
  Karman c.
  Klein c.
  Leon c.
  Leon cobra c.
  liposuction c.
  Mercedes c.
  motorized c.
  oscillating c.
  Pinto superficial dissection c.
  pyramid c.
  reciprocating c.
  Robles cutting point c.
  Shark-tip c.
  single-holed suction c.
  single-lumen c.
  small-bore c.
  soft tissue shaving c.
  spatula tip c.
  standard single port c.
  suction c.

cannula *(continued)*
  Toledo V-dissector c.
  Toomey angled c.
  Toomey G-bevel c.
  Toomey standard c.
  Tulip c.
  tumescent infiltrator c.
  ultrasonic c.

cannulate

cannulation
  duct c.

cannulization

CANS
  computer-assisted neurosurgical navigational system

cant
  c. of mandible
  occlusal c.
  c. of occlusal plane of mandible
  c. of upper lip

canthal
  c. drift
  c. lift
  medial c. tendon

canthectomy

canthitis

cantholysis
  inferior c.
  lateral c.
  superior c.

canthomeatal
  c. flap
  c. line

canthopexy
  bilateral c.
  lateral c.

canthoplasty
  Agnew c.
  Ammon c.
  arrowhead c.

canthoplasty *(continued)*
    inferior retinacular lateral c.
    lateral c.
    medial c.
    provisional c.
    tarsal strip c.

canthorrhaphy

canthotomy
    lateral c.

canthus *pl.* canthi
    external c.
    inner c.
    internal c.
    lateral c.
    medial c.
    nasal c.
    outer c.
    temporal c.

cantilever
    c. graft

cantilevered bone graft

cap
    chin c.
    skull c.
    c. splint
    c. technique

capacity
    cranial c.

capillary
    alveolar c.
    c. angioma
    c. arcade
    c. bed
    c. drainage
    c. flames
    c. hemangioma
    lymph c.
    c. lymphangioma
    lymphatic c.
    c. malformation
    c. nevus
    c. plexus
    c. pressure
    c. refill

capillary *(continued)*
    c. vascular malformation

capitate
    c. bone
    c. fracture
    c. papillae

capitolunate
    c. articulation
    c. joint
    c. ligament

capitonnage
    c. sutures

capitulum
    c. mandibulae
    c. processus condyloidei

Caplan nasal bone scissors

Capner boutonnière splint

Capset bone graft barrier

capsula
    c. adiposa
    c. articularis articulationis temporomandibularis
    c. articularis mandibulae

capsular
    c. calcification
    c. contracture
    c. flap pyeloplasty

capsule
    adherent c.
    adipose c.
    articular c.
    fibrous c.
    lateral c.
    midcarpal c.
    nasal c.
    parotid c.
    periprosthetic fibrous c.
    radiocarpal joint c.
    salivary gland c.
    temporomandibular joint c.
    c. of temporomandibular joint
    thyroid c.
    tumor c.

capsulectomy

capsulitis

capsulopalpebral fascia

capsuloplasty

capsulorrhaphy

capsulotomy
 closed c.
 open c.

caput *pl.* capita
 c. angulare musculi quadrati labii superioris
 c. infraorbitale musculi quadrati labii superioris
 c. mandibulae
 c. medusae
 c. progeneum
 c. quadratum
 c. ulnae syndrome
 c. zygomaticum musculi quadrati labii superioris

Carapace disposable face shield

carbolic acid

carbon

carbonaceous material

carbon dioxide (CO_2)
 c. d. laser

carbuncle

carbuncular

carbunculoid

carcinoembryonic antigen (CEA)

carcinogen

carcinogenesis

carcinogenic

carcinoid
 laryngeal c.
 oncocytoid c.

carcinoma (CA)
 acinar c.
 acinic cell c.
 acinous c.
 acinous cell c.
 adenocystic c.
 adenoid cystic c.
 adenoid cystic c. of head and neck (ACCHN)
 adenoid squamous cell c.
 c. adenomatosum
 adenopapillary c.
 ameloblastic c.
 amphicrine c.
 anaplastic c.
 basal cell c. (BCC)
 basaloid c.
 basal squamous cell c.
 c. basocellulare
 basosquamous c. (BSC)
 branchiogenic c.
 central mucoepidermoid c.
 clear cell c.
 colloid c.
 cribriform c.
 cribriform salivary c. of the excretory duct
 c. cutaneum
 cystic c.
 ductal c.
 ductal c. in situ
 epidermoid c.
 c. epitheliale adenoides
 epithelial-myoepithelial c.
 exophytic c.
 c. ex pleomorphic adenoma
 fibroepithelioma basal cell c.
 follicular c.
 follicular thyroid c.
 gelatiniform c.
 gelatinous c.
 giant cell c.
 glandular c.
 glottic c.
 glottic squamous cell c.

carcinoma *(continued)*
    hair-matrix c.
    hematoid c.
    hypopharyngeal c.
    hypopharyngeal squamous
      cell c.
    infiltrating c.
    infiltrative basal cell c.
    inflammatory c.
    infraglottic c.
    infraglottic squamous
      cell c.
    c. in situ
    in situ squamous cell c.
    intermediate c.
    intraductal c.
    intraepidermal c.
    intraepithelial c.
    intraosseous c.
    invasive c.
    invasive lobular c.
    juvenile c.
    keratinizing squamous
      cell c.
    laryngeal c.
    laryngeal neuroendo-
      crine c.
    latent c.
    lateral aberrant thyroid c.
    lenticular c.
    lingual thyroid c.
    lobular c.
    lobular c. in situ
    lymphoepithelial c.
    maxillary sinus c.
    medullary c.
    melanotic c.
    Merkel cell c.
    metaplastic c.
    metastatic c.
    metastatic basal cell c.
    metatypical c.
    microcystic adnexal c.
    moderately differentiated
      neuroendocrine c.
    morbilliform basal cell c.
    morpheaform basal cell c.
    mucinous c.

carcinoma *(continued)*
    mucoepidermoid c. (MEC)
    mucoepidermoid c. of pa-
      rotid
    mucoepidermoid c. of the
      tongue
    mucus-producing adenopa-
      pillary c. (MPAPC)
    nasopharyngeal c. (NPC)
    c. of nasopharynx (types
      a–c)
    neuroendocrine c.
    nevoid basal cell c.
    nodular basal cell c.
    nodular ulcerative basal
      cell c.
    noninfiltrating lobular c.
    nonkeratinizing c.
    oat cell c.
    occult c.
    oncoplastic c.
    oral squamous c.
    oral squamous cell c.
    papillary c.
    papillary squamous c.
    papillary thyroid c.
    parotid c.
    pigmented basal cell c.
    pilomatrixoma c.
    preinvasive c.
    prickle-cell c.
    primary c.
    primary neuroendocrine c.
      of the skin
    recurrent basal cell c.
    recurrent squamous cell c.
    reserve cell c.
    salivary duct c. (SDC)
    salivary gland c. (SGC)
    sarcomatoid c.
    Schmincke-Regaud lym-
      phoepithelial c.
    schneiderian c.
    scirrhous c.
    sclerosing basal cell c.
    sebaceous c.
    secondary c.
    secretory c.

carcinoma *(continued)*
  c. simplex
  small cell c.
  small cell neuroendocrine c.
  spheroidal cell c.
  spindle cell c.
  squamous cell c. (SCC)
  squamous cell c. of head
    and neck (SCCHN)
  subglottic squamous cell c.
  subungual squamous cell c.
  superficial basal cell c.
  supraglottic c.
  supraglottic squamous
    cell c.
  sweat gland c.
  c. telangiectaticum
  thyroid c.
  trabecular c.
  transglottic squamous
    cell c.
  tuberous c.
  tubular c.
  undifferentiated c.
  undifferentiated c. of naso-
    pharyngeal type
  verrucous c.
  well-differentiated c.

carcinomatosis

carcinosis
  miliary c.

Carhart notch

carina

Carlens mediastinoscope

Carmault hemostat

Carmody
  C.-Batson elevator
  C.-Batson operation

carotenemia

carotenoderma

caroticotympanic

carotid
  c. air cell
  c. aneurysm

carotid *(continued)*
  c. arterial beds
  c. artery
  c. bifurcation
  c. body
  c. body tumor
  c. canal
  c.–cavernous sinus fistula
    (CCSF)
  common c. artery
  external c. artery
  c. genu
  ipsilateral common c. ar-
    tery
  c. isolation
  c. nerve
  c. plexus
  c. sheath
  c. sinus
  c. sinus reflex
  c. space

carotodynia

carpal
  c. bones
  c. boss
  c. canal
  c. compression test
  c. dislocation
  endoscopic c. tunnel de-
    compression
  endoscopic c. tunnel re-
    lease (ECTR)
  c. height measurement
  c. height ratio
  c. instability
  proximal c. row
  c. row bones
  c. tunnel compression
  c. tunnel decompression
  c. tunnel release (CTR)
  c. tunnel release system
    (CTRS)
  c. tunnel syndrome (CTS)

Carpenter syndrome

carp mouth

carpometacarpal (CMC)
  c. articulations

carpometacarpal *(continued)*
    c. joint
    c. ligament

Carpue
    C. method
    C. operation
    C. rhinoplasty

carpus
    columnar c. theory
    greater arc injury of the c.
    lesser arc injury of the c.

CarraSmart foam

Carrasyn hydrogel

carrier
    miniature c.

Carrington dermal wound gel

Carroll skin hook

Carter
    C. intranasal splint
    C. pillow
    C.-Thomason suture passer

cartilage
    accessory c.
    accessory nasal c.
    accessory c. of nose
    accessory quadrate c.
    alar c.
    alar batten c.
    alar dome and c.
    alisphenoid c.
    annular c.
    articular c.
    arytenoid c.
    auricular c.
    beveled septal c.
    bovine c.
    c.-breaking technique
    calcified c.
    conchal c.
    condylar c.
    convex c. graft
    corniculate c.
    costal c.
    cricoid c.
    cuneiform c.

cartilage *(continued)*
    cuneiform c. of Wrisberg
    ear c.
    c. edge
    epactal c's
    floating c.
    c. graft
    greater alar c.
    Huschke c.
    hyaline c.
    hyaline articular c.
    hyoid c.
    innominate c.
    c. island
    Jacobson c.
    laryngeal c.
    lateral c.
    lateral c. of nose
    lesser alar c.
    loose c.
    lower lateral c.
    Luschka c.
    mandibular c.
    Meckel c.
    Meyer c.
    c.-molding technique
    Morgagni c.
    morselized c.
    ossifying c.
    palpebral c.
    paraseptal c.
    permanent c.
    quadrangular c.
    quadrilateral c.
    rectangular c. graft
    rib c.
    sail of c.
    Santorini c.
    c. scaffolding
    c. scoring
    Seiler c.
    semilunar c.
    septal c.
    sesamoid c. of larynx
    sesamoid c. of nose
    soft c.
    splayed alar c.
    supra-arytenoid c.
    temporary c.

cartilage *(continued)*
 thyroid c.
 tissue-engineered c.
 tragal c.
 triangular c.
 tympanomandibular c.
 upper lateral nasal c.
 vomerine c.
 vomeronasal c.
 Wrisberg c.
 yellow c.

cartilaginous
 c. autologous thin septal
   graft
 c. collagen
 c. growth
 c. septum
 c. support

cartilago *pl.* cartilagines
 c. alaris major
 cartilagines alares minores
 c. arytenoidea
 c. auriculae
 c. corniculata
 c. costalis
 c. cricoidea
 c. cuneiformis
 c. epiglottica
 cartilagines laryngis
 c. meatus acustici
 cartilagines nasales
 cartilagines nasales acces-
   soriae
 cartilagines nasi
 c. sesamoidea laryngis
 c. thyroidea
 cartilagines tracheales
 c. triticea
 c. vomeronasalis

caruncle
 lacrimal c.
 Stensen duct c.
 sublingual c.
 submaxillary c.

caruncula *pl.* carunculae
 c. lacrimalis
 c. salivaris

caruncula *(continued)*
 c. sublingualis

carver
 acorn c.
 Vehe c.

cascade
 complementary c.

caseated tissue

caseating
 c. granuloma

caseation

caseous necrosis

Casser fontanelle

casserian fontanelle

cast
 diagnostic c.
 gnathostatic c.
 master c.
 modified c.
 preoperative c.
 short-arm thumb spica c.

Castallo lid retractor

Castanares
 C. bilateral blepharoplasty
 C. face-lift scissors

Castroviejo
 C. calipers
 C. dermatome
 C. forceps
 C. retractor
 C. scissors
 C. tenotomy scissors

cat
 c. cry syndrome
 c's ear
 c. epithelium
 c's paw retractor
 c. sneer exercise

catabasial

catarrh
 atrophic c.

catarrh *(continued)*
  hypertrophic c.
  nasal c.
  postnasal c.

catarrhal

catenating

caterpillar flap

catgut
  absorbable c.
  chromic c.
  fast-absorbing c.
  formaldehyde c.
  IKI c.
  c. ligature
  c. needle
  c. plain ties
  Rica surgical c.
  SMIC surgical c.
  c. suture (CGS)

catheter
  Abocath c.
  ARROWgard central ven-
    ous c.
  axillary c.
  Bivona epistaxis c.
  fine-bore c.
  Fogarty c.
  Foley c.
  Hickman c.
  indwelling c.
  nasotracheal c.
  pectoral c.
  red Robinson c.
  red rubber c.
  Robinson c.
  Schrötter c.
  sialographic c.
  silicone epistaxis c.
  c. technique for brachial
    plexus block
  transoral c.
  two-way c.
  VNUS Closure c.
  VNUS Restore c.

cauda
  c. equina
  c. helicis

caudad

caudal
  c. border
  c. condensation of the
    transverse fascial tissues
  c. displacement
  c. septal angle
  c. septal reduction
  c. septum

caudocranial view

cauliflower ear

causalgia
  facial c.

cause
  extra-articular c's of wrist
    pain

caustic
  c. acid
  alkali c.

cauterization

cautery
  bipolar c.
  chemical c.
  Colorado tip c.

Cavanaugh sphenoid bur

cave
  Meckel c.

cavernoma

cavernosum
  angioma c.
  corpus c.

cavernous
  c. angioma
  c. hemangioma
  c. lymphangiohemangioma
  c. lymphangioma
  c. sinus
  c. sinus syndrome

caviar lesion

Cavilon barrier ointment

cavitas *pl.* cavitates
  c. dentis
cavity
  abdominal c.
  alveolar c.
  bony c. of nose
  buccal c.
  c. of concha
  cranial c.
  faucial c.
  idiopathic bone c.
  infraglottic c.
  labial c.
  laryngeal c.
  laryngopharyngeal c.
  lingual c.
  mastoid c.
  Meckel c.
  nasal c.
  neovaginal c.
  nonseptate c.
  oral c.
  orbital c.
  pharyngeal c.
  pharyngonasal c.
  Rosenmüller c.
  thoracic c.
  wound c.
cavum *pl.* cava
  c. conchae
  c. conchal cartilage graft
  c. dentis
  c. nasi
  c. trigeminale
Cawood nasal splint

Cazenave vitiligo

C-bar web-spacer

CCA
  common carotid artery
CCB
  cancellous cellular bone
CCG
  costochondral graft

CCH
  circumscribed choroidal
    hemangioma
CCMS
  cerebrocostomandibular
    syndrome
CCRN
  congenital cartilaginous
    rest of the neck
CCS
  Composite Cultured Skin
CCSF
  carotid–cavernous sinus
    fistula
CEA
  carcinoembryonic antigen
cebocephaly
celiac
  c. artery
  c. dimple
celiorrhaphy
celiotomy
cell
  acinar c.
  c. adhesion molecule
    (CAM)
  anterior ethmoidal air c.
  basal epidermal c's
  basaloid c.
  Boll c's
  bowenoid c's
  carotid air c.
  collagen-producing c's
  cultured periosteal c.
  dendritic c.
  desquamated epithelial c.
  endothelial c.
  epithelial c.
  epithelioid c.
  ethmoid c.
  ethmoid air c.
  ethmoidal c.

cell *(continued)*
   ethmoidal air c.
   ethmoidal labyrinth c.
   fat c.
   foreign body giant c.
   c.-free zone
   Hürthle c.
   immunocompetent c.
   inflammatory c.
   infralabyrinthine air c.
   infundibular c.
   interdigitating dendritic c.
    (IDC)
   K c.
   Langerhans c's
   Langerhans-type giant c's
   macular hair c.
   malpighian c.
   mast c.
   mastoid tip c.
   meningothelial c.
   Merkel c.
   mesenchymal c.
   microvillar c.
   Mikulicz c's
   monocytoid c.
   mucous c.
   mucus-secreting c.
   multinucleated dentino-
    blastic c.
   multinucleated giant c.
   myoepithelial c.
   myofibroblast c.
   nerve c.
   Neumann c.
   neural crest c.
   oncocytic epithelial c.
   Paget c's
   c.-poor zone
   c.-rich zone
   Schultze c's
   Schwann c.
   spindle c.
   supporting c.
   supraorbital air c.
   transplanted fat c's
   Virchow c's

CellFriendly cannula

cell-mediated
   c.-m. immune response
   c.-m. immunity

cellular
   c. blue nevus
   c. debris
   c. pleomorphism

cellulite
   Chesterfield sofa c.
   c. phenomenon

cellulitic defect

cellulitis
   acute scalp c.
   anaerobic c.
   anaerobic clostridial c.
   demarcated c.
   dissecting c. of scalp
   orbital c.
   periorbital c.
   preseptal c.
   submaxillary c.
   synergistic necrotizing c.

cellulocutaneous flap

cement
   BoneSource HA c.
   modified zinc oxide-eugen-
    ol c.
   My-Bond Carbo c.

Cencit facial scanner

center-action forceps

central
   c. facial paralysis
   c. fat
   c. fibroma
   c. fibromatosis
   c. fossa
   c. giant cell granuloma
   c. giant cell tumor
   c. hemangioma
   c. mucoepidermoid carci-
    noma
   c. occlusion
   c. ossifying fibroma

central *(continued)*
c. resorption
c. vermilion

centric
c. checkbite
c. jaw relation
c. maxillomandibular
  record
Myo-monitor c.
c. occlusion
c. position
c. relation
retruded c.

centrically balanced occlusion

centriciput

centrofacial

cephalad

cephalalgia
pharyngotympanic c.
quadrantal c.

cephalgia

cephalhematoma
calcified c.
c. deformans

cephalic

cephalocaudad

cephalocaudal

cephalocele
basal c.
frontal c.
frontoethmoidal c.
occipital c.
parietal c.
sincipital c.

cephalodactyly
Vogt c.

cephalogram
lateral c.

cephalography

cephalomegaly

cephalomelus

cephalometer
radiographic c.

cephalometric
c. analysis
c. correction
c. landmark
c. plane
c. radiograph
c. radiography
c. relationship
c. standards
c. tracing

cephalometrics

cephalometry

cephalonia

cephalo-oculocutaneous telangiectasia

cephalopagus

cephalopolysyndactyly syndrome

cephalostat
portable c.
Porta-Stat c.

cephalothoracopagus
c. disymmetros
c. monosymmetros

CeraMed bone grafting material

ceramic
machinable apatite-free
  glass c.

cerclage

cerebellopontile angle

cerebellopontine
c. angle
c. angle syndrome
c. angle tumor

cerebellum

cerebral
c. anoxia
c. cortex

cerebral *(continued)*
    c. gigantism
    c. palsy
    c. reference line

cerebri
    falx c.
    pseudotumor c.

cerebriform tongue

cerebrocostomandibular syndrome (CCMS)

cerebrospinal
    c. fluid (CSF)
    c. fluid fistula
    c. fluid leak
    halo test for c. fluid (CSF) leak
    halo test for c. fluid (CSF) rhinorrhea
    c. rhinorrhea

cerumen inspissatum

ceruminoma

cervical
    c. abrasion
    c. actinomycosis
    c. anchorage
    c. cyst
    c. fascia
    c. flap
    c. ganglion
    c. humeral flap
    c. hydrocele
    c. hygroma
    c. hyperesthesia
    c. line (CL)
    c. midline pterygium
    c. muscle contraction
    c. patagium
    c. plexus
    c. plexus anesthesia
    c. rib
    c. rotational flap
    c. spondylolysis
    c. sympathetic nerve
    c. visor flap

cervicoaxial (CA)

cervicobrachial

cervicobregmatic diameter

cervicodynia

cervicofacial
    c. actinomycosis
    c. contour
    c. fat
    c. flap
    c. liposurgery
    c. rhytidectomy
    c. sling

cervicomental angle

cervico-occipital

cervicopectoral flap

cervicoplasty

cervix
    c. dentis
    implant c.

cevitamic acid

C-flap

CFM
    chemotactic factor for macrophage

CGS
    catgut suture

Chagas disease

chagoma

chain
    spinal sympathetic c.

Chajchir dissector

chalazion *pl.* chalazia
    c. clamp
    c. curet
    c. excision
    c. forceps
    c. knife

chalazodermia

chalinoplasty

chamaecephalic

chamaecephalous

chamaecephaly

chamaeprosopic

chamaeprosopy

chamber
    bone growth c's
    hyperbaric c.

chamois yellow appearance

Champy miniplate rigid fixation
    system

chancre

chancriform

change
    actinic skin c's
    fibrocystic c.
    oncocytoid c.
    bony pathologic c.
    pigmentary c's
    postpeel pigmentary c's

channel
    blood c's
    lymph c's
    perineural c's

channel shoulder pin technique

Charcot
    C. arthropathy
    C. joint
    C. sign
    C.-Marie-Tooth atrophy
    C.-Marie-Tooth disease

char-free carbon-dioxide laser

CHARGE
    coloboma, heart anomaly,
        choanal atresia, retarda-
        tion, and genital and ear
        anomalies

Charlin syndrome

chart
    Lund and Browder c. for
        burn estimation

Charters method

Chassaignac space

Chaston eye pad

Chaussier areola

Chayes method

checkbite
    centric c.

cheek
    c. advancement flap
    c. augmentation
    c. bag
    c. biting
    c. bone
    cervical c.
    cleft c.
    collapsed c.
    c. compression
    c. flap
    c. hollows
    c. implant
    c. mucous-muscle flap
    c. muscle
    c. pad
    postmaxillectomy col-
        lapsed c.
    c. pouch
    c. retractor
    c. rotation flap
    c. tone
    c. and tongue retractor
    c. tooth
    vestibule of c.

cheek-lip flap

cheilalgia

cheilectomy
    Sage-Clark c.

cheilectropion

cheilion

cheilitis
    actinic c.
    acute c.
    angular c.
    apostematous c.

cheilitis *(continued)*
  candidal angular c.
  commissural c.
  contact c.
  c. exfoliativa
  c. glandularis
  c. glandularis apostema-
    tosa
  c.-glossitis-gingivitis syn-
    drome
  c. granulomatosa
  granulomatous c.
  impetiginous c.
  solar c.
  c. venenata
  Volkmann c.

cheiloalveoloschisis

cheiloangioscopy

cheilocarcinoma

cheilognathoglossoschisis

cheilognathopalatoschisis

cheilognathoprosoposchisis

cheilognathoschisis

cheilognathouranoschisis

cheiloncus

cheilophagia

cheiloplasty
  Abbe stage I c.
  Abbe stage II c.
  Abbe-Estlander c.
  Bernard-Burow c.
  Burow c.
  Chopart c.
  Cronin c.
  Hagedorn c.
  Simon c.
  Stein c.
  Tennison c.
  Webster c.
  Webster modification of
    Bernard-Burow c.
  Wolfe c.

cheilorrhaphy

cheiloschisis

cheilosis

cheilostomatoplasty

cheilotomy
  Garceau c.

cheirology

cheiroplasty

chemabrasion

chemexfoliation

chemical
  c. agent
  c. burn
  c. dermatitis
  c. face peeling
  c. peel
  c. peeling

chemodectoma

chemosurgery
  Mohs c.

chemosurgical superficial der-
  matologic peel

chemotactic factor
  c. f. for macrophage (CFM)

chemotaxis

chemotherapeutic agent

chemotherapy
  adjuvant c.
  combination c.

cherry
  c. angioma
  c. hemangioma
  c. spot

cherubic facies

cherubism

chessboard graft

chest
  anterior c. wall flap
  caved-in c.
  c. flap
  foveated c.

chest *(continued)*
    funnel c.
    keeled c.
    pigeon c.
    c. wall
    c. wall anomaly
    c. wall reconstruction

Chesterfield sofa cellulite

Chevalier Jackson laryngeal
    speculum

chevron
    c. incision
    c. marking technique

CHI
    closed head injury

Chiari
    adult C. malformation
    C. malformation (*types I, II,
    III, IV*)

chiasm
    Camper c.
    c. of digits of hand
    tendinous c. of flexor digi-
        torum sublimis muscle

chilblain

Chill Tip cooling handpiece

chin
    asymmetric c.
    c. augmentation
    double c.
    extended anatomical c.
    galouche c.
    c. implant
    c. lift
    c. muscle
    c. point
    c. protuberance
    ptosis of the c.
    senile c.
    c. support
    c. tuck
    weak c.
    witch's c.

chin-contouring procedure

Chinese flap

chink
    glottal c.
    glottic c.

chin-nose view

chip
    Dembone demineralized
        cancellous c's
    Dembone demineralized
        cortical c's
    Dembone demineralized
        corticocancellous c's
    c. graft

chisel
    bilevel c.
    binangle c.
    Blair nasal c.
    bone c.
    cartilage c.
    contra-angle c.
    Converse guarded c.
    Converse nasal c.
    Cottle c.
    Freer bone c.
    Freer lacrimal c.
    Freer nasal c.
    Hajek septal c.
    monoangle c.
    Rubin nasal c.
    sinus c.
    Skoog nasal c.
    submucous c.
    Wedelstaedt c.

chloasma
    c. bronzinum
    c. gravidarum
    melanoderma c.

choana *pl.* choanae
    bony choanae
    c. narium
    choanae osseae
    primary c.
    secondary c.

choanal
    c. atresia

choanal *(continued)*
  c. opening
  c. polyp
  c. stenosis

chocolate cyst

choke vessel

cholangiopancreatography
  endoscopic c.

cholelithiasis
  occult c.

cholesteatoma
  acquired c.
  congenital c.
  iatrogenic c.

cholesterol
  c. cleft
  c. granuloma cyst

chondral

chondrectomy

chondrification

chondritis
  costal c.

chondroblast

chondroblastoma

chondrocalcinosis
  hydroxyapatite c.

chondrocarcinoma

chondrocutaneous flap

chondrocranium

chondrocyte

chondrodermatitis
  c. helicis nodularis
  c. nodularis chronica helicis

chondrodynia

chondrodysplasia
  hereditary deforming c.

chondroectodermal dysplasia

chondrodystrophia
  c. calcificans congenita
  c. congenita punctata
  c. fetalis
  c. fetalis calcificans

chondrodystrophy
  familial c.
  hyperplastic c.
  hypoplastic c.

chondroendothelioma

chondrofibroma

chondrogenesis

chondrogenic sarcoma

chondroglossus muscle

chondroid

chondrolipoma

chondroma
  benign c.
  condylar c.
  extraskeletal c.
  juxtacortical c.
  laryngeal c.
  malignant c.
  nasal c.

chondromalacia
  c. fetalis
  generalized c.
  c. of larynx
  systemic c.

chondromatosis

chondromatous

chondromucosal graft

chondromyxoma

chondromyxofibroma

chondronecrosis

chondro-osseous

chondro-osteodystrophy

chondropharyngeal muscle

chondroplasia

chondroplastic blade

chondroplasty
    c. Beaver blade

chondroporosis

chondroradionecrosis
    laryngeal c.

chondrosarcoma
    central c.
    extraosseous c.
    extraskeletal c.
    mesenchymal c. (MC)

chondrosarcomatosis

chondrosis

chondrosternal

chondrosternoplasty

chondrotomy

Chopart
    C. amputation
    C. articulation
    C. cheiloplasty
    modified C. amputation
    C. operation

chordee
    correction of c.
    c. release

chorditis
    c. vocalis inferior

chordoma *pl.* chordomas
    craniocervical c.
    dedifferentiated c.
    skull base c.

chorea
    laryngeal c.

choreoathetosis

choriomeningitis
    lymphocytic c.

choristoma
    neuromuscular c.

choroidal hemangioma

Chow technique

Christoudias fascial closure device

chromic
    c. catgut sutures
    c. catgut mattress sutures

chromicized catgut sutures

chromomycosis

chronic
    c. actinic dermatitis
    c. allograft rejection
    c. cystic mastitis
    c. fibrocystic disease
    c. graft-versus-host disease
    c. granulomatous disease
    c. hyperplastic candidiasis
    c. inflammation
    c. nerve compression
    c. pain syndrome

Churg-Strauss vasculitis

Ciaccio glands

Cica-Care silicone gel sheeting

cicatricial
    c. alopecia
    c. entropion

cicatrix *pl.* cicatrices
    hypertrophic c.
    vicious c.

cicatrization
    epithelial c.
    exuberant c.

ciliary

ciliectomy

ciliogenesis

ciliotomy

cilium *pl.* cilia
    olfactory cilia

cinch suture

cingulum dentis

circle
    Haller c.
    c. of Willis

circuit
    neuronal c.

circular
    c. subcutaneous island flap

circumareolar
    c. incision
    c. scar

circumferential
    c. fracture

circumflex
    c. iliac artery
    c. scapular artery
    c. scapular flap
    c. scapular pedicle
    c. vessel

circummandibular
    c. fixation
    c. wiring

circumocular

circumoral

circumorbital

Circumpress chin strap

circumscribed
    c. choroidal hemangioma
        (CCH)
    c. lesion
    c. precancerous melanosis
        of Dubreuilh

circumscripta
    alopecia c.
    calcinosis c.
    osteoporosis c.

circumzygomatic
    c. fixation
    c. wiring

Citelli sphenoid rongeur

citric acid

Civinini spine

CL
    cervical line
    cleft lip

CLA
    cleft lip/alveolus

clamp
    Acland c.
    Adair breast c.
    Allis c.
    approximator c.
    atraumatic bowel c.
    Berke ptosis c.
    Blair cleft palate c.
    blepharostat c.
    Brown lip c.
    bulldog c.
    calvarial c.
    chalazion c.
    columella c.
    Cottle columella c.
    D'Assumpçao c.
    David-Baker c.
    David-Baker lip c.
    Desmarres lid c.
    Erhardt lid c.
    Ewing lid c.
    fine-toothed c.
    Frazier-Adson osteoplastic
        flap c.
    Green lid c.
    Hunt c.
    Joseph c.
    Karamar-Mailatt tarsorrha-
        phy c.
    Khan-Jaeger c.
    Ladd lid c.
    Lahey c.
    Millard c.
    mosquito c.
    nerve-approximating c.
    O'Connor lid c.
    pedicle c.
    plate-holding c.
    serrefine c.

clamp *(continued)*
 shape memory c.
 Wadsworth lid c.

Clapton line

Clark
 C. classification of malignant melanoma *(Clark levels I–IV)*
 C. nevi
 C.-Elder classification of
 malignant melanoma
 C.-McGovern classification
 of malignant melanoma

Clarke-Fournier glossitis

clasp
 arrow c.
 embrasure c.
 extended c.
 infrabulge c.
 lingual c.
 mesiodistal c.
 movable-arm c.
 multiple c.

class
 c. I, II, III, IV malocclusion
 c. I, II, III occlusion
 c. III ring avulsion injury
 pattern

classification
 Ackerman-Proffitt c.
 Ackerman-Proffitt c. of mal-
 occlusion
 Altmann c. of congenital
 aural atresia
 Angle c. of malocclusion
 Antoni c. of schwannoma
 morphology
 Baker c. of capsular con-
 tracture *(Grades I–IV)*
 Blauth c. of hypoplasia of
 thumb *(types I, II, IIIA, IIIB,
 IV, V)*
 Breslow c. for malignant
 melanoma
 Broders tumor c. *(grades
 1–4)*

classification *(continued)*
 Clark c. of malignant melanoma *(Clark levels I–IV)*
 Clark-Elder c. of malignant
 melanoma
 Clark-McGovern c. of malignant melanoma
 cleft palate c.
 Coleman c. of congenital
 aural atresia
 Cormack-Lamberty c. of
 fasciocutaneous flaps
 (types A–C)
 de la Cruz c. of congenital
 aural atresia
 Elder c. of malignant melanoma
 Fitzpatrick c. of sun-reac-
 tive skin types *(types
 I–VI)*
 Gell and Coombs c.
 Glogau c. for photoaging
 (groups I–IV)
 Gustilo-Anderson c.
 Hanna c. of head and neck
 defects *(classes A, B, C)*
 Herbert alphanumeric c.
 system for scaphoid frac-
 tures *(types A1, A2, B1–4,
 C, D1, D2)*
 House-Brackmann c.
 House-Brackmann c. for fa-
 cial nerve function
 Kazangia and Converse fa-
 cial fracture c.
 Kazangia and Converse
 mandibular fracture c.
 Kernahan and Elsahy
 striped Y c. for cleft lip
 and palate
 Lichtman c. of Kienböck
 disease *(stages I, II, IIIA,
 IIIB, IV)*
 Knight and North c. of ma-
 lar fractures *(groups I–VI)*
 Le Fort c. of maxillary frac-
 tures *(I, II, III)*
 Marx c. of microtia

classification *(continued)*
  Mathes and Nahai c. for muscle circulation *(types I–V)*
  Millard modification of Kernahan and Elsahy striped Y c. for cleft lip and palate
  modified Pulvertaft c. for mutilating injuries *(categories 1–5)*
  Munro c. of orbital hypertelorism *(types A–D)*
  Nahai-Mathes c. of fasciocutaneous flaps *(types A–C)*
  Pairolero c. of sternotomy wound infection *(types I–III)*
  Pulec and Freedman c. of congenital aural atresia
  Reid c. for mutilating injuries *(groups 1–6)*
  Salter-Harris c. of epiphyseal fractures
  Schuknecht c. of congenital aural atresia
  Seddon c. for nerve injuries *(types 1–3)*
  Simons c. of malocclusion
  Spaulding c.
  Steele c. of intra-articular fractures *(types I–III)*
  Sunderland c. for nerve injuries *(grades I–V)*
  surgical c. of gynecomastia *(grades 1, 2A, 2B, 3)*
  Tessier c.
  Tessier c. of craniofacial clefts *(Tessier numbers 0–14)*
  tic-tac-toe c. for mutilating injuries of the hand *(types I–VII; subtypes A–C; vascular status 0–1)*
  Veau c.
  Wei c. for mutilating injuries *(types I, II)*

classification *(continued)*
  Wolfe c. of breast dysplasia

claudication
  venous c.

claw
  burn c.
  c. deformity
  devil's c.
  c. hand
  c. hand deformity
  lobster c. deformity
  ulnar c. hand

clawing
  c. deformity
  rheumatoid c.
  c. of ring and little fingers

claypipe cancer

cleanser
  SAF-Clens chronic wound c.
  Sea-Clens wound c.
  Shur-Clens wound c.
  SilqueClenz skin c.

clear
  c. cell acanthoma
  c. cell carcinoma

clearance
  interocclusal c.
  occlusal c.

Clear Away Disc

ClearSite
  C. bandage
  C. borderless dressing
  C. Hydro Gauze dressing
  C. wound dressing

cleft
  alveolar c.
  c. anomaly
  asymmetric bilateral c.
  atypical c.
  bilateral c.
  bilateral c. lip and palate (BCLP)
  bony c.
  Boo-Chai craniofacial c.

cleft *(continued)*
    cholesterol c.
    c. cheek
    complete bilateral c.
    congenital earlobe c.
    craniofacial c.
    c. earlobe
    c. face
    facial c.
    Facial Impairment Scales
      for c's
    fascial c.
    c. foot
    gluteal c.
    c. hand
    c. high points
    hyomandibular c.
    incomplete c.
    incomplete c. of earlobe
    isolated naso-ocular c.
    isolated unilateral c. lip/al-
      veolus (UCLA)
    c. jaw
    labial c.
    laryngeal c.
    laryngotracheoesopha-
      geal c.
    lateral facial c.
    c. of lateral aspect of nose
    laterofacial c.
    c. lip (CL)
    c. lip/alveolus (CLA)
    c. lip deformity
    c. lip nose
    c. lip and palate (CLP)
    c. margin flap
    c. maxillary segment
    medial c. of lip
    medial c. of palate
    median facial c.
    median c. of lower lip and
      mandible
    median maxillary anterior
      alveolar c.
    mesenchymal c.
    naso-ocular c.
    natal c.
    nose c.
    oblique facial c.

cleft *(continued)*
    oculofacial c.
    olfactory c.
    operated c.
    oral c.
    oronaso-ocular c.
    oro-ocular c.
    osseous c.
    palatal c.
    palatomaxillary c.
    pharyngeal c.
    postalveolar c. palate fistu-
      lation
    prealveolar c.
    prepalatal c.
    primary c.
    c. of primary palate
    secondary c.
    soft palate c.
    stenotic c.
    sternal c.
    Stillman c.
    submucosal c. palate
    submucous c.
    submucous c. palate
    symmetrical bilateral c.
    Tessier c.
    Tessier craniofacial c.
    thenar c.
    c. tongue
    transverse facial c.
    type II earlobe c.
    unilateral c.
    unilateral c. lip nose
    unilateral c. of lip and pal-
      ate
    unoperated c.
    c. uvula

clefting
    facial c.
    midline cranio-orbital c.
    suprabasal c.

cleft palate
    c. p. classification
    c. p. elevator
    c. p. forceps
    c. p. impression
    c. p. knife

cleft palate *(continued)*
  c. p. and lateral synechia
    syndrome (CPLS)
  c. p. prosthesis
  c. p. repair
  c. p. sharp hook
  c. p. tenaculum

cleidocranial
  c. dysostosis
  c. dysplasia
  c. dystrophia

Cleland ligament

clenched fist deformity

Clerf laryngeal saw

click
  temporomandibular joint c.

clicking

climate
  occlusal c.

climactericum
  keratoderma c.
  keratosis c.

clinocephaly

clinodactyly

clinoid process

clip
  Adson scalp c.
  Backhaus towel c.
  blepharoplasty c.
  Feldstein blepharoplasty c.
  hemostasis scalp c.
  hemostatic c.
  microvascular c.
  Raney c.
  Zimmer c.

clitoridauxe

clitorimegaly

clitoroplasty

clival
  c. lesion
  lower c. region

clivus

Cloquet ganglion

closed
  c. capsulotomy
  c. degloving injury
  c. disruption of digital artery
  c. head injury (CHI)
  c. in anatomic layers
  c. osteotomy
  c. reduction
  c. reduction and internal
    fixation
  c. skull fracture

closed-bite malocclusion

closure
  anatomic c.
  circular with Passavant
    ridge pattern of c.
  compression skull cap c.
  Dorrance c.
  early hard palate c.
  facial compression skull
    cap c.
  first intention wound c.
  Furlow c.
  glottic c.
  Gore-Tex c.
  inconsistent velopharyn-
    geal c.
  Marlex mesh c.
  maxillary antrum c.
  palatal c.
  palatopharyngeal c.
  primary wound c.
  secondary wound c.
  secondary c. of wound
  second intention wound c.
  sinus c.
  Steri-Strip skin c.
  Steritapes c.
  supraglottic c.
  SutureStrip Plus wound c.
  tension-free c.
  tertiary wound c.
  third intention wound c.
  vacuum-assisted closure
    (VAC)

closure *(continued)*
    Veau straight-line c.
    velopharyngeal c.
    von Langenbeck palate c.
    V-Y c.
    V-to-Y fashion c.
    watertight c.
    watertight skin c.
    Y configuration c.

clothesline
    c. evulsion of maxilla
    c. injury

clotting factor

cloverleaf skull

CLP
    cleft lip and palate

clubbed finger

clubbing

clubfoot

clubhand

CMC
    carpometacarpal
        CMC joint

CMD
    craniomandibular dysfunction

CO_2
    carbon dioxide
        continuous wave CO_2
            laser
        esthetic CO_2 laser
        CO_2 FeatherTouch
            SilkLaser
        25 Gold portable CO_2
            laser
        CO_2 laser
        CO_2 laser blepharoplasty
        Luxar NovaPulse CO_2
            laser
        NovaPulse CO_2 laser
        Sharplan CO_2 laser
        CO_2 SilkLaser

CO_2 *(continued)*
        SilkLaser aesthetic CO_2
            laser
        Surgipulse XJ 150 CO_2
            laser
        Tru-Pulse CO_2 skin resurfacing laser
        UltraPulse CO_2 laser
        Unilase CO_2 laser

coagulate

coagulation
    cutaneous protein c.
    disseminated intravascular c.
    c. factor
    laser c.
    c. meshwork
    c. necrosis
    sepsis-induced disseminated intravascular c.

coagulator
    argon beam c.
    ASSI Polar-Mate bipolar c.
    bipolar c.
    Coherent argon laser photocoagulator

coagulopathy

Coakley nasal speculum

coalescence

coapt

coaptation
    c. splint

coarse
    c. breath sound
    c. facial feature

coat
    mucosal c.

coated
    c. suture
    c. tongue
    c. Vicryl suture

coating
    Calcitite hydroxyapatite c.

Coban
  C. bandage
  C. elastic dressing
  C. wrap

Cobb syndrome

Cobbett skin graft knife

cobblestone tongue

cobblestoning

Cobelli glands

Coblation

Cobra
  C. cannula
  C. cannula tip
  C. K+ cannula tip
  C. K tip

coccidioidomycosis
  cutaneous c.
  c. tenosynovitis

cocked hat procedure
  Gillies c. h. p.

cockleshell ear

Codman Cranioplastic

Coffin
  C. split plate
  C. spring
  C. transpalatal wire
  C.-type transpalatal wire
  C.-Lowry syndrome
  C.-Siris syndrome

Cogan syndrome

Cohen analysis

Coherent
  C. argon laser
  C. argon laser photocoagu-
    lator
  C. UltraPulse 5000C laser
  C. Versapulse device

coil
  helical c.

cold
  c. abscess
  c. beam laser
  c. dissection
  c. gangrene
  c. injury
  c. intolerance after finger-
    tip injury
  c.-knife dissection
  c. urticaria

Coleman
  C. aspiration cannula
  C. classification of congeni-
    tal aural atresia

Colin STBP-780 stress test
  blood pressure monitor

CollaCote
  C. bovine collagen
  C. wound dressing

collagen
  c. absorbable suture
  Avitene fibrillar c.
  c. antibody
  autologous human c.
  Bio-Oss c.
  bovine c.
  cartilaginous c.
  CollaCote bovine c.
  c. deposition
  Dermalogen human c.
  c. fibers
  Fibrel c.
  c. graft
  c. hemostatic material for
    wounds
  human c.
  c. implant
  injectable c.
  c. injection
  Isolagen human c.
  microfibrillar c.
  purified bovine c.
  remodeling of c.
  c. skin test
  sterilized fibrillar bovine c.
  subepidermal c.

collagen *(continued)*
 c. sutures
 c. synthesis
 c. type
 c. vascular disease
 Zyderm I c.
 Zyderm II c.
 Zyplast c.
 Zyplast injectable c.

collagenase

collagenation

collagenesis

collagenolysis

collagenosis
 reactive perforating c.

collagenous fibers

collagen-producing cells

collagen vascular disease

Collagraft bone graft matrix

CollaPlug wound dressing

collapse
 alar rim c.
 bony vault c.
 cardiovascular c.
 circulatory c.
 nasal valve c.
 scapholunate advanced c.
  (SLAC)

collapsed cheek

collar
 mucosal c.
 thyroid c.

collar-button abscess

collarette

Collastat
 C. OBP microfibrillar collagen hemostat material

CollaTape

collateral
 accessory c. ligament

collateral *(continued)*
 c. ligament
 true c. ligament
 c. vessel

Colles
 C. fascia
 C. fracture
 C. ligament

colliculus *pl.* colliculi
 c. of arytenoid cartilage
 fascial c.
 inferior c.

collimated beam handpiece for
 laser surgery

Collins-Mayo retractor

colliquative
 c. degeneration
 c. necrosis

collodion
 hemostatic c.

colloid
 c. acne
 c. cyst
 c. milium

collum *pl.* colla
 c. dentis
 c. mandibulae

coloboma *pl.* colobomas, colo-
 bomata
 atypical c.
 c. lentis
 c. lobuli
 c. palpebrae
 typical c.

colony-stimulating factor (CSF)

Colorado
 C. electrocautery tip
 C. microdissection needle
 C. tip cautery

colpocleisis
 Simon c.

columella *pl.* columellae
 bifidity of the c.

columella *(continued)*
- c. clamp
- hanging c.
- midline of the c.
- c. nasi
- retracted c.

columellar
- c. base
- c. crease
- c. deformity
- c. flap
- c. jut of nose
- c. implant
- c. reconstruction
- c. repair
- c. strut
- c. subluxation stabilization

column
- philtral c.

combination
- c. chemotherapy
- c. gel and inflatable mammary prosthesis
- c. skin

combined upper blepharoplasty

comedo *pl.* comedones
- c. acne
- comedones epidermal nevus

comedocarcinoma

comedonal acne

COM/MAND mandibular fixation system

comminuted fracture

comminution
- mandibular symphysis c.

commissural
- c. cheilitis
- c. pit

commissure
- anterior c. of labia
- labial c.

commissure *(continued)*
- laryngeal c.
- lateral c. of eyelids
- lateral oral c.
- lateral palpebral c.
- c. of lips of mouth
- medial c. of eyelids
- medial palpebral c.
- palpebral c.

commissuroplasty
- oral c.

commissurorrhaphy

commissurotomy

common
- c. anterior facial vein
- c. blue nevus
- c. canal
- c. carotid artery (CCA)
- c. carotid plexus
- c. facial vein
- c. iliac artery
- c. nevus

commune
- crus c.

compactor
- McSpadden c.
- Micro-Flow c. (MFC)

compartment
- decompressed c.
- extraconal fat c.
- intraconal fat c.
- c. pressure
- released c.
- scrotal c.
- c. syndrome
- thenar c.
- tissue c's

compensating curve

compensatory
- c. bone resorption
- c. periosteal bone apposition

competence
- immunological c.

competence *(continued)*
    velopharyngeal c. (VPC)
    venous valvular c.

competency
    lip c.
    velopharyngeal c.

complement
    serum c. *(C1–C9)*

complete
    c. bilateral cleft
    c. bilateral deformity
    c. cleft lip
    c. cleft palate
    c. facial rejuvenation
    c. subperiosteal implant
    c. syndactyly

complex
    areolomammary c.
    avidin-biotin-peroxidase c.
      (ABC)
    brow-upper lid c.
    craniofacial c.
    DAE c.
    dentofacial c.
    exstrophy/epispadias c.
    forehead-brow c.
    HLA c.
    immune c.
    junctional c.
    levator c.
    major histocompatibility c.
      (MHC)
    malar ligament c.
    maxillozygomatic c.
    modified junctional c.
    nipple-areola c. (NAC)
    ostiomeatal c.
    peripheral triangular fibro-
      cartilage c.
    c. polysyndactyly
    c. regional pain syndromes
      (CRPS)
    SMAS (superficial muscu-
      loaponeurotic system) c.
    teardrop-shaped nipple-
      areola c.

complex *(continued)*
    triangular fibrocartilage c.
      (TFCC)
    zygomatic c. fracture
    zygomatic malar c. (ZMC)
    zygomatic maxillary c.
      (ZMC)
    zygomaticomaxillary c.

complication
    implant-related c's (IRC)

component
    anterior c.
    anterior c. of force

composite
    c. bilateral infrastructure
      maxillectomy
    c. chondrocutaneous flap
    c. dressing
    c. flap
    c. graft
    c. inlay
    c. mandibular reconstruc-
      tion
    c. material
    c. onlay
    c. osteomyocutaneous pre-
      formed flap
    c. rhytidectomy

Composite Cultured Skin (CCS)

composition
    modeling c.

compound
    c. apertognathia
    c. cyst
    c. dislocation
    c. flap
    c. fracture
    c. melanocytoma
    Microfil silicone-rubber in-
      jection c.
    modeling c.
    c. nevus
    c. skin flap
    c. skull fracture
    triangular fibrocartilage c.

compress
  cool c.
  cribriform c.
  fenestrated c.
  wet c.

compression
  c. bandage
  c. binder
  carpal tunnel c.
  cheek c.
  chronic nerve c.
  c. dressing
  c. earring
  facial c. skull cap closure
  c. garment
  c. girdle
  Jobst c. garment
  nerve c.
  neurovascular cross c.
   (NVCC)
  c. plate
  radial sensory c.
  c. skull cap closure
  suprascapular nerve c.
  thoracic outlet c.
  tissue c.

compressive
  c. plastic splint
  c. strength

compressor
  c. muscle of naris

computed tomography (CT)
  axial c. t. scan
  coronal c. t. scan
  c. t. laser mammography
  spiral c. t.
  three-dimensional c. t. (3D
   CT)
  three-dimensional c. t.
   scans

computer-assisted
  c.-a. design/c.-a. manufacturing (CAD/CAM)
  c.-a. neurosurgical navigational system (CANS)

concavity
  macroscopic c.

concha *pl.* conchae
  c. auriculae
  c. bullosa
  c. of cranium
  cavum c.
  c. of ear
  highest c.
  inferior c.
  inferior ethmoidal c.
  inferior nasal c.
  inferior turbinate c.
  medial nasal c.
  middle nasal c.
  Morgagni c.
  nasal c.
  nasoturbinal c.
  Santorini c.
  c. Santorini
  sphenoidal c.
  sphenoidal nasal conchae
  superior nasal c.
  supreme nasal c.

conchal
  c. bowl
  c. cartilage
  c. cartilage graft
  c. contraction
  c. crest of maxilla
  c. flap
  c. fossa
  c. mucosa
  c. retrodisplacement
  c. show

conchal-mastoid angle

conchoscaphoid angle

conchotome
  Hartmann nasal c.
  Henke-Stille c.
  Olivecrona c.
  Stille c.
  Struyken c.
  Watson-Williams c.
  Weil-Blakesley c.

Concorde
    C. disposable skin stapler
    C. suction cannula

concrement

concrescence

concrete burn

concussion (*grades 1–3*)

condensation
    caudal c. of the transverse
        fascial tissues

condenser
    McShirley electromallet c.
    mechanical c.

condylar
    c. aplasia
    c. axis
    bilateral c. fracture
    c. canal
    c. cartilage
    c. chondroma
    c. deformation
    c. displacement
    c. dysplasia
    c. emissary vein
    c. fragment
    c. guide
    c. head
    c. hinge position
    c. hyperplasia
    c. hypoplasia
    c. lag screw plate
    c. neck
    c. path
    c. process fracture
    c. process fracture axial an-
        chor screw fixation
    progressive c. resorption
        (PCR)
    unilateral c. fracture

condyle
    displaced c.
    lateral c.
    c. of mandible
    mandibular c.

condyle (*continued*)
    neck of c.
    occipital c.
    protrusive c.
    c. rod

condylectomy

condylion

condyloid
    c. fossa
    c. process

condyloma
    c. acuminatum
    flat c.
    giant c. acuminatum

condyloplasty

condylotomy

condylus

cone
    master c.

confirmation
    intraoperative spatial c.

congenita
    arthrogryposis multiplex c.
    aplasia cutis c.
    cutis marmorata telangiec-
        tatica c.
    dyskeratosis c.
    hyperkeratosis c.
    melanosis diffusa c.
    pachyonychia c.

congenital
    c. alveolar synechia syn-
        drome
    c. amputation
    c. anomaly
    c. camptodactyly
    c. carpal synchondrosis
    c. cholesteatoma
    c. circumscribed hypome-
        lanosis
    c. defect
    c. earlobe cleft
    c. ectodermal dysplasia
    c. facial diplegia

congenital *(continued)*
    c. fibromatosis
    c. generalized lipodystrophy
    c. hand anomaly
    c. hand duplication
    c. malformation
    c. nevus
    c. sebaceous hyperplasia
    c. subglottic hemangioma
    c. synchondrosis
    c. telangiectatic erythema
    c. thumb duplication
    c. tufted angioma

conical
    c. flap

coning of areola

conjoined twins

conjoint extensor digitorum brevis muscle and dorsalis pedis osteocutaneous island flap

Conley incision

connective tissue
    c. t. augmentation
    c. t. disease (CTD)
    c. t. graft
    c. t. neoplasm
    c. t. nevus

connector
    ACMI light source c.
    implant superstructure c.
    linguoplate major c.
    Machida light source c.
    major c.
    minor c.
    palatal c.
    Y-port c.

conservative subtraction-addition rhinoplasty (CSAR)

consistency
    doughy c.
    lesion c.

constraint

constriction
    nares c.
    c. ring syndrome

constrictor
    inferior pharyngeal c.
    middle pharyngeal c.
    c. muscle of pharynx
    c. naris
    superior pharyngeal c.

construction
    absolute c.
    costochondral graft mandibular ramus c.
    Gillies c. of replacement thumb

contact
    c. area
    balanced c. between the cusps
    centric c.
    c. cheilitis
    deflective occlusal c.
    c. dermatitis
    faulty c.
    initial occlusive c.
    interceptive occlusal c.
    linguopalatal c.
    point of proximal c.
    premature c.
    retruded c.

contact-layer wound dressings

contamination
    bacterial c.

Contigen Bard collagen implant

continuity
    axonal c.

continuous
    c. running sutures
    c. wave laser

contour
    breast c.
    c. of the brow
    buccal c.

contour *(continued)*
    cervicofacial c.
    c. defect
    c. deformity
    c. irregularities
    mandibular c.

contouring
    abdominal c.
    body c.
    facial c.
    implant c.
    occlusal c.

Contour Profile Natural saline
  breast implant

contracting scar

contraction
    cervical muscle c.
    cicatricial c.
    conchal c.
    muscle c.
    myofibroblast c.
    palmar c.
    primary c. of skin graft
    secondary c. of skin graft
    wound c.
    wound matrix c.

contracture
    axillary c.
    Baker capsular c.
    Baker classification of cap-
      sular c.
    burn scar c. (BSC)
    capsular c.
    Dupuytren c.
    elbow flexion c.
    false Dupuytren c.
    fibrous capsular c.
    finger c.
    flexion c.
    c. of interosseous muscles
    ischemic c.
    joint c.
    c. of joint capsule
    scar c.
    soft tissue c.
    spherical c.

contracture *(continued)*
    thumb-index c.
    tight c.
    Volkmann c.
    Volkmann ischemic c.

contralateral
    c. breast
    c. ear
    c. face
    c. musculature

contrast
    maximal c.

contrecoup
    c. contusion
    c. injury

control
    anchorage c.
    musculoaponeurotic c.

contusion
    brain c.
    contrecoup c.
    scalp c.

conventional SMAS (superficial
  musculoaponeurotic system)
  face-lift

converging triangular flap

Converse
    C. alar elevator
    C. alar retractor
    C. bistoury
    C. blade retractor
    C. button-end bistoury
    C. curet
    C. double-end curet
    C. double-ended retractor
    C. flap
    C. fracture-wiring button
    C. guarded chisel
    C. guarded osteotomy
    C. hinged skin hook
    C. method
    C. nasal chisel
    C. nasal retractor
    C. nasal rongeur
    C. nasal root rongeur

Converse *(continued)*
    C. nasal saw
    C. nasal speculum
    C. nasal tip scissors
    C. needle holder
    C. operation
    C. osteotome
    C. periosteal elevator
    C. plastic surgery scissors
    C. rasp
    C. raspatory
    C. retractor
    C. rongeur
    C. saw
    C. scalping flap
    scalping flap of C.
    C. scissors
    C. splint
    C. sweeper curet
    C. technique
    C.-Gillies needle holder
    C.-Lange rongeur
    C.-MacKenty elevator

convex
    c. forehead

convexity
    forehead c.

convexobasia

Conway
    C. lid retractor
    C. technique

cookie
    Gelfoam c.

Cooper
    C. ligaments
    C. nasal ganglia guide
    C.-Rand intraoral artificial
      larynx

co-ossify

copper-beaten finding

copula
    c. linguae

core
    mesodermal c.

corium

Cormack
    C.-Lamberty classification
      of fasciocutaneous flaps
      (types A–C)
    C.-Lamberty fasciocuta-
      neous flap *(types A–C)*

cornea
    apex c.

corneal
    c. abrasion
    c. opacification
    c. surface
    c. ulceration

corneoblepharon

corneous

corner mouth lift

corneum
    stratum c. epidermidis

corniculate
    c. cartilage
    c. tubercle

cornification
    disorder of c.

cornified
    c. cell envelope
    c. layer
    c. epithelium

cornoid lamella

cornu *pl.* cornua
    c. cutaneum
    ethmoid c.
    cornua of thyroid cartilage

corona *pl.* coronae, coronas
    c. ciliaris
    c. dentis
    c. seborrheica
    c. veneris

coronal
    bilateral c. synostosis
    c. brow lift

coronal *(continued)*
- c. incision
- c. lift
- c. plane
- c. synostosis
- unilateral c. synostosis

coronale

coronion

coronocanthopexy

coronoid
- c. flap
- c. hyperplasia
- c. process of mandible

coronoidectomy
- bilateral c's

coronoplasty

coronoradicular stabilization

corpus *pl.* corpora
- c. adiposum buccae
- c. adiposum orbitae
- c. cavernosum
- c. ciliare
- c. ciliaris
- c. costae
- erectile corpora
- c. linguae
- c. mammae
- c. mandibulae
- c. maxillae
- c. ossis sphenoidalis
- corpora santoriana
- c. unguis

corpuscle
- axis c.
- cartilage c.
- Golgi c's
- Golgi-Mazzoni c's
- Krause c.
- lingual c.
- Meissner c's
- Meissner tactile c.
- Merkel c's
- Pacini c's
- pacinian c's
- Ruffini c's
- Schwalbe c.

corpuscle *(continued)*
- tactile c's
- tendon c's
- Vater c's
- Vater-Pacini c's
- Virchow c's
- Wagner-Meissner c.

correction
- Berke ptosis c.
- Berke-Motais ptosis c.
- Blaskovics ptosis c.
- cephalometric c.
- c. of chordee
- notch c.
- presurgical orthopedic c. (POC)
- occlusal c.
- one-stage esthetic c.
- Whitlow and Constable alar cartilage c.

corrugator
- c. frown
- c. muscle
- c. muscle resection
- c. removal
- c. supercilii muscle

corset platysmaplasty

cortex
- cerebral c.
- mastoid c.

cortical
- c. anchoring screw
- c. bone allograft
- c. bone graft
- c. bone plate
- c. fracture
- c. freeze-dried allograft
- c. necrosis

corticocancellous
- c. bone
- c. graft

corticosteroid
- intralesional c.
- oral c.
- c. rosacea
- systemic c.
- topical c.

Coschwitz duct

CoSeal fibrin glue

Cosmetech cannula

cosmetic
   c. camouflage
   c. reconstruction
   c. surgery

costal
   c. cartilage
   c. cartilage graft

CoStasis fibrin glue

costochondral
   c. graft (CCG)
   c. graft mandibular ramus
     reconstruction
   c. graft reconstruction

costosternoplasty

Cottle
   C. alar elevator
   C. alar protector
   C. alar retractor
   C. bone guide
   C. bulldog nasal scissors
   C. calipers
   C. cartilage guide
   C. chisel
   C. columella clamp
   C. cartilage guide
   C. dorsal scissors
   C. double hook
   double-pronged C. hook
   C. dressing scissors
   C. elevator
   C. heavy septal scissors
   C. knife
   C. knife guide
   C. knife guide and retractor
   C. knife handle
   C. maneuver
   C. modified knife handle
   C. nasal-biting rongeur
   C. nasal hook
   C. nasal knife
   C. nasal saw
   C. nasal scissors

Cottle *(continued)*
   C. nasal speculum
   C. pronged retractor
   C. protected knife handle
   C. rasp
   C. rhinoplasty
   C. septal elevator
   C. single-prong tenaculum
   C. skin elevator
   C. skin hook
   C. soft palate retractor
   C. tenaculum hook
   C. thumb hook retractor
   C. Universal nasal saw
   C. upper lateral retractor
   C.-Arruga cartilage forceps
   C.-Jansen rongeur forceps
   C.-Joseph hook
   C.-Joseph retractor
   C.-Joseph saw
   C.-Kazanjian bone-cutting
     forceps
   C.-Kazanjian forceps
   C.-Kazanjian nasal-cutting
     forceps
   C.-Kazanjian nasal forceps
   C.-Kazanjian rongeur
   C.-MacKenty elevator
   C.-MacKenty elevator rasp
   C.-Medicon osteotome
   C.-Neivert retractor
   C.-Walsham septal straight-
     ener
   C.-Walsham septum-
     straightening forceps
   C.-Walsham straightener

Cotton
   C. cartilage graft
   C. cartilage graft to crico-
     laryngeal area

cotton
   absorbent c.
   c. bolster dressing
   c. pledget
   salicylated c.
   styptic c.

cotton-wool
   c.-w. appearance
   c.-w. exudate

cotton-wool *(continued)*
    c.-w. patch
    c.-w. spot

Cottony-Dacron suture

Cotunnius
    nerve of C.

count
    quantitative microbiologic
      bacterial c.

counter
    joule c.

counterincision

counteropening

coup
    contre c.
    c. de sabre
    en c. de sabre

Covaderm composite wound
  dressing

coverage
    c. flap

covering
    allograft wound c.
    Biobrane wound c.
    biosynthetic wound c.
    fibroelastic c.
    fibrous c.
    titanium mini bur hole c.
    wound c.
    xenograft wound c.

Coverlet adhesive dressing

Cover-Roll
    C. adhesive gauze
    C. stretch bandage

Cover-Strip wound closure strip

Cowden disease

cow face

Cox
    C. II ocular laser shield
    C. regression analysis of
      partially edentulous jaw

Coxsackie virus

CP
    cleft palate

CPLS
    cleft palate and lateral sy-
      nechia syndrome

cracked-pot sound

crackling jaw

cramp
    laryngeal c.

Crandall syndrome

cranial
    c. anchorage
    anterior c. fossa
    c. arteritis
    c. autografts
    c. base defect
    c. base landmark
    c. base neoplasm
    c. base surgery
    c. bur
    c. capacity
    c. coronal ring articulation
    c. flap fixation
    c. fossa defect
    c. growth
    middle c. fossa
    c. nerves (I–XII)
    posterior c. fossa
    c. prosthesis
    c. sutures
    c. suture joint
    c. suture synostosis
    c. vault suture

cranialization
    sinus c.

craniamphitomy

craniectomy
    anterior c.
    endoscopic strip c.
    frontal bone advancement
      with strip c.
    linear c.
    sagittal c.
    strip c.
    suboccipital c.

cranioaural

craniobuccal

craniocaudad

craniocaudal

craniocervical
    c. chordoma

cranioclasis
    fetal c.

craniodentofacial deformity

craniofacial
    c. anomaly
    c. appliance
    c. cleft
    c. complex
    c. deformity
    c. disorder
    c. disjunction
    c. dysmorphism
    c. dysostosis
    c. dysplasia
    c. fixation
    c. fracture appliance
    LactoSorb c. plate fixation
        system
    c. microsomia
    c. morphology
    c. notch
    c. osteogenic sarcoma
    c. pathology
    c. reconstruction
    c. resection
    c. surgery
    c. suspension wiring
    c. syndromes

craniofaciocervical

craniofenestria

craniolacunia

craniomalacia

craniomandibular dysfunction
    (CMD)

craniomaxillofacial
    c. callus distraction
    c. surgery

craniomedial

craniometry

cranio-orbital
    c. neurofibromatosis

craniopagus

craniopharyngeal duct tumor

craniopharyngioma

Cranioplastic
    C. acrylic cranioplasty ma-
        terial
    Codman C.
    C. material dressing
    C. powder

cranioplasty

craniorachischisis

cranioschisis

craniosclerosis

craniostenosis

craniostosis

craniosynostosis pl. craniosy-
    nostoses
        common c.
        Crouzon c.
        kleeblattschädel c.
        metopic c.
        Saethre-Chotzen c.
        secondary c.
        single-suture c.
        syndromic c.

craniotabes

craniotomy
    attached c.
    bifrontal c.
    detached c.
    c. flap
    frontal c.
    osteoplastic c.
    posterior fossa c.
    retromastoid c.
    c. scissors

cranium pl. crania
    bifid c.

cranium *(continued)*
    c. bifidum
    c. bifidum occultum
    cerebral c.
    dysmorphic c.
    visceral c.

crater
    alveolar process c.
    bone c.
    bony c.
    c. formation
    interalveolar bone c.

craterization

crater-shaped erosion

cream
    Aqua Glycolic c.
    autolytic débridement c.
    BioMedic Micro-
      Encapsulated retinol c.
    bleaching c.
    enzymatic débridement c.
    Massé breast c.
    Maximum Strength Dese-
      nex antifungal c.
    topical c.

crease
    alar c.
    columellar c.
    earlobe c.
    flexion c.
    glabellar c.
    helical c.
    inframammary c.
    labiocolumellar c.
    lateral neck c.
    palmar c.
    preauricular c.
    simian c.
    submammary c.
    Sydney c.
    vertical glabellar c.

creed
    Millard c.

creep
    biologic c. of skin
    mechanical c. of skin
    c. recovery

creep *(continued)*
    skin c.
    web c.

cremaster muscle

crenation of tongue

crepitation
    c. in the lower eyelids
    c. of mandible on manual
      palpation

crepitus
    c. at fracture site

crescent
    Heidenhain c's
    sublingual c.
    traumatic c.

crest
    alveolar c.
    c. of alveolar ridge
    anterior lacrimal c.
    buccinator c.
    cerebral c's of cranial bone
    conchal c.
    conchal c. of maxilla
    conchal c. of palatine bone
    ethmoidal c.
    external frontal c.
    external mental c.
    iliac c.
    inferior turbinal c. of max-
      illa
    inferior turbinal c. of pala-
      tine bone
    infratemporal c.
    infrazygomatic c.
    jugular c. of great wing of
      sphenoid bone
    malar c. of great wing of
      sphenoid bone
    mandibular c.
    marginal c.
    nasal c.
    nasal c. of maxilla
    nasal c. of palatine bone
    c. of palatine bone
    posterior lacrimal c.
    c. of ridge
    sagittal c.
    sphenoidal c.

crest *(continued)*
    superficial temporal c.
    superior turbinal c. of max-
      illa
    superior turbinal c. of pala-
      tine bone
    supramastoid c.
    triangular c.
    vomeropremaxillary c.
    zygomatic c.
    zygomatic c. of great wing
      of sphenoid bone

Crete-Manche implant

cretinism

crib
    allogeneic c.
    allogeneic bone c.
    alloplastic c.
    bone c.
    Jackson c.
    lip-sucking habit c.

cribriform
    c. pattern
    c. plate
    c. plate of alveolar process
    c. salivary carcinoma of the
      excretory duct
    transverse widening of c.
      plate

cribroethmoid foramen

cricoarytenoid
    c. ankylosis
    c. joint
    c. muscle

cricoid
    c. cartilage
    c. ring
    c. split

cricoidynia

cricopharyngeus muscle

cricothyroid
    c. angle
    c. artery
    c. muscle

cricothyroidectomy

cricotomy

cri du chat syndrome

Crile
    C. nerve hook
    C. retractor

crisis
    anaphylactic c.
    anaphylactoid c.
    laryngeal c.

crista *pl.* cristae
    c. ampullaris
    c. buccinatoria
    c. conchalis maxillae
    c. conchalis ossis palatini
    c. dentalis
    c. ethmoidalis maxillae
    c. ethmoidalis ossis pala-
      tini
    c. frontalis
    c. galli
    c. helicis
    c. lacrimalis
    c. marginalis
    c. nasalis maxillae
    c. occipitalis
    c. palatina
    c. temporalis

criteria *plural of* criterion
    Ellenbogen c. for ideal eye-
      brow position and con-
      tour
    Highet and Sander modi-
      fied c. of MacKinnon and
      Dellon for sensory recov-
      ery following nerve repair
    Highet and Sander modi-
      fied c. of Zachary and
      Holmes for sensory re-
      covery following nerve re-
      pair
    Mark May sinus disease c.

Criticare
    C. 507N noninvasive blood
      pressure monitor
    C. 507O pulse oximeter/
      NIBP monitor

Criticare *(continued)*
  C. 507S vital sign monitor
  C. comprehensive vital sign
    monitor
  C. monitor
  C. POET TE end-tidal CO2
    respiration monitor

Cronin
  C. cheiloplasty
  C. cleft palate elevator
  C. implant
  C. mammary implant
  C. method
  C. palate elevator
  C. palate knife
  C. Silastic mammary pros-
    thesis

crossbite
  anterior c.
  buccal c.
  lingual c.
  posterior c.
  scissors-bite c.
  telescoping c.

cross-facial
  c.-f. technique

cross-finger flap

cross-hatch incision

cross-hatching undermining

cross-leg
  c.-l. flap
  c.-l. skin flap

cross-lid flap

crossover
  facial nerve c.

cross-sectional projection

cross-tunneling incision

croton oil

Crouzon
  C. craniostenotic defect
  C. craniosynostosis
  C. disease
  C. syndrome

Crouzon *(continued)*
  C. syndromic synostosis

crowding
  mandibular incisor c.

Crowe
  C. pilot point
  C.-Davis mouth gag
  C.-Davis mouth retractor

crow's feet

CRPS
  complex regional pain syn-
    dromes

crural
  c. feet

crus *pl.* crura
  crura of anthelix
  c. commune
  helical c.
  c. helicis
  inferior c. of lateral canthal
    tendon
  internal c. of greater alar
    cartilage of nose
  lateral c.
  lateral c. of greater alar
    cartilage
  medial c.
  medial c. of lower lateral
    cartilage
  posterior c.
  superior c. of antihelix

crusher
  spur c.

crushing
  Adams c. of nasal septum

crush injury

cryoprecipitate

cryosurgery

cryotherapy

cryptococcosis
  labyrinthine c.

cryptophthalmia

cryptophthalmos

cryptorchidism

cryptotia

crystal
    myxoid c.
    Virchow c's

CSAR
    conservative subtraction-
        addition rhinoplasty

CSF
    cerebrospinal fluid
        halo test for CSF rhi-
            norrhea
        CSF rhinorrhea
    colony-stimulating factor

CT
    computed tomography
        CT-guided fine-needle
            aspiration
        CT laser mammogra-
            phy
        CT scan
        three-dimensional CT

CTD
    connective tissue disease

CTR
    carpal tunnel release

CTRS
    carpal tunnel release sys-
        tem

CTS
    carpal tunnel syndrome

cubital
    c. artery
    c. tunnel syndrome

cuboidal epithelium

cuff
    epithelial c.

culture
    anaerobic c.

cultured
    c. autograft
    c. autologous keratinocyte
    c. autologous melanocyte
    c. epithelial autografting
    c. mucosal graft
    c. periosteal cell

cuneiform
    c. cartilage
    c. osteotomy

cup ear

Cupid's bow
    high point of C. b.
    C. b. peak

Curaderm hydrocolloid dress-
    ing material

Curafil hydrogel dressing

Curafoam wound dressing

Curagel hydrogel dressing

Curasorb calcium alginate
    dressing

curet (spelled also curette)
    aspirating c.
    Ballenger ethmoid c.
    biopsy suction c.
    chalazion c.
    Converse c.
    Converse double-end c.
    Converse sweeper c.
    dermal c.
    Fox dermal c.
    frontal sinus c.
    Goldman c.
    Halle ethmoidal c.
    Halle sinus c.
    Lucas alveolar c.
    McCall c.
    Moult c.
    Piffard dermal c.
    Read facial c.
    serrated c.
    Synthes facial c.
    Volkmann bone c.
    Wolff dermal c.

curettage
    c. of basal cell carcinoma
    infrabony pocket c.
    soft tissue c.

curette (*variant of* curet)

curtain
    lip c.

curvature
    buccolingual c.
    occlusal c.

curve
    alignment c.
    anteroposterior c.
    buccal c.
    compensating c.
    dose-response c.
    labial c.
    marked falling c.
    Monson c.
    occlusal c.
    c. of occlusion
    saddle c.
    spherical three-dimension-
      al c.
    c. of Spee
    von Spee c.
    c. of von Spee
    U-shaped c.
    c. of Wilson

curvilinear incision

Cushing
    C. nerve retractor
    C.-Landolt transsphenoidal
      speculum

cushion
    Passavant c.

cuspid
    mandibular c.
    maxillary c.

cutaneoperiosteal flap

cutaneous
    c. blue nevus
    c. capillary formation

cutaneous (*continued*)
    c. fibrous histiocytoma
    c. flap
    c. hyperpigmentation
    c. hypopigmentation
    c. meningioma
    c. metastasis
    c. nodule
    c. vascular abnormality
    c. vascular lesion

cutaneous-subcutaneous nod-
    ule

cutaneum
    cornu c.
    sebum c.

cut-as-you-go technique

cut-back
    rotation flap c.-b.

cuticle of hair

cuticula
    c. dentis

Cutinova
    C. Cavity wound filling ma-
      terial
    C. Hydro dressing

cutis
    c. graft
    c. laxa
    c. marmorata telangiecta-
      tica congenita
    c. neuroma
    c. osteoma
    c. verrucosa

Cutler
    C.-Ederer life-table method-
      ology

Cutler
    C.-Beard bridge flap
    C.-Beard bridge flap proce-
      dure
    C.-Beard flap
    C.-Beard reconstruction
    C.-Beard technique

cutter
    bone c.

cutter *(continued)*
  Lindeman bone c.

cyanoacrylate
  c. glue
  c. tissue adhesive

Cyano-Dent material

cyanosis

Cybex test

cycle
  biphasic growth c.

cycloplegia

Cyclops procedure

cylinder
  Bodenham dermabrasion c.

cymba
  c. conchae
  c. conchae auriculae
  c. conchal cartilage graft
  midconcha c.

cymbiform

Cymetra

Cynosure laser

Cyrano nose

cyst
  adventitious c.
  air c.
  aneurysmal bone c. (ABC)
  antral mucosal c.
  apical c.
  apocrine retention c.
  Blandin-Nuhn c.
  bone c.
  Boyer c.
  branchial c.
  branchial cleft c.
  buccal c.
  calcifying c.
  calcifying and keratinizing
    odontogenic c.
  calcifying odontogenic c.
  cervical c.
  chocolate c.

cyst *(continued)*
  cholesterol granuloma c.
  colloid c.
  compound c.
  daughter c.
  dentigerous c.
  dentoalveolar c.
  dermoid c.
  dermoid inclusion c.
  desmoid c.
  enteric c.
  enterogenous c.
  epidermal c.
  epidermal inclusion c.
  epidermoid c.
  epithelial c.
  eruption c.
  false c.
  Favre-Racouchot c.
  fissural c.
  follicular c.
  follicular infundibular c.
  follicular isthmus c.
  follicular odontogenic c.
  ganglion c.
  glandular odontogenic c.
  globulomaxillary c.
  Gorlin c.
  hemorrhagic c.
  implantation c.
  inclusion c.
  inflammatory c.
  intralingual c. of foregut or-
    igin
  intraoral c.
  intraosseous ganglion c.
  keratinizing epithelial
    odontogenic c.
  keratinous c.
  laryngeal saccular c.
  lateral c.
  lingual c.
  lymphoepithelial c.
  mandibular c.
  mandibular median c.
  maxillary c.
  maxillary median anter-
    ior c.
  maxillary sinus c.

cyst *(continued)*
    median alveolar c.
    median anterior maxil-
        lary c.
    median mandibular c.
    median palatal c.
    milia c.
    mucinous c.
    mucosal c.
    mucous c.
    mucous retention c.
    multilocular c.
    nasoalveolar c.
    nasolabial c.
    nasopalatine c.
    nasopalatine duct c.
    nasopharyngeal c.
    nonepithelial bone c.
    palatine papilla c.
    papillary c.
    parakeratinized c.
    parasitic c.
    parotid c.
    periosteal c.
    preauricular c.
    proliferating pilar c.
    retention c.
    saccular c.
    salivary duct c.

cyst *(continued)*
    salivary gland c.
    salivary gland retention c.
    Sampson c.
    sebaceous c.
    sequestration c.
    simple bone c.
    sinus tract c.
    soft tissue c.
    solitary bone c.
    sphenoidal c.
    Stafne bone c.
    subchondral c.
    sublingual c.
    tarsal c.
    thyroglossal duct c.
    Tornwaldt c.
    unilocular c.
    vestibular c.

cystadenoma
    c. lymphomatosum
    papillary c. lymphomato-
        sum
    serous c.

cytology
    aspiration biopsy c.
    fine-needle aspiration c.
        (FNAC)

D
deciduous
dentin
D-shaped implant

Dacron
D.-backed implant
D. batting
D. netting
thick-walled D.-backed implant

dacryocystorhinostomy (DCR)
endonasal d.
endoscopic d.
d. procedure

dacryocystotomy
Ammon d.

dacryon

dacryorhinocystostomy

dacryostenosis

dactinomycin

dactyl
d. speech

dactylitis
septic d.

dactylology

dactylolysis spontanea

D.A.D. mattress

DAE complex

daisy
oxeye d.

Dakin solution

Dalbo
D. extracoronal attachment
D. extracoronal unit
D. stud attachment
D. stud unit

Dale
D. abdominal binder
D. Foley catheter holder

Dale *(continued)*
D. oxygen cannula support
D. tracheostomy tube holder
D. ventilator tubing support

Dalgan

Dalla Bona
Dalla B. attachment
Dalla B. ball and socket abutment

Dall-Miles cable grip system

dam
post d.
rubber d.
rubber punch d.

damage
actinic d.
axonal d.
epidermal actinic d.

Damascus Disk

Damason-P

damiana

Dandy-Walker malformation

Daniel EndoForehead instrument

dappen dish

d'Arcet metal

Dardour
D. flap
D. lateral flap
superiorly based D. lateral flap

Darier
D. disease
D. sign
D.-White disease

dark lateral

Darrach procedure

dartos
  d. fascia
  d. fasciocutaneous flap
  d. muscle
  d. musculocutaneous flap

Darwin
  auricular tubercle of D.

darwinian
  d. ear
  d. tubercle

DASE
  Denver Articulation Screen-
    ing Examination

D'Assumpçao clamp

Datascope pulse oximeter

Daubenton angle

daughter cyst

daunorubicin

David-Baker
  D.-B. clamp
  D.-B. eyelid retractor
  D.-B. lip clamp

David Letterman sign

Davis
  D. graft
  D. rhytidectomy scissors
  D.-Crowe mouth gag
  D.-Crowe tongue blade
  D.-Kitlowski procedure

Davol dermatome

DCP
  dynamic compression plate

DCR
  dacryocystorhinostomy

3D CT
  three-dimensional com-
    puted tomography

DDR
  direct digital radiography

deafferentation
  bilateral vestibular d.
  total unilateral vestibular d.
  vestibular d.

deaffrication

deafness
  Mondini d.

deamination

Dean
  D. fluorosis index
  D. periosteal elevator
  D. rongeur
  D. scissors
  D. tonsil hemostat

Deaver retractor

debanding

deblocking

debonding
  d. pliers (DP)

débride

débridement
  accurate d.
  autolytic d.
  enzymatic d.
  epithelial d.
  revision and d.
  serial d.
  single-stage d.
  surgical d.
  triangular fibrocartilage
    complex (TFCC) d.
  wide d.
  wound d.

debris
  cellular d.
  Malassez d.

Debrisan

Debrox Otic

debulking
  secondary d.

debulking *(continued)*
   surgical d.

decalcified
   d. freeze-dried bone allo-
      graft (DFDBA)
   d. freeze-dried cortical
      bone (DFDCB)

decannulation

decay
   bone d.

decentration

deciduous (D)

decision
   Bates d.

decompression
   carpal tunnel d.
   endolymphatic sac d.
   endoscopic carpal tun-
      nel d.
   endoscopic orbital d.
   facial nerve d.
   gastric d.
   jugular bulb d.
   microvascular d. (MVD)
   orbital d.
   sac-vein d.
   subfascial carpal tunnel d.
   suboccipital d.
   three-wall orbital d.
   transantral orbital d.
   transconjunctival endo-
      scopic orbital d.
   wide d.

Decon
   Par D.

deconditioning

Deconsal
   D. II
   D. Sprinkle

decontamination

decorative tattoo

decorticated flap

decruitment

decubitus
   d. ulcer

decuspation

decussate

decussation

dedentition

dedifferentiated chordoma

Dedo laryngoscope

deep
   d. bite
   d. cervical fascia
   d. facial lymph node
   d. hemangioma
   d. inferior epigastric artery
   d. inferior epigastric vein
   d. lateral node
   d. lobectomy
   d.-lobe parotid tumor
   d. muscular aponeurotic
      system (DMAS)
   d. overbite
   d. palmar arch
   d. parotid lobe
   d. parotid node
   d. peroneal nerve
   d. petrosal nerve
   d.-plane face-lift
   d.-plane rhytidectomy
   d. plantar arch
   d. scaler
   d. scaling
   d. space
   d. structure
   d. subdermal
   d. suspension suture
   d. temporal fascia (DTF)
   d. vertical overlap

Deep Test of Articulation

deepening
   d. pocket
   web space d.

Deepep-Hard

deepithelialization
    periareolar d.
    vertical rhomboid d.

deepithelialized
    d. local flap
    d. revascularized lateral in-
        tercostal flap

deepithelization (*variant of* de-
    epithelialization)

Deesix

Deetwo

defatted

defatting
    internal d.
    d. the umbilical stalk

defect
    acquired d.
    alveolar bone d.
    alveolar ridge d.
    birth d.
    bone d.
    buccal d.
    buccal mucosal d.
    calvarial d.
    cellulitic d.
    congenital d.
    contour d.
    cranial base d.
    cranial fossa d.
    Crouzon craniostenotic d.
    extirpative d.
    extraoral d.
    full-thickness d.
    fascial d.
    heminasal d.
    hernia d.
    intercalated d.
    interradicular osseous d.
    intrabony d.
    intraoral mucosal d.
    mandibular d.
    Mohs d.
    one-buttress d.

defect (*continued*)
    orbitomaxillary d.
    oromandibular d.
    oropharyngeal d.
    osteoporotic marrow d.
    pars flaccida d.
    periodontal d.
    periodontal bony d.
    periodontal intrabony d.
    pharyngoesophageal d.
    pitting d.
    postablation d.
    postresection d.
    repair of alveolar ridge d.
    resorptive d.
    sacrococcygeal d.
    saddle d.
    saddle nose d.
    segmental bone d.
    segmental continuity d.
    septal d.
    speech d.
    suboccipital dural d.
    three-buttress d.
    through-and-through d.
    two-buttress d.

Defen-LA

deficiency
    acquired immunoglobulin
        A d.
    arch length d.
    immune d.
    intraoral lining d.
    iron d.
    malar d.
    mandibular d.
    mandibular sagittal d.
    maxillary d.
    premaxilla peripyriform d.
    submalar d.
    vitamin d.
    volar plate d.

deficit

defined
    d. frequency
    d. sterilization

definitive prosthesis

deflation
   implant d.

deflective
   d. malocclusion
   d. occlusal
   d. occlusal contact

deformation
   condylar d.
   dentinoblastic d.
   elastic d.
   permanent d.
   viscoelastic d.

deformational frontal plagiocephaly

deformity
   Andy Gump d.
   bathtub d. of facial fat
   bilateral flexion d.
   bishop collar d.
   bony d.
   boutonnière d.
   Burow triangle d.
   calvarial d.
   chin d.
   claw d.
   claw hand d.
   clawing d.
   cleft lip d.
   clenched fist d.
   columellar d.
   complete bilateral d.
   contour d.
   craniodentofacial d.
   craniofacial d.
   dentofacial d.
   dish-face d.
   dorsal intercalated segmen-
     tal instability (DISI) d.
   double-bubble breast d.
   d. of earlobe
   facial d.
   facial contour d.
   flexion d.
   fusiform d.

deformity *(continued)*
   gibbous d.
   gibbus d.
   gingival d.
   halo d.
   harlequin d.
   hourglass nasal d.
   humpback d. of scaphoid
   iatrogenic d.
   inverted teardrop areola d.
   ipsilateral hand d.
   lambdoid synostosis d.
   lateral facial cleft d.
   lobster claw d.
   lobster hand d.
   mallet finger d.
   maxillary d.
   middle vault d.
   Mondini d.
   nasal tip d.
   parrot beak d.
   Pinocchio tip d.
   Poland chest wall d.
   polly beak d.
   polly beak nasal d.
   postmaxillectomy d.
   pseudo-boutonnière d.
   pseudomallet d.
   residual d.
   ripple d.
   Romberg facial d.
   rotational d.
   rotational d. of finger
   saddle d.
   saddle nose d.
   scaphocephalic d.
   septal d.
   skeletal d.
   soft tissue d.
   stairstep d.
   step d.
   supratip d.
   swan neck d.
   thumb-in-palm d.
   Treacher Collins d.
   ulnar deviation d.
   unesthetic contour d.
   unilateral cleft lip nose d.
   uni-tip d.

deformity *(continued)*
    Volkmann claw hand d.
    whistling d.
    witch's chin d.

Defourmental
    D. nasal rongeur
    D. rongeur forceps

DEFS
    Detailed Evaluation of Facial Symmetry

degassing

degeneration
    calcific d.
    colliquative d.
    fatty d.
    granular d.
    hyaline d.
    myxomatous d.
    wallerian d.

degenerative
    d. joint disease
    d. joint disease of wrist
    d. zone

deglove

degloved amputation

degloving
    d. injury
    midfacial d.

deglutition
    d. apnea
    d. maneuver
    d. reflex

deglutitory disturbance

degradation

degrease the skin

degree
    Juri II, III d. of male pattern baldness

dehiscence
    alveolar d.
    congenital tympanic d.
    intimal d.

dehiscence *(continued)*
    Killian d.
    levator d.
    d. of mandibular canal
    root d.
    soft tissue d.
    sternotomy d.
    wound d.
    Zuckerkandl's d.

dehydration
    d. of gingivae

dehydrogenase
    glucose 6-phosphate d.
    11-hydroxysteroid d.
    lactic d.
    malic d.
    succinate d.
    succinic d.

dehydrosterone

deictic

Deiters nucleus

Dejerine syndrome

de la Cruz classification of congenital aural atresia

de la Plaza transconjunctival retractor

delay
    d. maneuver
    d. of muscle/musculocutaneous flap

delayed
    d. dentition
    d. distally based total sartorius flap
    d. echolalia
    d. expansion
    d. flap
    d. graft
    d. hypersensitivity
    d. reflex
    d. wound healing

Delcort

Delerm and Elbaz technique

delivery
   d. assistance sleeve
   d. hose

Delphian node

deltoid flap

deltopectoral flap

deltoscapular flap

delusion
   somatic d.

demarcate

demarcation
   areolar d.

Dembone
   D. demineralized cancel-
      lous chips
   D. demineralized cortical
      chips
   D. demineralized cortico-
      cancellous chips
   D. graft

demecarium

demineralized
   d. bone (DMB)
   d. bone graft
   d. bone matrix
   d. cortical bone powder
   d. flexible laminar bone
      strip
   d. freeze-dried bone
      (DFBD)
   d. freeze-dried bone allo-
      graft (DFDBA)

De Morgan spots

demucosation

demyelinating disease

demyelination
   segmental d.

Denar
   D. articulator
   D.-Witzig articulator

dendrite

dendritic
   d. cell

Denholz appliance

Denis Browne clubfoot splint

Dennie
   D. infraorbital fold
   D.-Morgan infraorbital fold

Denonvilliers aponeurosis

denotation
   lexical d.

de novo tumor

Denquel

dens pl. dentes
   d. angularis
   d. bicuspis
   d. caninus
   d. cuspidatus
   d. deciduus
   d. in dente
   d. incisivus
   d. invaginatus
   d. invaginatus gestant
      odontoma
   d. lacteus
   d. molaris
   d. permanens
   d. premolaris
   d. sapientiae
   d. serotinus
   d. succedaneus

densification

Densite

densitometer
   Victoreen digital d.

densitometric
   d. analysis

densitometry

density
   alveolar bone d.

density *(continued)*
     bone mineral d. (BMD)
     calcific d.
     cohesive site d.
     microvessel d. (MVD)
     d. radiograph
     radiographic d.
     shadow d.

dent *(Fr.)*
     d's de Chiaie

dentagra

dental
     d. alveolus
     d. analysis
     d. occlusion

dentalis
     alveolus d.
     crista d.
     odontalgia d.

dente
     dens in d.

dentes *(plural of* dens)
     d. acustici
     d. acuti
     d. bicuspides
     d. canini
     d. cuspidati
     d. decidui
     d. incisivi
     d. molares
     d. permanentes
     d. premolares

dentigerous
     d. cyst

dentilabial

dentilingual

dentin (D)
     mantle d.
     mature d.

dentinogenesis
     d. hypoplastica hereditaria
     d. imperfecta
     radicular d.

dentinogenic
     d. fiber

dentinoid
     d. formation

dentinoma
     immature d.

dentinosteoid

dentinum

dentiparous

dentis *genitive of* dens
     apex radicis d.
     cavitas d.
     cavum d.
     cervix d.
     cingulum d.
     collum d.
     corona d.
     cuticula d.
     ebur d.
     facies contactus d.
     facies distalis d.
     facies facialis d.
     facies lingualis d.
     facies mesialis d.
     facies occlusalis d.
     facies vestibularis d.
     foramen apicis d.
     gubernaculum d.
     iter d.
     pulpa d.
     radix d.
     tuberculum d.

dentistry
     esthetic d.

dentition
     delayed d.
     mandibular d.
     maxillary d.
     mixed d.

dentium
     iter d.
     stridor d.

dentoalveolar
     d. abscess

dentoalveolar *(continued)*
    d. cyst
    d. dysplasia
    d. fracture
    d. ligament

dentoalveolitis

dentoaural

dentoepithelial
    d. junction

dentofacial
    d. anomaly
    d. complex
    d. deformity
    d. dysplasia
    d. esthetics
    d. orthopedics
    d. surgery
    d. zone

Dentofacial Planner software

dentoform

dentogenic
    d. movement

dentogingival
    d. fiber
    d. junction
    d. lamina

dentography

dentolabial
    d. dysplasia

dentonomy

dentoperiosteal
    d. fiber

dentopulmonary
    d. syndrome

dentoskeletal

dentosurgical

dentotropic

dentulism

dentulous
    d. dental arch

denture
    esthetic d.
    d. esthetics
    maxillary removal implant-
      retained d.
    d. sore mouth

denude

denuded
    d. finger
    d. furca
    d. furcation
    d. tissue

Denver
    D. Articulation Screening
      Examination (DASE)
    D. nasal splint

depalatalization

depigmentation
    skin d.

depigmenting
    d. skin

deposit
    fatty d's

deposition
    bone d.
    collagen d.
    silicone d.

depot
    fat d.

depression
    lingual salivary gland d.
    prejowl d.
    trochanteric d.

depressor
    d. anguli oris muscle
    d. epiglottidis
    d. labii inferioris muscle
    d. labii oris muscle
    d. muscle of angle of
      mouth
    d. septi
    d. septi muscle
    tongue d.

depth
      mandibular d.
      maxillary d.
      oral vestibular d.
      pocket d.
      probing d. (PD)
      vestibular d.

DePuy nerve hook

de Quervain
      de Q. granulomatous thy-
         roiditis
      de Q. syndrome
      de Q. tenosynovitis

derangement
      alveolar arch d.
      internal d. (ID)

Derm

Derma
      D. K combination laser
      D. 20 laser

dermabrader
      sandpaper d.

dermabrasion (also dermoabrasion)
      spot d.
      therapeutic d.

dermacarrier
      Tanner mesh graft d.

Dermacerator handpiece

Dermaflex Gel

dermal
      d. analogue tumor
      d. atrophy
      d. brassiere technique
      d. curet
      d. fat free flap
      d. fat free tissue transfer
      d. fat graft
      d. fat pedicle flap
      d. graft
      d. grafting
      d. melanosis
      d. network

dermal (continued)
      d. orbicular pennant tech-
         nique
      d. overgrafting
      d. pedicle technique
      d. pouch
      d. pouch reconstruction
      d. pyramidal flap
      d. vascularized pedicle
      d. vascular plexus

Dermalogen human collagen

Dermamesh graft expander

Dermanet wound contact layer

dermaplaning

Derma-Smoothe/FS

Dermastat dermatology handpiece

Derma-Tattoo surgical tattoo

dermatitis
      acneiform d.
      atopic d.
      berlock d.
      blastomycetic d.
      chemical d.
      chronic actinic d.
      contact d.
      d. herpetiformis (DH)
      d. medicamentosa
      papulosquamous d.
      perioral d.
      radiation d.
      retinoid d.
      Schamberg d.
      seborrheic d.
      solar d.
      stasis d.
      tinea d.
      d. venenata
      vesicular d.
      weeping d.
      x-ray d.

dermatoalloplasty

dermatoautoplasty

dermatocele

dermatochalasis
  true d.

dermatofibroma
  d. protuberans

dermatofibrosarcoma protuberans

dermatoheteroplasty

dermatohomoplasty

dermatome
  Brown d.
  Brown-Blair d.
  Brown electric d.
  Castroviejo d.
  Davol d.
  drum d.
  electric d.
  Hall d.
  Padgett d.
  Padgett-Hood d.
  Reese d.
  Reuse Expanda-graft d.
  Tanner-Vandeput mesh d.

dermatomyositis

Dermatop

dermatopathologist

dermatoplastic

dermatoplasty

dermatosis *pl.* dermatoses
  benign papular acantholytic d.
  Bowen precancerous d.
  d. papulosa nigra
  radiation d.
  Schamberg progressive pigmented purpuric d.
  temperature-dependent d.

dermatoxenoplasty

Dermedex
  Donell D.

DERMED

DERMESS

Dermicel tape

DermiCort

dermis
  activated d.
  AlloDerm preserved human d.
  d. fascia
  fresh autologous deepidermalized d.
  new d.
  reticular d.
  superficial d.

dermoabrasion (*variant of* dermabrasion)

dermoadipose
  d. flap
  d. tissue

dermoepidermal Gillies stitch

dermofasciectomy

dermofat
  d. flap
  d. graft
  d. technique

dermoid
  d. cyst
  d. inclusion cyst
  sequestration d.

Dermo-Jet
  D.-J. high pressure injector
  D.-J. injector

Dermolate

dermolipectomy
  abdominal d.
  brachial d.

dermoplasty
  d. procedure

descending necrotizing mediastinitis (DNM)

Desenex
  Maximum Strength D. antifungal cream

desiccation

Desmarres
    D. eye speculum
    D. lid clamp
    D. lid retractor

desmolysis

desmolytic
    d. stage

desmoplasia
    stromal d.

desmoplastic
    d. ameloblastoma
    d. fibroma
    d. melanoma

desmosome
    modified d.

desquamate

desquamated
    d. epithelial cell

desquamating
    d. epithelium

desquamation
    branny d.
    erosion d.

destruction
    bony d.
    deep d.
    SLAC (scapholunate advanced collapse) d.
    superficial d.

Detailed Evaluation of Facial Symmetry (DEFS)

devascularization

developer
    All-Pro automatic film d.

deviated
    d. nasal septum
    d. septum

deviation
    lateral d. on opening
    mandibular d.

deviation *(continued)*
    radial d.
    septal d.
    ulnar d.
    wrist radial d.
    wrist ulnar d.

device
    Agee d.
    angled delivery d. (ADD)
    blade-form d.
    Christoudias fascial closure d.
    Coherent Versapulse d.
    distraction d.
    Handisol phototherapy d.
    Hoffman external fixation d.
    Lewy suspension d.
    3M CTRS d.
    3M microvascular anastomotic coupling d.
    Magna-Finder locating d.
    magnetic jaw tracking d.
    Medicamat ultrasound d.
    Medicon ultrasonic liposuction d.
    Medicon US liposuction d.
    Mentor ultrasound d.
    Morwel ultrasound d.
    rapid palatal expansion d.
    Sebbin ultrasound d.
    SkinTech medical tattooing d.
    SMEI ultrasound d.
    subcutaneous tunneling d.
    Surgitron 3000 ultrasound d.
    Vitallium d.

devil
    d's claw
    d's incision mammaplasty

Devine-Millard-Aufricht retractor

devitalized
    d. skin
    d. soft tissue

Dexon
    D. surgically knitted mesh
    D. suture

DF
    distal fossa

DFBD
    demineralized freeze-dried
        bone

DFDBA
    decalcified freeze-dried
        bone allograft
    demineralized freeze-dried
        bone allograft

DFDCB
    decalcified freeze-dried
        cortical bone

diabetes
    d. mellitus

diameter
    aerodynamic equivalent d.
        (AED)
    cervicobregmatic d.
    fetal cranial d's
    suboccipitobregmatic d.

Diamond-Edge Supercut scissors

diapedesis

diaphanoscopy

diaphragm
    d. of mouth
    oral d.
    styloid d.

diastemata (*plural of* diastema)
    multiple d.

die
    metal-plated d.

Dieffenbach method

Differin Gel

digastric
    d. fossa
    d. muscle
    d. muscle flap
    d. ridge
    d. space
    d. triangle

DiGeorge syndrome

digit
    sausage d.
    supernumerary d.

dilation
    Anel lacrimal duct d.

dilator
    Anthony quadrisected
        minigraft d.
    bisected minigraft d.
    hydrostatic d.
    implant site d.
    Jackson triangular brass d.
    Marritt d.
    micrograft d.
    minigraft d.
    d. naris
    d. naris muscle
    Porges Neoflex d.
    quadrisected graft d.
    quadrisected minigraft d.
    tracheoesophageal d.

dimension

dimple
    celiac d.
    müllerian d.
    palatal d.
    philtral d.
    vaginal d.

Dingman
    D. flexible retractor
    D. forceps
    D. mouth gag
    D. zygoma hook
    D. zygoma hook retractor
    D.-Denhardt mouth gag

DIP
    distal interphalangeal
        DIP joint

diplegia
    congenital facial d.

diplopia

direct
    d. crease excision

direct *(continued)*
    d. digital radiography
      (DDR)
    d. supraciliary excision

dirhinic

disarticulation

Disc
    Clear Away D.

discharge
    wound d.

discontinuous
    d. neck dissection

discontinuity
    bony d.

discorraphy

discrepancy
    anterior-posterior d.
    arch d.
    envelope of d.
    posterior occlusal d.
    transverse d.

discrimination
    moving two-point d.

disease
    Addison d.
    Albers-Schönberg d.
    Albright d.
    Anders d.
    Apert d.
    Apert-Crouzon d.
    arteriosclerotic occlu-
      sive d.
    arteriosclerotic peripheral
      vascular d.
    Baelz d.
    Barlow d.
    Basedow d.
    Bazin d.
    Besnier-Boeck-Schau-
      mann d.
    Bloch-Sulzberger d.
    Bowen d.
    Breda d.
    Brill-Symmers d.

disease *(continued)*
    brittle bone d.
    Brooke d.
    Buerger d.
    Caffey d.
    Caffey-Silverman d.
    central Recklinghausen d.,
      type II
    Chagas d.
    Charcot-Marie-Tooth d.
    chronic fibrocystic d.
    chronic graft-versus-host d.
    chronic granulomatous d.
    collagen vascular d.
    connective tissue d. (CTD)
    Cowden d.
    Crouzon d.
    Darier d.
    Darier-White d.
    degenerative d.
    degenerative joint d.
    degenerative joint d. of
      wrist
    demyelinating d.
    Dupuytren's d.
    Engman d.
    extramammary Paget d.
    Fabry d.
    fibrocystic d.
    Fordyce d.
    Garré d.
    Gilchrist d.
    Goldscheider d.
    graft-versus-host d. (GVH)
      (grades 1–4)
    granulomatous d.
    Hand-Schüller-Christian d.
    Heck d.
    Hopf d.
    Hutchinson-Gilford d.
    iatrogenic d.
    inclusion d.
    inflammatory d.
    Kawasaki d.
    Kienböck d.
    Korsakoff d.
    Leri-Weill d.
    Magitot d.
    marble bone d.

disease *(continued)*
  Meige d.
  Ménétrier d.
  Meniere d.
  Meyenburg d.
  micrometastatic d.
  Mikulicz d.
  Möller d.
  Mondor d.
  mycotic d.
  Ollier d.
  Paget d.
  Paget d. of bone
  Paget d. of nipple
  Preiser d.
  Recklinghausen d.
  Romberg d.
  salivary gland virus d.
  Schimmelbusch d.
  Senear-Usher d.
  Simmonds d.
  Sneddon-Wilkinson d.
  Stickler d.
  Sutton d.
  undifferentiated connective
    tissue d.
  Unna d.
  van Buchem disease
  van Buren d.
  vanishing bone d.
  vascular occlusive d.
  Vincent d.
  Virchow d.
  von Meyenburg d.
  Wagner d.
  Weber-Christian d.
  Werdnig-Hoffmann d.
  Werther d.
  Winkler d.
  Wohlfart-Kugelberg-Welan-
    der d.
  Woringer-Kolopp d.

dish
  dappen d.
  d. face
  d.-face deformity

disharmony
  facial d.

disharmony *(continued)*
  maxillomandibular d.
  midline d.
  occlusal d.

dished-in face

DISI
  dorsal intercalated segmen-
    tal instability
    DISI deformity

disinsertion
  levator d.

disjunction
  craniofacial d.
  Le Fort III craniofacial d.

disk
  articular d.
  Damascus D.
  interarticular d. of tempo-
    romandibular joint
  Ranvier tactile d's

dislocation
  carpal d.
  compound d.
  fracture d.
  mandibular d.
  perilunate d.
  prosthetic d.
  simple d.
  subglenoid d.
  temporomandibular joint d.
  tendon d.

dislodger
  Tessier d.

disorder
  autoimmune d.
  bipolar d.
  body dysmorphic d.
  body image d.
  d. of cornification
  craniofacial d.
  endonasal d.
  fibrocystic d.
  fibrocystic breast d.
  lymphoproliferative d.
  motor d.

disorder *(continued)*
    myofascial pain-dysfunction d.
    temporomandibular pain-dysfunction d. (TMPD)

displaced
    d. fracture
    d. malar fracture
    d. sideburn
    d. zygomatic fracture

displacement
    anterior d. (AD)
    anterior d. no reduction (ADNR)
    caudal d.
    condylar d.
    cross-head d.
    eye d.
    locked septal d.
    septal d.

disproportion
    skeletal d.

disruption
    closed d. of digital artery
    scapholunate d.

dissatisfaction
    body image d.

dissection
    axillary node d.
    balloon d.
    bilateral neck d.
    blunt d.
    blunt and sharp d.
    cold d.
    cold-knife d.
    discontinuous neck d.
    elective lymph node d. (ELND)
    elective neck d. (END)
    electrosurgical d.
    extended supraplatysmal plane (ESP) d.
    facial nerve d.
    functional neck d.
    hydraulic d.
    mediastinal d.
    modified neck d. (MND)

dissection *(continued)*
    neck d.
    plane of d.
    radical neck d.
    retrograde d.
    selective neck d. (SND)
    sharp d.
    skin-subcutaneous d. with SMAS manipulation
    d. snare
    subgaleal d.
    submucosal d.
    submucous d.
    subperichondrial d.
    subperiosteal d.
    suprahyoid neck d.
    supraomohyoid neck d.
    supraperichondrial d.
    tongue-jaw-neck d.
    two-team d.
    Wookey radical neck d.

dissector
    10 d.
    aspirating d.
    ASSI breast d. angulated
    ASSI breast d. spatulated
    Chajchir d.
    endoscopic d.
    Freer d.
    Gorney d.
    Hajek-Ballenger septal d.
    Hurd d.
    Resposable Spacemaker surgical balloon d.
    Stallard d.
    submammary d.
    submucous d.
    synovial d.
    Toledo d.

dissociation
    scapholunate d.

distal
    d. angle
    d.-based flap
    d.-based island flap
    d. end
    d. force (DF)
    d. fossa

distal *(continued)*
 d. interphalangeal (DIP)
 d. interphalangeal (DIP) joint
 d. movement
 d. oblique groove (DOG)
 d. occlusion
 d. pedicle flap
 d. pedicle flap technique
 d. phalanx
 d. surface
 d. triangular fossa (DTF)

distally based fasciocutaneous flap (DBFF)

distal-occlusal

distance
 inframammary d.
 interalveolar d.
 interarch d.
 interincisal d.
 maximum interincisal d. (MID)
 orbito-temple d.

distant flap

distraction
 callus d.
 craniomaxillofacial callus d.
 d. device
 forward mandibular d.
 d. lengthening
 mandibular d.
 d. osteogenesis (DO)
 d. osteosynthesis
 palatal d.
 d. pin
 rigid external d. (RED)
 simple mandibular d.
 skeletal d.
 d. TRAM

distractor
 mandibular d.
 Molina mandibular d.
 multidirectional d.
 MULTIGUIDE mandibular d.
 RED system rigid external d.

distribution
 asymmetric d.

disturbance
 deglutitory d.
 occlusal d.

divergence
 anterior d.

diversion
 laryngeal d.
 laryngotracheal d.

diverticulum
 pharyngoesophageal d.

division
 maxillary d.

divot
 liposuction d.

Dix-Hallpike maneuver

DMAS
 deep muscular aponeurotic system

DMB
 demineralized bone

DNM
 descending necrotizing mediastinitis

DO
 distraction osteogenesis

DOG
 distal oblique groove

dog ear
 d. e. of anastomosis
 lateral d. e's
 medial d. e's

domain
 abdominal d.

dome
 alar d. and cartilage
 nasal d.

Donders
 space of D.

Donell Dermedex

donor
   autologous d.
   d. bone marrow engraft-
      ment
   cadaveric d.
   d. incision
   d. nipple
   d. site
   d. site dressing
   d. size

Doppler
   color flow D. scanner

Dorello canal

Dorrance
   D. closure
   D. palatal pushback

dorsa (*pl.* of dorsum)

dorsal
   d. antebrachial cutaneous
      nerve
   d. artery
   d. artery of foot
   d. artery of nose
   d. artery of penis
   d. back roll
   d. condylar surface
   d. cross-finger flap
   d. digital artery
   d. intercalated segmental
      instability (DISI) defor-
      mity
   d. lingual artery
   d. lingual mucosa
   d. metacarpal artery
   d. metatarsal artery
   d. mutilation
   d. thoracic fascia free flap
   d. vein
   d. wrist syndrome

dorsalis
   d. pedis artery
   d. pedis-FDMA system
   d. pedis flap
   tabes d.

dorsonasal

dorsum *pl.* dorsa
   d. linguae
   nasal d.
   d. nasi
   d. of nose
   d. sella
   d. sellae
   d. of tongue

dose
   maximum accumulated d.
      (MAD)
   maximum permissible d.
      (MPD)
   radiation absorbed d.
   roentgen absorbed d. (rad)

Dott
   D. mouth gag
   D.-Kilner mouth gag

double
   d.-barreled fibular bone
      graft
   d.-bubble breast deformity
   d. cross-lip flap
   d.-end graft
   d. gloving
   d. jaw surgery
   d. lip
   d. lumen implant
   d.-lumen suction irrigation
      tube
   d. opposing Z-plasty
   d.-paddle flap
   d.-paddle island flap
   d.-paddle peroneal tissue
      transfer
   d. papilla graft
   d. papilla pedicle graft
   d. pedicle flap
   d. pedicle technique
   d.-pedicle transverse rec-
      tus abdominis musculo-
      cutaneous flap
   d. pendulum flap
   d. protrusion
   d. rectus harvest

double *(continued)*
 d. skin paddle fibular flap
 d.-spoon biopsy forceps
 d. tunnel
 d. V-Y flap
 d. V-Y plasty with paired
   inverted Burow triangle
   excisions

double-cross-plasty

double-eyelid plasty

Douglas
 D. graft
 D. mesh skin graft
 D. nasal scissors

dovetail
 lingual d.

Downes nasal speculum

downgrafting
 maxillary d.

Doyle
 D. nasal splint
 D. II silicone stent

DP
 debonding pliers

DPM
 dual-pedicle dermoparen-
   chymal mastopexy

Dragstedt graft

drain
 Blake d.
 Blake silicone d.
 Hemovac d.
 Jackson-Pratt d.
 Shirley wound d.
 Sof-Wick d.

drainage
 capillary d.
 incision and d. (I&D)
 lumbar d.
 lymphatic d.
 retrograde venous d.
 sanguineous d.
 suction d.

drainage *(continued)*
 venous d.
 wound d.

drapery swag of cheek

dressing
 Abdopatch Gel Z Adhe-
   sive d.
 Ace elastic d.
 Adaptic d.
 air pressure d.
 Alldress multilayered
   wound d.
 Alvogyl surgical d.
 amniotic membrane d.
 Aquaplast d.
 bacitracin d.
 Band-Aid d.
 binocular d.
 binocular eye d.
 Biobrane d.
 Biobrane glove d.
 Biobrane wound d.
 Biopatch antimicrobial d.
 BlisterFilm transparent
   wound d.
 bolus d.
 bulky pressure d.
 Bunnell d.
 ClearSite borderless d.
 ClearSite Hydro Gauze d.
 ClearSite wound d.
 cotton bolster d.
 Coban elastic d.
 CollaCote wound d.
 CollaPlug wound d.
 composite d.
 compression d.
 contact-layer wound d's
 Covaderm composite
   wound d.
 Coverlet adhesive d.
 Cranioplastic material d.
 Curafil hydrogel d.
 Curafoam wound d.
 Curagel hydrogel d.
 Curasorb calcium algin-
   ate d.
 Cutinova Hydro d.

dressing *(continued)*
  donor site d.
  Fibracol collagen-alginate d.
  fine-mesh d.
  Flexzan d.
  Flexzan foam wound d.
  Flexzan topical wound d.
  Gentell alginate wound d.
  Gentell foam wound d.
  GraftCyte gauze wound d.
  GraftCyte moist d.
  Hueter perineal d.
  hyCURE collagen hemostatic wound d.
  Hydrasorb foam wound d.
  hydrocolloid d.
  HydroDerm transparent d.
  hydrogel d.
  hydrophilic polymer d.
  hydrophilic semipermeable absorbent polyurethane foam d.
  HyFil hydrogel d.
  Hypergel wound d.
  LaserSite wound d.
  Mammopatch gel self-adhesive d.
  Medipatch Gel Z adhesive d.
  Mepitel d.
  Mepitel nonadherent silicone d.
  Mesalt sodium chloride impregnated d.
  Micropore d.
  moustache d.
  nonocclusive d.
  occlusive d.
  open d.
  polyurethane foam d.
  pressure d.
  Reston foam d.
  SAF-Gel hydrogel d.
  saline d.
  semicompressive d.
  semiocclusive d.
  semiopen d.
  semipermeable d.

dressing *(continued)*
  semipermeable membrane d.
  semipressure d.
  SignaDRESS d.
  Silastic foam d.
  Silastic gel d.
  silicone d.
  Silon-TSR wound d.
  Silon wound d.
  Siloskin d.
  SkinTegrity hydrogel d.
  SofSorb absorptive d.
  SoftCloth absorptive d.
  Sof-Wick d.
  Sommers compression d.
  sterile compression d.
  super-absorptive polymer d.
  synthetic barrier d.
  Tegaderm d.
  Tegaderm occlusive d.
  Tegaderm semipermeable d.
  Tegaderm transparent d.
  Telfa d.
  Telfa island d.
  Telfa plastic film d.
  Thera-Boot compression d.
  tie-over d.
  Ventex d.
  Vigilon gel d.
  Vigilon semipermeable nonocclusive d.
  Vigilon synthetic occlusive d.
  wet-to-dry d.
  Woun'Dres hydrogel d.
  Wound-Span Bridge II d.
  Xeroform d.

drift
  canthal d.

drill
  Hall surgical d.
  MicroMax speed d.

drop
  d. finger
  wrist d.

drug
  second-line d.
drum
  d. dermatome
drumhead
drumstick finger
dry eye syndrome
D-shaped implant
DTF
  deep temporal fascia
  distal triangular fossa
dual-chambered
  d.-c. implant
  d.-c. prosthesis
DualMesh biomaterial graft
dual-pedicle dermoparenchy-
  mal mastopexy (DPM)
duck lips exercise
duct
  acoustic d.
  alveolar d.
  Bartholin d.
  d. cannulation
  cochlear d.
  Coschwitz d.
  endolymphatic d.
  excretory d.
  frontonasal d.
  guttural d.
  Hensen's d.
  intercalated d.
  interlobular d.
  intralobular d.
  lacrimal d.
  lingual d.
  mammary d.
  müllerian d.
  nasofrontal d.
  nasolacrimal d.
  nasopalatine d.
  parotid d.
  perilymphatic d.
  periotic d.

duct (continued)
  pharyngoinfraglottic d.
  Rivinus d's
  saccular d.
  sacculoutricular d.
  salivary d.
  secretory d.
  semicircular d's
  semicircular d., anterior
  semicircular d., lateral
  semicircular d., posterior
  semicircular d., superior
  Stensen d.
  striated d.
  sublingual d.
  submandibular d.
  submaxillary d.
  tear d.
  thoracic d.
  utricular d.
  utriculosaccular d.
  vestibulo-infraglottic d.
  Wharton d.
ductal
  d. carcinoma
  d. carcinoma in situ
  d. obstruction
  d. stricture
ductus
  d. cochlearis
  d. endolymphaticus
  d. perilymphatici
  d. perilymphaticus
  d. reuniens
  d. semicirculares
  d. semicircularis anterior
  d. semicircularis lateralis
  d. semicircularis posterior
  d. semicircularis superior
  d. utriculosaccularis
Dufourmental flap
Dumbach
  D. mandibular reconstruction system
  D. mini mesh
  D. regular mesh
  D. titanium mesh

Dumbo ear

Dumon silicone stent

Duplay-Lynch nasal speculum

duplication
    central d.
    congenital hand d.
    congenital thumb d.
    postaxial d. of the fifth ray
        (*types I–III*)
    preaxial thumb d. (*types I–
        VII*)
    thumb d.
    thumb d. correction

Dupuy-Dutemps operation

Dupuytren
    D. contracture
    D's disease
    false D. contracture
    D. fascia
    D. sign

Dura

Durafill dental restorative material

dural
    d. grafting
    d. venous sinus injury

durapatite

duraplasty

Dur-A-Sil ear impression material

Durette external laser shield

duration
    maximum d. of phonation
    maximum d. of sustained
        blowing

durum
    palatine d.

dwarf
    bird-headed d.

dwarf (*continued*)
    Seckel bird-headed d.

dwarfism
    Robinow d.
    Seckel d.

DWS
    dorsal wrist syndrome

DynaGraft granule

dynamic compression plate
    (DCP)

Dynamic Mesh craniomaxillofacial pre-angled connecting bar

dysarthria
    flaccid d.
    neurogenic d.

dyscephaly
    mandibulo-oculofacial d.

dyschromia *pl.* dyschromias
    pigmentary d.

dysesthesia
    palmar d.

dysfunction
    craniomandibular d. (CMD)
    dental d.
    facial neuromuscular d.
    minimal brain d. (MBD)
    myofascial pain-d. (MPD)
    nasolacrimal d.
    neurological d.
    temporomandibular d.
        (TMD)
    temporomandibular joint d.
        (TMD, TMJ)
    temporomandibular pain-d.
        (TMPD)

dysgenesis
    mixed gonadal d.
    pure gonadal d.

dysjunction (*variant of* disjunction)

dyskeratoma
  warty d.

dyskeratosis
  benign intraepithelial d.
  d. congenita
  intraepithelial d.

dysmetria
  ocular d.

dysmorphic cranium

dysmorphism
  craniofacial d.
  facial d.

dysmorphology
  facial d.
  orbital d.

dysostosis
  acrofacial d.
  clcidocranial d.
  craniofacial d.
  faciomandibular d.
  mandibulofacial d.
  maxillonasal d.
  d. multiplex
  Nager acrofacial d.
  orodigitofacial d
  otomandibular d.

dysphagia
  d. lusoria
  neurogenic d.

dysplasia
  anteroposterior d.
  anteroposterior facial d.
  brachycephalofronto-
    nasal d.
  chondroectodermal d.
  cleidocranial d.
  condylar d.
  congenital ectodermal d.

dysplasia *(continued)*
  craniofacial d.
  dentoalveolar d.
  dentofacial d.
  dentolabial d.
  ectodermal d.
  familial fibrous d.
  familial white folded d.
  fibromuscular d.
  fibro-osseous d.
  fibrous d. of jaws
  florid osseous d.
  focal osseous d.
  frontonasal d.
  hereditary bone d.
  Holt-Oram atriodigital d.
  internasal d.
  maxillomandibular d.
  Mondini d.
  monostotic fibrous d.
  nasal d.
  nasomaxillary d.
  oculodento-osseous d.
  Robinow mesomelic d.
  sphenoid d.
  vertical d.
  Wolfe breast d.
  Wolfe classification of
    breast d.

dystonia
  oromandibular d.

dystopia
  globe d.
  ocular d.

dystrophia
  cleidocranial d.

dystrophy
  mucopolysaccharide kera-
    tin d.
  muscular d.
  reflex sympathetic d. (RSD)

E

EAC
    external auditory canal

Eagle-Barrett syndrome

EAP
    endoscopic access port

ear
    artificial e.
    aviator's e.
    Aztec e.
    bat e.
    Blainville e's
    e. bowl
    bowl of e.
    boxer's e.
    Cagot e.
    e. canal
    e. cartilage
    cat's e.
    cauliflower e.
    cockleshell e.
    constricted e.
    contralateral e.
    cup e.
    darwinian e.
    dog e.
    dog e. of anastomosis
    Dumbo e.
    external e.
    helix of e.
    inner e.
    lateral dog e's
    e. lobe (*variant of* earlobe)
    e. lobule
    lop e.
    medial dog e's
    middle e.
    Morel e.
    Mozart e.
    outer e.
    persistent lop e.
    prominent e.
    protruding e.
    question mark e.
    e. reconstruction
    e. replantation
    scroll e.

ear (*continued*)
    e. shape
    Stahl e.
    e. surgery
    swimmer's e.
    telephone e.
    Wildermuth e.

earlobe
    e. adipose tissue
    cleft e.
    e. composite graft
    incomplete cleft of e.
    e. keloid
    ptotic e.

early
    e. hard palate closure

earmold
    e. lab
    nonoccluding e.
    open e.
    perimeter e.
    shell e.
    skeleton e.
    standard e.
    vented e.

earring
    Brent pressure e. for keloid
        surgery
    compression e.

EBL
    endoscopic band ligation

Ebner glands

ebur dentis

eboris
    membrana e.

ecchymosis

echolalia
    delayed e.
    immediate e.
    mitigated e.

Ecker fissure

ECRL
    extensor carpi radialis longus
        ECRL tendon

ectasia (*also* ectasis)
    mammary duct e.
    papillary e.
    skyrocket capillary e.

ectocanthus

ectocranial

ectocyst

ectoderm

ectodermal
    e. dysplasia
    e. tumor

ectopic
    e. parts surgery

ECTR
    endoscopic carpal tunnel release

ectropion

ECU
    extensor carpi ulnaris
        ECU tendon

eczema
    stasis e.
    weeping e.

EDB
    extensor digitorum brevis

edema
    angioneurotic e.
    brawny e.
    cerebral e.
    facial e.
    e. glottidis
    inflammatory e.
    labial e.
    laryngeal e.
    palatal e.
    penoscrotal e.
    purulent e.

edema (*continued*)
    Reinke e.
    retropharyngeal e.
    stasis e.
    Yangtze e.

edge
    cartilage e.
    cutting e.
    feathered e.
    gaping wound e's
    incisal e.
    labioincisal e. (LIE)
    linguoincisal e. (LIE)
    shearing e.
    e. strength

EDGE coated blade

Edlan
    E. vestibulotomy
    E.-Mejchar operation

effect
    Karoli e.

effusion
    middle ear e. (MEE)
    mucopurulent hemorrhagic e.

EGF
    epidermal growth factor

Ehlers-Danlos syndrome

Ehrenritter ganglion

Eicken method

EIE 150F operating microscope

EIP
    extensor indicis proprius
        EIP tendon

ELAFF
    extended lateral arm free flap

elastic
    maxillomandibular e.

Elasticon bandage

Elastikon elastic tape

elastomer
  silicone e.

Elastoplast bandage

elastosis
  e. perforans serpiginosa
  senile e.
  solar e.

elastotic tissue

elder
  marsh e.

Elder classification of malignant
  melanoma

elective
  e. lymph node dissection
    (ELND)
  e. neck dissection (END)
  e. neck irradiation

electric
  e. dermatome
  e. irritability
  e. nerve stimulator

electrocoagulation
  bipolar e.

electrode
  MegaDyne arthroscopic
    hook e.

electromallet
  McShirley e.

electrosurgery
  bipolar e.

electrosurgical
  e. current intensity
  e. dissection
  e. scaling
  e. scalpel

element
  neural e.

elephantiasis
  filarial e.
  e. gingivae
  scrotal e.

elevation
  blanched cutaneous e.
  FAME midface e.
  flap e.
  forehead e. and fixation
    with percutaneous mi-
    croscrews
  medial e.
  mucoperichondrial e.
  periosteal e.
  philtral column e.
  sinus e.
  subgaleal e.
  subperiosteal e.
  transblepharoplasty sub-
    periosteal midface e.

elevator
  angled e.
  angular e.
  Aufricht e.
  Baron palate e.
  Barsky e.
  Blair cleft palate e.
  Boies nasal e.
  Boies nasal fracture e.
  Boies plastic surgery e.
  Bristow zygomatic e.
  Cameron e.
  Carmody-Batson e.
  cleft palate e.
  Converse alar e.
  Converse periosteal e.
  Converse-MacKenty e.
  Cottle e.
  Cottle alar e.
  Cottle septal e.
  Cottle skin e.
  Cottle-MacKenty e.
  Cronin cleft palate e.
  Cronin palate e.
  Dean periosteal e.
  Freer nasoseptal e.
  Freer septal e.
  Freer single-ended e.
  Gillies zygomatic e.
  Goldman septal e.
  Gorney septal suction e.
  Hajek e.

elevator *(continued)*
  Hajek-Ballenger septal e.
  Halle nasal e.
  Halle septal e.
  Hurd septal e.
  lip e.
  MacKenty septal e.
  malar e.
  Molt No. 4 e.
  periosteal e.
  septal e.
  soft tissue e.
  Suraci zygoma hook e.
  Tenzel double-end periosteal e.
  Tenzel periosteal e.
  Tessier e.
  Veau e.
  zygoma e.

elfin facies

Ellenbogen criteria for ideal eyebrow position and contour

Elliot flap

elliptical flap

Ellison fixation staple

Ellis-van Creveld syndrome

ELND
  elective lymph node dissection

Elschnig lid retractor

Ely's procedure

Elysee Lasercare

EMA
  epithelial membrane antigen

embolism
  air e.

embolus
  air e.

embrasure
  buccal e.

embrasure *(continued)*
  e. clasp
  gingival e.
  e. hook
  incisal e.
  interdental e.
  labial e.
  lingual e.
  occlusal e.
  e. space

emergency free flap

eminectomy

eminence
  arcuate e.
  articular e.
  articular e. of temporal bone
  canine e.
  hypobranchial e.
  hypopharyngeal e.
  hypophysial e.
  hypothenar e.
  malar e.
  pyramidal e.
  retromylohyoid e.
  temporomandibular joint articular e.
  thenar e.
  triangular e.
  zygomatic e.

eminentia
  e. arcuata
  e. triangularis

EMLA
  eutectic mixture of local anesthetics

Emory EndoPlastic retractor

empyema
  mastoid e.

emulsification
  fat e.

encephalitis
  mumps e.

encephalocele
  spheno-occipital e.

END
elective neck dissection

end
distal e.

ending
nerve e.
Ruffini papillary e's

endocarditis
bacterial e.
infective e.

endoforehead
e. lift
e.-endomidface lift
e.-periorbital-cheek lift

endoforeheadplasty
laser e.

endolymphatic duct

EndoMax endoscopic instrumentation

endometriosis

endomidface
e. lift

endomolare

endomysium

endonasal
e. approach
e. dacryocystorhinostomy
e. disorder
e. fenestration
e. incision
e. rhinoplasty

Endopore implant

endoscope
fiberoptic e.
Hopkins rod e.
Padgett e.

endoscope-assisted
e.-a. rectus abdominis muscle flap harvest
e.-a. suction extraction

endoscopic
e. access port (EAP)

endoscopic *(continued)*
e. band ligation (EBL)
e. brow lift
e. brow lift with simultaneous carbon dioxide laser resurfacing
e. carpal tunnel release (ECTR)
e. cholangiopancreatography
e. dacryocystorhinostomy
e. dissector
e. ethmoidectomy
e. face-lift
e. forceps
e. forehead-brow rhytidoplasty
e. forehead lift
e. guidance
e. harvest
e. intranasal frontal sinusotomy
e. medial maxillectomy
e. muscle plication
e. orbital decompression
e. procedure
e. sinus surgery
e. sphenoethmoidectomy with septoplasty
e. subperiosteal forehead lift
e. subperiosteal forehead and midface lift
e. subperiosteal midface lift
e. transaxillary submuscular augmentation mammaplasty
e. variceal ligation (EVL)
e. variceal sclerotherapy (EVS)

endoscopically
e. assisted abdominoplasty
e. assisted brow lift
e. harvested tissue

endoscopic-assisted facial implant insertion

endoscopy
e. browpexy
flexible fiberoptic e.

endoscopy *(continued)*
  fluorescein e.
  nasal e.
  peroral e.

endotemporal
  e. lift
  e.-endomidface lift

endothelial
  e. cell
  e. relaxing factor
  e. sarcoma

endothelioma

endothelium
  vascular e.

Endotrac retractor

Endotron-Lipectron ultrasonic
  scalpel

endplate
  motor e.

end-to-end
  e.-to-e. anastomosis
  e.-to-e. microvascular anas-
    tomosis
  e.-to-e. venous anastomosis

end-to-side
  e.-to-s. anastomosis

engine
  Acrotorque hand e.

engineering
  tissue e.
  tissue-graft e.

Engman disease

engorgement
  venous e.

engraftment
  donor bone marrow e.

enhancement
  lip e.
  penile girth e.
  vermilion e.

enlargement
  idiopathic e.

enlargement *(continued)*
  salivary gland e.

enteric
  e. cyst

enterocutaneous
  e. fistula

enterogenous
  e. cyst

enteroplasty

entomophthoramycosis
  e. conidiobolae
  rhinofacial e.

entrance
  wound e.

entrapment
  suprascapular nerve e.
  sural nerve e.

entropion
  cicatricial e.
  congenital e.
  involuntary e.

envelope
  cornified cell e.
  e. of discrepancy
  e. flap
  shriveled skin e.
  skin e.
  viral e.

environment
  neurotropic e.

ENZA laser skin care program

enzyme
  mitochondrial oxidative e.

epaulet flap

EpDRF
  epithelium-derived relax-
    ation factor

epiblepharon

epicanthal fold

epicanthoplasty
  medial e.

epicanthus
    congenital e.

epidemiology

epidermal
    e. actinic damage
    e. atrophy
    e. cyst
    e. growth factor (EGF)
    e. growth factor receptor
    e. inclusion cyst
    e. necrosis
    e. nevus
    e. sliding

epidermatoplasty

epidermic graft

epidermis
    hyperkeratotic e.
    hyperplastic e.

epidermization

epidermoid
    e. carcinoma
    e. cyst
    e. resection
    e. tumor

epidermolysis
    e. bullosa
    e. bullosa dystrophica
    e. bullosa simplex
    generalized atrophic be-
        nign e. bullosa (GABEB)
    e. simplex

epidermolytic vesicant

Epi-Derm silicone gel sheeting

epididymoplasty

epigastric
    e. artery
    e. flap

epiglottis
    bifid e.

epiglottitis
    suprahyoid e.

EpiLaser
    E. hair removal laser
    E. system

epilepsy
    laryngeal e.

EpiLight hair removal system

epiloia

epimyoepithelium

epiphora

epithelia (*pl.* of epithelium)

epithelial
    e. adaptation
    e. attachment
    e. atypia
    e. cell
    e. cicatrization
    e. cuff
    e. débridement
    e. granuloma
    e. inlay
    e. invagination
    e. marker
    e. membrane antigen
        (EMA)
    e. migration
    e.-myoepithelial carcinoma
    e. neoplasm
    e. pearl
    e. peg
    e. proliferation
    e. rest
    e. rete peg
    e. ridge
    e. sarcoma (ES)
    e. seam
    e. sheath
    e. strand
    e. turn-in flap

epithelialization
    e. technique
    vaginal e.

epithelial-myoepithelial (EME)

epithelioid
    e. cell

epithelioid *(continued)*
 e. sarcoma

epithelioid-cell sialadenitis

epithelioma
 e. adenoides cysticum
 basal cell e. (BCE)
 Borst-Jadassohn type in-
  traepidermal e.
 Brooke e.
 calcifying e. of Malherbe
 cystic adenoid e.
 Ferguson-Smith e.
 e. of Malherbe
 superficial basal cell e.

epithelium *pl.* epithelia
 attachment e.
 autologous-cultured e.
  (ACE)
 buccal e.
 cat e.
 cornified e.
 crevicular e.
 cuboidal e.
 desquamating e.
 e.-derived relaxation factor
  (EpDRF)
 follicular e.
 hornified e.
 junctional e.
 keratinized e.
 noncornified e.
 nonhornified e.
 nonkeratinized e.
 parakeratinized e.
 pocket e.
 squamous e.
 stratified squamous e.
 sulcal e.
 sulcular e.
 urethral e.
 vestibular e.

epithelization *(variant of* epithelialization)

EpiTouch
 E. Alex laser hair removal
  system
 E. Ruby SilkLaser

EpiTouch *(continued)*
 E. Ruby SilkLaser hair removal system

EPL
 extensor pollicis longus
  EPL tendon

eponychial fold

eponychium

Epoxy Die material

Epstein-Barr virus (EBV)

ePTFE
 expanded polytetrafluoroethylene
  ePTFE implant

equilibration
 mandibular e.
 occlusal e.

equivalent
 migraine e.

Erb
 E. palsy
 E.-Duchenne palsy

erbium CrystaLase laser

erectile corpora

Erhardt lid clamp

Erich
 E. alar cartilage relocation
 E. arch bar
 E. facial fracture appliance
 E. maxillary splint
 E. nasal splint

erosion
 bony e.
 crater-shaped e.
 notch-shaped e.
 saucer-shaped e.
 V-shaped e.

eruption
 acneiform e.
 hypopigmented macular e.
 Kaposi varicelliform e.

eruption *(continued)*
    nonfebrile-associated vesicular e.
    sclerodermalike e.
    skin e.
    vesicopustular e.
    vesicular e.

erythema
    atypical e. multiforme
    bullous e. multiforme
    congenital telangiectatic e.
    facial e.
    e. migrans
    e. multiforme
    e. simplex
    telangiectatic e.

erythroderma
    Sézary e.

erythroplakia
    precancerous e.

erythroplakic lesion

erythroplasia of Queyrat

ES
    epithelial sarcoma

eschar
    black e.
    burn e.
    constricting e.

escharotomy

ESI
    ESI light-weight, narrow mammaplasty retractor
    ESI Lite-Pipe fiberoptic instrument
    ESI Lite-Pipe plastic surgery instrument
    ESI long, narrow mammaplasty retractor
    ESI narrow mammaplasty retractor

Esmarch bandage

esophagectomy
    Lewis-Tanner e.

esophagoscope
    fiberoptic e.
    Jackson e.

esophagus
    Barrett e.
    bird-beak distal e.

esotropia

ESP
    extended supraplatysmal plane
        ESP dissection
        ESP face-lift technique

Esser
    E. graft
    E. operation

Essig-type splint

esthetic *(spelled also* aesthetic*)*
    e. appearance
    e. breast reconstruction
    e. CO_2 laser
    e. dentistry
    e. denture
    e. laser system
    e. restoration
    e. rhinoplasty
    e. septorhinoplasty
    e. surgery
    e. Taylor mandibular angle implant

esthetically pleasing

esthetician *(also spelled* aesthetician*)*

esthetics *(spelled also* aesthetics*)*
    dentofacial e.
    denture e.
    facial e.
    gingival e.
    profile e.

Estlander
    E. flap
    E. operation

Ethicon
E. SAS (synthetic absorbable suture)
E. suture

Ethilon suture

ethmoid
e. air cell
anterior e.
e. bone
e. bulla
e. cell
e. plate
posterior e.
e. punch forceps
e. registration point
supraorbital e.

ethmoidal
e. air cell
e. artery
c. bulla
e. cells
e. fissure
e. infundibular system
e. infundibulum
e. labyrinth
e. labyrinth cell
e.-lacrimal fistula
e. mucosa
e. nerve
e. notch
e. ostium
e. periostitis
e. prechamber
e. sinus
e. sinusitis

ethmoidale

ethmoidalis
bulla e.
bulla e. cava nasi
bulla e. ossis ethmoidalis
fovea e.

ethmoidectomy
anterior e.
endoscopic e.
external e.
internal e.

ethmoidectomy *(continued)*
intranasal e.
partial e.
Riedel frontal e.
total e.
transantral e.

ethmoidomaxillary
e. plate
e. suture

eutectic mixture of local anesthetics (EMLA)

evacuation
hematoma e.

evaluation
Detailed E. of Facial Symmetry (DEFS)

everter
Berke double-end lid e.

EVL
endoscopic variceal ligation

EVS
endoscopic variceal sclerotherapy

evulsion
clothesline e. of maxilla
nerve e.

Ewing
E. lid clamp
E. sarcoma
E. sign

examination
Denver Articulation Screening E. (DASE)
radial wrist e.
Wood light e.

excementosis
intraepithelial e.

excess
bony e.
mandibular e.
marginal e.
maxillary e.

excess *(continued)*
    e. overhang
    vertical maxillary e. (VME)

excessive
    e. lip support
    e. nasality
    e. overbite
    e. spacing

exchange
    air e.
    saline implant e.

excimer ultraviolet laser

excision
    alar rim e.
    alar wedge e.
    anterior port scalp e.
    Arlt pterygium e.
    chalazion e.
    direct crease e.
    direct supraciliary e.
    double V-Y plasty with
      paired inverted Burow
      triangle e.
    Feldman e.
    Fergusson e. of maxilla
    flared-W e.
    fusiform e.
    interdental e.
    inverted-T skin e.
    local e.
    L-shaped skin e.
    lunate e.
    modified fishtail e.
    Mohs e.
    mucosal e.
    neuroma e.
    osteocartilaginous e.
    radical e.
    regional e.
    retroorbicularis ocular fat
      pad e.
    serial scar e's
    serial e's of skin lesion
    shave e.
    subtotal e.
    tangential e.
    through-and-through but-
      tonhole fashion e.

excision *(continued)*
    U-shaped skin e.
    vertical skin e.
    V-shaped skin e.
    wedge e.
    Weir e.
    wide e.
    wound e.

excisional biopsy

excretory duct

excursion
    eyelid e.
    lateral e.
    left lateral e.
    protrusive e.
    retrusive e.
    right lateral e.

exercise
    cat sneer e.
    duck lips e.
    rabbit sniffing e.

exfoliated

exfoliation
    skin e.

exfoliator
    Bi-Phasic e.

exostosis
    multiple e's of jaw
    osteocartilaginous e.
    subungual e.

expanded
    e. free scalp flap
    e. polytetrafluoroethylene
      (ePTFE) implant

expander
    AccuSpan tissue e.
    Becker tissue e.
    BioDIMENSIONAL tissue e.
    Biospan anatomical tis-
      sue e.
    blood e.
    Dermamesh graft e.
    Heyer-Schulte subcutane-
      ous tissue e.
    Heyer-Schulte tissue e.

expander *(continued)*
    Integra tissue e.
    e. pocket
    Radovan subcutaneous tissue e.
    Radovan tissue e.
    saline-filled e.
    Silastic HP tissue e.
    slow palatal e.
    soft tissue e.
    subperiosteal tissue e. (STE)
    Surgitek T-Span tissue e.
    tissue e.
    T-Span tissue e.
    Versafil tissue e.

expansible
    e. infrastructure endosteal implant
    e. osseous neoplasm

expansion
    balloon e.
    delayed e.
    intraoperative skin e.
    maxillary e.
    mercuroscopic e.
    palatal e.
    rapid maxillary e.
    scalp e.
    scalp tissue e.
    serial e.
    skin e.
    slow maxillary e.
    surgical-assisted rapid palatal e. (SA-RPE)
    tissue e.

explantation
    mammary prosthesis e.

exposure
    Nissenbaum surgical e.

expression
    facial e.
    nonvolitional facial e.

Exprin DQI biopsy instrument

exstrophy
    e./epispadias complex
    e. reconstruction

extended
    e. anatomical chin
    e. clasp
    e. frontal approach
    e. lateral arm free flap (ELAFF)
    e. lateral arm free flap for head/neck reconstruction
    e. liposuction
    e. mesh technique
    e. multiplanar multivector face-lift
    e. open-tip rhinoplasty
    e. posterior rhytidectomy
    e. shoulder flap
    e. sub-SMAS face-lift
    e. supraplatysmal plane (ESP)
    e. supraplatysmal plane (ESP) dissection
    e. supraplatysmal plane (ESP) face-lift technique

extender
    autograft e.

extensibility
    inherent e. of skin

extension
    resisted radial wrist e.
    scalp e.
    wrist e.

extensor
    e. brevis flap
    e. carpi radialis brevis muscle
    e. carpi radialis longus (ECRL) muscle
    e. carpi radialis longus (ECRL) tendon
    e. carpi ulnaris (ECU) muscle
    e. carpi ulnaris (ECU) tendon
    e. digiti minimi muscle
    e. digiti minimi tendon
    e. digitorum brevis (EDB)
    e. digitorum communis tendon
    e. digitorum longus flap

extensor *(continued)*
    e. digitorum longus muscle
    e. digitorum muscle
    e. hallucis longus muscle
    e. indicis muscle
    e. indicis proprius (EIP)
        tendon
    e. pollicis brevis muscle
    e. pollicis longus (EPL)
        muscle
    e. pollicis longus (EPL) ten-
        don

external
    e. artery of nose
    e. auditory canal (EAC)
    e. bevel incision
    e. carotid artery
    e. ear
    e. ethmoidectomy
    e. jugular vein
    e. ligament of mandibular
        articulation
    e. ligament of temporoman-
        dibular articulation
    e. ligament of temporoman-
        dibular joint
    e. mammary artery
    e. maxillary artery
    e. nasal nerve
    e. nose
    e. oblique aponeurosis
    e. oblique line
    e. oblique ridge
    e. paralateronasal skin inci-
        sion
    e. pharyngotomy approach
    e. pudendal artery

extraconal fat

extraction
    endoscope-assisted suc-
        tion e.
    foreign body e.
    suction e.

extrafollicular

extralaryngeal
    e. approach
    e. muscle
    e. skeleton

extramammary Paget disease

extraperitoneal fat

extravelar muscle bundle

exudate
    cotton-wool e.

exudative calcifying fasciitis

eye
    appendages of the e.
    bagginess of e's
    e. pad
    raccoon e's
    sphincter of e.

eyebrow
    e. height
    high e.
    e. lift
    e. ptosis
    ptotic e.

eyebrowpexy

eye-ear plane

eyelid
    e. crease suture
    double e. operation
    e. excursion
    gray line of upper e.
    inelastic lower e.
    e. invagination
    e. laxity
    e. margin
    e. operation
    e. ptosis
    e. redundancy
    e. sphincter
    e. sulcus placement
    e. tightening

eye shield
    Barraquer e. s.
    Buller e. s.
    Fox aluminum e. s.
    protective e. s.
    Stevanovsky metal e. s.

E-Z Flap cranial flap fixation

Fabry disease
face
    acromegalic f.
    adenoid f.
    bird-f.
    bovine f.
    cleft f.
    contralateral f.
    cow f.
    dish f.
    dished-in f.
    frog f.
    f. lifting
    masklike f.
    sunken-in f.
face-bow
    adjustable axis f.-b.
    Asher high-pull f.-b.
face-lift (*written also* face lift,
  facelift)
    composite f.-l.
    conventional SMAS (super-
      ficial musculoaponeurotic
      system) f.-l.
    deep-plane f.-l.
    endoscopic f.-l.
    extended multiplanar multi-
      vector f.-l.
    extended sub-SMAS f.-l.
    extended supraplatysmal
      plane (ESP) f.-l.
    FAME f.-l.
    f.-l. hematoma
    midface suspension f.-l.
      surgery
    mini–f.-l.
    open f.-l.
    f.-l. scissors
    secondary skin-only f.-l.
    sloughed f.-l.
    SMAS (superficial muscu-
      loaponeurotic system)
      deep-plane f.-l.
    SMAS (superficial muscu-
      loaponeurotic system) im-
      brication f.-l.

face-lift (*continued*)
    SMAS (superficial muscu-
      loaponeurotic system)
      platysma f.-l.
    SMAS (superficial muscu-
      loaponeurotic system)
      platysma deep-tissue f.-l.
    SMAS (superficial muscu-
      loaponeurotic system)
      plication f.-l.
    SMILE (subperiosteal mini-
      mally invasive laser endo-
      scopic) f.-l.
    subcutaneous temporofa-
      cial f.-l.
    subcutaneous temporoma-
      lar f.-l.
    subperiosteal f.-l.
    subperiosteal minimally in-
      vasive f.-l.
    subplatysmal f.-l.
    vertical f.-l.

facial
    f. aging
    f. alloplastic implant
    f. analysis
    f. angle
    f. animation
    f. artery
    f. artery musculomucosal
      (FAMM) flap
    f. asymmetry
    bilateral f. paralysis
    f. bone
    f. canal
    f. causalgia
    f. cleft
    f. compression skull cap
      closure
    f. contour deformity
    f. contouring
    f. danger zones
    F. Disability Index (FDI)
    f. disharmony
    f. dysmorphism
    f. dysmorphology

facial *(continued)*
    f. edema
    f. erythema
    f. esthetics
    f. fascial layer
    f. fracture
    F. Grading System (FGS)
    F. Grading System voluntary movement (FGSM)
    f. growth
    f. hamartoma
    f. harmony
    f. height
    f. hemihypertrophy
    f. hemiplegia
    f. implant
    f. landmark
    f. lipodystrophy
    f. mimetic musculature
    f. moulage
    f. muscle
    f. neuralgia
    f. neuromuscular dysfunction
    f. node
    f. paralysis
    f. paralysis reconstruction with free muscle transfer
    f. paralysis reconstruction with gracilis free muscle transfer
    f. paralysis reconstruction with pectoralis minor muscle transfer
    f. paralysis reconstruction with rectus abdominis muscle transfer
    f. plane
    f. plane angle
    f. profile
    f. prosthesis
    f. reanimation
    f. recess
    f. reconstruction
    f. rejuvenation
    f. restructuring
    f. retaining ligaments
    f. sling

facial *(continued)*
    f. subcutaneous lift
    f. symmetry
    f. triangle

facial nerve
    f. n. branches
    f. n. crossover
    f. n. decompression
    f. n. dissection
    f. n. latency
    f. n. palsy
    f. n. paralysis
    f. n. preservation
    f. n. resection
    f. n. sacrifice
    f. n. weakness

facies *pl.* facies
    adenoid f.
    Andy Gump f.
    f. anterior corporis maxillae
    f. anterior palpebrarum
    f. anterior partis petrosae
    f. antonina
    f. articularis arytenoidea cricoideae
    f. articularis cartilaginis arytenoideae
    f. articularis ossis temporalis
    f. articularis thyroidea cricoideae
    f. bovina
    cherubic f.
    f. contactus dentis
    f. cranii
    f. distalis dentis
    elfin f.
    f. externa
    f. externa ossis frontalis
    f. externa ossis parietalis
    f. facialis dentis
    hound-dog f.
    Hutchinson f.
    f. inferior linguae
    f. inferior partis petrosae
    f. infratemporalis maxillae

facies *(continued)*
- f. interna
- f. interna ossis frontalis
- f. interna ossis parietalis
- f. labialis
- f. lateralis ossis zygomatici
- leonine f.
- f. lingualis dentis
- masklike f.
- f. maxillaris alae majoris
- f. maxillaris ossis palatini
- f. medialis cartilaginis arytenoideae
- f. mesialis dentis
- myasthenic f.
- myopathic f.
- f. nasalis maxillae
- f. nasalis ossis palatini
- f. occlusalis dentis
- f. orbitalis
- f. orbitalis alae majoris
- f. palatina
- f. posterior cartilaginis arytenoideae
- f. posterior palpebrarum
- f. posterior partis petrosae
- Potter f.
- f. scaphoidea
- f. temporalis
- f. vestibularis dentis

faciocervical

faciocraniosynostosis

faciolingual

faciomandibular dysostosis

facioplasty

facioplegia

facioscapulohumeral

faciostenosis

FACT-HN
- functional assessment of cancer therapy—head and neck

factor
- angiogenesis f.

factor *(continued)*
- antinuclear f. (ANF)
- autologous growth f. (AGF)
- basic fibroblastic growth f. (bFGF)
- blood coagulation f.
- chemotactic f.
- chemotactic f. for macrophage (CFM)
- clotting f.
- coagulation f.
- colony-stimulating f. (CSF)
- endothelial relaxing f.
- epidermal growth f. (EGF)
- epithelium-derived relaxation f. (EpDRF)
- fibroblast growth f. (FGF)
- granulocyte colony-stimulating f. (G-CSF)
- growth hormone–releasing f. (GHRF)
- human fibroblast growth f.-1 (FGF-1)
- insulin-like growth f.
- macrophage-activating f. (MAF)
- macrophage-inhibiting f. (MIF)
- melanocyte-stimulating hormone–inhibiting f.
- migration-inhibiting f. (MIF)
- mitogenic f. (MF)
- nerve f.
- nerve growth f. (NGF)
- neurogenic f.
- osteoclast-activating f.
- platelet f.
- platelet-activating f. (PAF)
- platelet-aggregating f. (PAF)
- platelet-derived growth f. (PDGF)
- platelet tissue f.
- recombinant human insulin-like growth f. (rhIGF)
- rheumatoid f. (RF)
- squamous cell carcinoma–inhibitory f. (SSCIF)
- sun protection f. (SPF)

factor *(continued)*
    thyrotoxic complement-fixation f.
    transforming growth f. (TGF)
    transforming growth f. beta (TGF-β)
    tumor angiogenic f. (TAF)
    tumor lysis f.
    tumor necrosis f.
    vascular endothelial growth f. (VEGF)

failure
    flap f.
    mixed f.
    f. to thrive

falciform

falling palate

fallopian
    f. aqueduct
    f. canal
    f. hiatus
    f. neuritis

Fallopio
    foramen of F.

false
    f. cyst
    f. Dupuytren contracture
    f. suture

falx
    f. cerebri
    f. of maxillary antrum

FAME
    FAME face-lift
    FAME midface elevation
    FAME midface lift

familial
    f. atypical multiple mole melanoma syndrome (FAMMM)
    f. chondrodystrophy
    f. fibrous dysplasia
    f. neurilemmatosis
    f. osteochondrodystrophy
    f. white folded dysplasia

family
    multicultural f.

FAMM
    facial artery musculomucosal
        FAMM flap

FAMMM
    familial atypical multiple mole melanoma syndrome

FANA
    fluorescent antinuclear antibody test

fan flap

fan-shaped flap

farcy
    button f.

Farnham nasal-cutting forceps

Farrior
    F. flap exposure instruments
    F. graft augmentation
    F. otoplasty knife
    F. septal cartilage stripper knife
    F.-Joseph nasal saw

Fasanella
    F. lacrimal cannula
    F.-Servat blepharoptosis operation
    F.-Servat operation for lid ptosis

fascia *pl.* fasciae
    alar f.
    anterior rectus f.
    aponeurotic f.
    aryepiglottic f.
    axillary f.
    brachial f.
    buccinator f.
    buccopharyngeal f.
    Buck f.
    Camper f.

fascia *(continued)*
    f. of Camper
    capsulopalpebral f.
    cervical f.
    Colles f.
    coracocostal f.
    dartos f.
    deep f.
    deep cervical f.
    deep temporal f. (DTF)
    dermis f.
    diseased f.
    dorsal thoracic f.
    Dupuytren f.
    endoabdominal f.
    external oblique f.
    f. flap
    f. of Gallaudet
    gluteal f.
    f. graft
    innominate f.
    intermediate f.
    internal abdominal f.
    internal oblique f.
    interposing f.
    lacrimal f.
    f. lata
    f. lata graft
    masseteric f.
    mastoid f.
    orbital fasciae
    palmar f.
    palpebral f.
    parotid f.
    pharyngeal f.
    pharyngobasilar f.
    preparotid f.
    pretracheal f.
    rectus f.
    Scarpa f.
    SMAS (superficial musculoaponeurotic system) f.
    sternocleidomastoid f.
    subcutaneous f.
    subgaleal f.
    subserous f.
    superficial f.
    superficial abdominal f.
    superficial facial f.

fascia *(continued)*
    superficial perineal f.
    superficial temporal f.
    suprasternal f.
    temporalis f.
    temporalis superficialis f.
    temporoparietal f.
    tensor fasciae latae
    thyrolaryngeal f.
    transversalis f.
    visceral f.
    volar interosseous f.

fascial
    f. anchoring
    f. anchoring technique
    f. cleft
    f. defect
    f.-fatty layer
    f. grafting
    f. layer
    f. perforator
    f. plane
    f. plication
    f. sheath
    f. sling
    f. sling for facial paralysis
    f. space
    superficial f. system (SFS)
    f. turnover flap

fasciaplasty

fascicle
    inferior alveolar nerve f.
    muscle f.
    nerve f.

fascicular
    f. graft

fasciculation

fasciculus *pl.* fasciculi

fasciectomy
    Skoog f.

fasciitis
    exudative calcifying f.
    infiltrative f.
    necrotizing f. (NF)
    nodular f.

fasciitis *(continued)*
    palmar f.
    proliferative f.
    pseudosarcomatous f.

fasciocutaneous
    arc of rotation of f. flap
    bilobed f. flap
    Cormack-Lamberty f. flap
      (*types A–C*)
    distally based f. flap
    f. flap
    f. free flap
    f. island flap
    Nahai-Mathes f. flap (*types
      A–C*)
    f. perforator
    retrograde perfused f. flap
    f. vessel

fascio-osteocutaneous flap

fascioplasty

fasciotomy

fasciovascular pedicle

fast-twitch fibers

FAT
    function, appearance, time
      FAT compromise

fat
    f. atrophy
    atrophy of f.
    f. augmentation
    autologous f. transplanta-
      tion
    brown f.
    buccal f.
    f. cell
    f. cell graft
    central f.
    cervicofacial f.
    f. depot
    f. emulsification
    extraconal f.
    extraperitoneal f.

fat *(continued)*
    f. flap
    f. graft
    harvested f.
    f. hypertrophy
    f. injection
    intraconal f.
    jowl f.
    laminar f.
    f. necrosis
    orbital f.
    parapharyngeal f.
    periorbital f.
    preaponeurotic f.
    preplatysmal f.
    reserve f. of Illouz
    retroorbicularis ocular f.
      (ROOF)
    subcutaneous f.
    subcuticular f.
    suborbicularis oculi f.
      (SOOF)
    subplatysmal f.
    superficial f.
    transplanted f. cells
    volumetric f. reduction
    white f.

fat pad
    Bichat f. p.
    buccal f. p.
    herniated f. p.
    malar f. p.
    masticatory f. p.
    ptotic malar f. p.
    scaphoid f. p.
    submental f. p.

fatty
    f. atrophy
    f. ball of Bichat
    f. degeneration
    f. deposits
    f. hypertrophy
    f. tumor

fauces
    anterior pillar of f.
    pillar of f.

faucial
  f. arch
  f. paralysis
  f. reflex

faun tail nevus

Favre-Racouchot cyst

FDDB
  freeze-dried demineralized
    bone

FDFG
  free dermal-fat graft

FDI
  Facial Disability Index

FDP
  flexor digitorum profundus
    FDP muscle
    FDP tendon

FDS
  flexor digitorum superfici-
    alis
    FDS muscle
    FDS tendon

feather
  f.-edged proximal finishing
    line
  f. the peel
  f. the transition

feathered
  f. edge
  f.-edge proximal finishing
    line
  f. extended malar implant

FeatherTouch SilkLaser

feature
  coarse facial f.
  extravascular granuloma-
    tous f's
  nondistinctive f.

feeding vessels

feet
  crow's f.

feet *(continued)*
  crural f.

Feldman excision

Feldstein blepharoplasty clip

felon
  aseptic f.

FEM
  finite element method

female hypospadias

femoral
  f. artery–saphenous bulb
    region
  f. cutaneous nerve
  lateral circumflex f. artery

fence
  ligamentous facial f.

fenestration
  apical f.
  endonasal f.
  intercellular f.
  labyrinthine f.
  tracheal f.

Ferguson-Smith
  F.-S. epithelioma
  F.-S. keratoacanthoma

Fergusson
  F. excision of maxilla
  F. incision
  F. knife

Fermit-N occlusal hole blockage
  material

Ferrein
  F. canal
  F. foramen
  F. ligament

fester

festoon
  McCall f.

festooning
  periocular f.

FET
  finger extension test

fetal
  f. alcohol syndrome
  f. cranial diameters
  f. cranioclasis
  f. face syndrome
  f. head constraint
  f. hydantoin syndrome
  f. valproate syndrome

fetalization

fetor
  f. ex ore
  f. oris

fever
  aseptic f.
  drug f.
  Malta f.
  Mediterranean f.
  rheumatic f.
  septic f.
  traumatic f.
  uveoparotid f.
  wound f.

FGF
  fibroblast growth factor

FGS
  Facial Grading System

FGSM
  Facial Grading System voluntary movement

fiber
  afferent nerve f.
  alveolar f's
  alveolar crest f's
  argyrophilic collagen f.
  f. bundle
  circular f's of ciliary muscle
  collagen f's
  collagenous f's
  dentinogenic f.
  dentogingival f.
  dentoperiosteal f.

fiber (continued)
  elastic f's
  fast-twitch f's
  Gerdy f's
  intermediate f.
  interradicular f.
  lattice f.
  medullated nerve f.
  Micro Link endoscope f.
  motor f's
  myelinated nerve f.
  myelinated sensory nerve f.
  nerve f.
  oblique f.
  orbiculociliary f's
  osteocollagenous f's
  osteogenetic f's
  reticular collagen f's
  Sappey f's
  Sharpey f's
  skeletal muscle f's
  slow-twitch f's
  sympathetic nerve f's
  unmyelinated nerve f.
  white f's
  yellow f's

FiberLase flexible beam delivery system for CO_2 surgical lasers

fiberoptic
  f. endoscope
  f. esophagoscope
  flexible f.
  f. laryngoscope
  f. lighted mirror

fiberoptics

Fibracol collagen-alginate dressing

Fibrel
  F. collagen
  F. gelatin matrix implant

fibril
  anchoring f.
  argyrophilic f.
  collagen f's
  interodontoblastic collagen f.

fibrin
    f. foam
    f. gel
    f. glue
    f. glue adhesive
    f. glue polymer
    f. matrix gel
    f. sealant

fibrinogen

fibrinogenesis

fibrinoid necrosis

fibrinous inflammation

fibroadenoma
    giant f. of the breast
    intracanalicular f.
    pericanalicular f.

fibroadenosis

fibroadipose tissue

fibroblast
    f. growth factor (FGF)
    scar f.
    wound f.

fibroblastic
    f. sarcoma
    f. tissue

fibroblastoma
    perineural f.

fibrocartilage
    semilunar f.
    triangular f. complex
    white f.

fibrochondroma

fibrocystic
    f. breast disorder
    f. change
    f. disease
    f. disorder
    f. nodules

fibrodysplasia ossificans progressiva

fibroepithelial papilloma

fibroepithelioma
    f. basal cell carcinoma
    premalignant f.

fibrofatty
    f. subcutaneous tissue
    f. tissue
    f. tumor

fibrofolliculoma

fibrogenic sarcoma

fibroglandular tissue

fibrogranuloma
    sublingual f.

fibrokeratoma

fibrolipoma

fibroma
    ameloblastic f.
    aponeurotic f.
    f. cavernosum
    cementifying f.
    central f.
    central ossifying f.
    f. cutis
    cystic f.
    desmoplastic f.
    giant cell f.
    intracanalicular f.
    juvenile ossifying f.
    malignant f.
    f. molle
    nasopharyngeal f.
    f. of nerve
    ossifying f.
    osteogenic f.
    f. pendulum
    peripheral ossifying f.
    f. sarcomatosum
    senile f.
    telangiectatic f.
    traumatic f.
    f. xanthoma

fibromatosis
    aggressive infantile f.
    central f.
    congenital f.

fibromatosis *(continued)*
    digital f.
    idiopathic f.
    palmar f.

fibromuscular dysplasia

fibromyxomatous
    f. connective tissue
    f. lesion

fibromyxosarcoma

fibronectin

fibro-osteoma

fibro-osseous
    f. ankylosis
    f. dysplasia
    f. flexor tendon canal
    f. lesion
    f. tunnel

fibro-ossification

fibropapilloma

fibroplasia
    papular f.

fibrosarcoma
    ameloblastic f.
    infantile f.
    odontogenic f.

fibrose

fibrosis
    nodular subepidermal f.
    subepidermal nodular f.
    submucous f.

fibrositis

fibrosus
    nevus f.

fibrotic

fibrous
    f. capsular contracture
    f. dysplasia of jaws
    f. nodule
    f. nonunion
    f. polly beak

fibrous *(continued)*
    f. thyroiditis
    f. xanthoma

fibrovascular
    f. aponeurosis
    f. hypertrophy

fibroxanthoma
    atypical f.

fibula
    f. donor site
    f. flap
    f. free flap
    f. osteoseptocutaneous flap

fibular
    f. head
    f. onlay strut graft
    f. osteocutaneous free flap
    f. tunnel syndrome

fiddler neck

field
    f. block
    f. block anesthesia
    bloodless f.
    narrow f.
    sterile f.
    wide f.

figure
    mitotic f.

figure-of-eight sutures

filament
    neural f.

fila olfactoria

filarial elephantiasis

Filatov
    F. flap
    F. spot
    F.-Gillies flap
    F.-Gillies tubed pedicle

file
    bone f.
    master apical f. (MAF)
    McXIM f.

filet *(variant of* fillet)

filiform
　　f. papilla
　　f. wart

filiformis
　　verruca f.

filler
　　Bio-Oss maxillofacial
　　　　bone f.
　　bovine-derived bone f.
　　f. graft
　　omental f.

fillet (spelled also filet)
　　f. flap
　　f. flap procedure
　　f. of foot free flap

film
　　measurement f.
　　scout f.

filopodium pl. filopodia

filter
　　labial f.

filtered flashlamp

filtrum
　　Merkel f. ventriculi
　　f. ventriculi

fimbriated fold

finding
　　copper-beaten f.

fine-bore catheter

fine-mesh dressing

fine-needle
　　f.-n. aspiration (FNA)
　　f.-n. aspiration biopsy
　　　　(FNAB)
　　f.-n. aspiration cytology
　　　　(FNAC)
　　f.-n. biopsy

fine-tipped mosquito hemostat

finger
　　avulsion of f.

finger (continued)
　　baseball f.
　　bolster f.
　　clubbed f.
　　dead f.
　　denuded f.
　　drop f.
　　drumstick f.
　　f. extension test (FET)
　　giant f.
　　hammer f.
　　hippocratic f's
　　index f.
　　index f. pollicization
　　index f. polydactyly
　　insane f.
　　lock f.
　　long f.
　　lumbrical-plus f.
　　mallet f.
　　f. pulp
　　rotational deformity of f.
　　sausage f.
　　snapping f.
　　spade f's
　　spider f.
　　stuck f.
　　trigger f.
　　waxy f.
　　webbed f's

fingertip
　　f. amputation
　　f. injury

finite element method (FEM)

Finkelstein sign

Finochietto-Bunnell test

first web flap

Fischer
　　F. aspirative lipoplasty
　　F. curet technique
　　F. nasal rasp

Fisher
　　F. exact test

fissura pl. fissurae
　　f. antitragohelicina

fissure
    abdominal f.
    antitragohelicine f.
    auricular f.
    auricular f. of temporal
       bone
    Ecker f.
    ethmoidal f.
    glaserian f.
    inferior orbital f.
    infraorbital f.
    interpalpebral f.
    longitudinal cerebral f.
    mandibular f.
    maxillary f.
    medial canthal f.
    orbital f.
    palatine bone f.
    palpebral f.
    petrosquamous f.
    petrotympanic f.
    pharyngomaxillary f.
    pterygoid f.
    pterygomaxillary f.
    pterygopalatine f.
    Santorini f's
    sphenoidal f.
    sphenomaxillary f.
    sphenopalatine f.
    sphenopetrosal f.
    squamotympanic f.
    superior orbital f.
    superior temporal f.
    tympanomastoid f.
    zygomatic f.
    zygomaticosphenoid f.

fissured
    f. fracture
    f. tongue

fissuring

fistula *pl.* fistulae
    abdominal f.
    alveolar f.
    arteriovenous f.
    f. auris congenita
    blind f.

fistula *(continued)*
    Blom-Singer tracheoeso-
       phageal f.
    branchial f.
    carotid–cavernous sinus f.
       (CCSF)
    cerebrospinal fluid f.
    cervical f.
    coccygeal f.
    complete f.
    craniosinus f.
    enterocutaneous f.
    esophagocutaneous f.
    ethmoidal-lacrimal f.
    high-flow arteriovenous f.
    incomplete f.
    internal lacrimal f.
    intralabyrinthine f.
    labyrinthine f.
    lacrimal f.
    lacteal f.
    lymphatic f.
    mammary f.
    orocutaneous f.
    orofacial f.
    oronasal f.
    palatal f.
    palatoalveolar f.
    pharyngeal f.
    pharyngocutaneous f.
    preauricular f.
    salivary f.
    submental f.
    f. takedown
    thyroglossal f.
    tracheocutaneous f.
    urethrocutaneous f.

fistulation
    postalveolar cleft palate f.
       (CPF)

fistulotomy

fistulous

Fitzpatrick classification of sun-
    reactive skin types (*types I–
    VI*)

fixation
    arch bar f.

fixation *(continued)*
  biodegradable plate f.
  biphase external pin f.
  circumalveolar f.
  circummandibular f.
  circumzygomatic f.
  closed reduction and internal f.
  composite wiring f.
  condylar process fracture axial anchor screw f.
  cranial flap f.
  craniofacial f.
  cricoarytenoid f.
  crossed K-wire f.
  dorsal plate and lag screw f.
  external pin f.
  E-Z Flap cranial flap f.
  Ilizarov internal f.
  interfragmentary wiring f.
  intermaxillary f. (IMF)
  internal f.
  interosseous wiring f.
  intramedullary device f.
  intraosseous f.
  Kirschner pin f.
  LactoSorb resorbable craniomaxillofacial f.
  lag screw f.
  McIndoe and Reese alar cartilage suture f.
  mandibulomaxillary f.
  maxillomandibular f. (MMF)
  medullary f.
  microplate f.
  miniplate f.
  nasomandibular f.
  nonresorbable f.
  open reduction and internal f. (ORIF)
  osseous f.
  plate and screw f.
  reduction and internal f.
  resorbable f.
  resorbable rigid f.
  rigid internal f. (RIF)
  rigid lag screw f.
  rigid plate f.

fixation *(continued)*
  Roger-Anderson pin f.
  f. screw
  semirigid f.
  skeletal f.
  skeletal pin f.
  tantalum f.
  tension-free scalp f.
  titanium rigid f.
  transcalvarial suture f.
  wire f.

fixator
  Hoffman external f.

fixed mandibular implant (FMI)

fixture
  implant f.

flaccid
  f. dysarthria
  f. skin

flaccidity
  abdominal f.

flag flap

flame
  capillary f's
  manometric f.

flammeus
  f. nevus
  nevus f.

flange
  Callahan f.
  labial f.
  lingual f.
  mandibular lingual f.

flank
  male f.

flap
  Abbe f.
  Abbe-Estlander f.
  abdominal axial subcutaneous f.
  abdominal axial subcutaneous pedicle f.
  abdominal wall f.
  abductor hallucis f.

flap *(continued)*

    access f. in osseous sur-
      gery
    adenoadipose f.
    adipofascial f.
    adipofascial axial pattern
      cross-finger f.
    adipofascial sural f.
    adipofascial turnover f.
    advancement f.
    allogenically vascularized
      prefabricated f.
    angiosomal f.
    Anita-Busch chondrocuta-
      neous f.
    antegrade island f.
    anterior chest wall f.
    anterior helical rim free f.
    anterior skin f.
    anterolateral thigh f.
    anterolateral thigh free f.
    apron f.
    Argamaso-Lewis compos-
      ite f.
    arterial f.
    arterialized f.
    Atasoy-Kleinert volar V-Y
      advancement f.
    autologous tissue f's
    axial f.
    axial advancement f.
    axial-based f.
    axial dorsal f.
    axial frontonasal f.
    axial pattern vascularized
      skin f.
    axial temporoparietal fas-
      cial f.
    Bakamjian f.
    Bakamjian pedicle f.
    Bakamjian tubed f.
    Banner f.
    Becker f.
    bell f.
    Berlin tulip f.
    Bernard f.
    biceps brachii f.
    bicoronal scalp f.

flap *(continued)*

    bilateral inferior epigastric
      artery f. (BIEF)
    bilateral pectoralis major
      muscle f.
    bilateral rotational f.
    bilobed f.
    bilobed fasciocutaneous f.
    bilobed skin f.
    bilobed transposition f.
    bipedicle f.
    bipedicled f.
    bipedicled delay f.
    bipedicle delay f.
    bipedicle digital visor f.
    bipedicle mucoperiosteal f.
    bipedicle TRAM f.
    bone f.
    boomerang-shaped rectus
      abdominis musculo-
      cutaneous free f.
    brachioradialis f.
    bridge f.
    broad-based type B Cor-
      mack-Lamberty pedicled
      fasciocutaneous f.
    buccal envelope f.
    buccal mucosal f.
    buccal musculomucosal f.
    buccinator myomucosal f.
    Bunnell f.
    Bunnell bipedicle f.
    Bunnell bipedicle digital vi-
      sor f.
    buried de-epithelialized lo-
      cal f.
    buried dermal f.
    Burow f.
    C-f.
    calvarium f.
    canthomeatal f.
    caterpillar f.
    cellulocutaneous f.
    cervical f.
    cervical humeral f.
    cervical rotational f.
    cervical visor f.
    cervicofacial f.

flap *(continued)*
  cervicopectoral f.
  cheek f.
  cheek advancement f.
  cheek-lip f.
  cheek mucous-muscle f.
  cheek rotation f.
  chest f.
  Chinese f.
  chondrocutaneous f.
  circular subcutaneous island f.
  circumflex scapular f.
  cleft margin f.
  columellar f.
  composite f.
  composite chondrocutaneous f.
  composite osteomyocutaneous preformed f.
  compound f.
  compound skin f.
  conchal f.
  conical f.
  conjoint extensor digitorum brevis muscle and dorsalis pedis osteocutaneous island f.
  converging triangular f.
  Converse f.
  Converse scalping f.
  Cormack-Lamberty fasciocutaneous f. *(types A–C)*
  coronoid f.
  coverage f.
  craniotomy f.
  cross-finger f.
  cross-leg f.
  cross-leg skin f.
  cross-lid f.
  cutaneoperiosteal f.
  cutaneous f.
  Cutler-Beard f.
  Cutler-Beard bridge f.
  Dardour f.
  Dardour lateral f.
  dartos fasciocutaneous f.
  dartos musculocutaneous f.

flap *(continued)*
  decorticated f.
  deepithelialized local f.
  deepithelialized revascularized lateral intercostal f.
  delayed f.
  delayed distally based total sartorius f.
  deltoid f.
  deltopectoral f.
  deltoscapular f.
  dermal fat free f.
  dermal fat pedicle f.
  dermal pyramidal f.
  dermoadipose f.
  dermofat f.
  digastric muscle f.
  distal-based f.
  distal-based island f.
  distally based fasciocutaneous f. (DBFF)
  distal pedicle f.
  distant f.
  dorsal cross-finger f.
  dorsalis pedis f.
  dorsal thoracic fascia free f.
  double cross-lip f.
  double-paddle f.
  double-paddle island f.
  double pedicle f.
  double-pedicle transverse rectus abdominis musculocutaneous f.
  double pendulum f.
  double skin paddle fibular f.
  double V-Y f.
  Dufourmental f.
  f. elevation
  Elliot f.
  elliptical f.
  emergency free f.
  envelope f.
  epaulet f.
  epigastric f.
  epithelial turn-in f.

flap *(continued)*
    Estlander f.
    expanded free scalp f.
    extended lateral arm free f.
      (ELAFF)
    extended lateral arm free f.
      for head/neck reconstruc-
      tion
    extended shoulder f.
    extensor brevis f.
    extensor digitorum lon-
      gus f.
    facial artery musculomu-
      cosal (FAMM) f.
    f. failure
    FAMM f.
    fan f.
    fan-shaped f.
    fascia f.
    fascial turnover f.
    fasciocutaneous f.
    fasciocutaneous free f.
    fasciocutaneous island f.
    fascio-osteocutaneous f.
    fat f.
    fibula f.
    fibula free f.
    fibula osteoseptocuta-
      neous f.
    fibular osteocutaneous f.
    fibular osteocutaneous
      free f.
    Filatov f.
    Filatov-Gillies f.
    fillet f.
    fillet of foot free f.
    first web f.
    flag f.
    fleur-de-lis f.
    fleur-de-lis forehead f.
    flexor carpi ulnaris f.
    forehead f.
    forked f.
    free f.
    free anterolateral thigh f.
    free arterialized venous
      forearm f.
    free bone f.

flap *(continued)*
    free f. for burn scar revi-
      sion
    free composite f.
    free cutaneous lateral
      arm f.
    free expanded f.
    free fascial f.
    free fasciocutaneous f.
    free fillet extremity f. for re-
      construction
    free forearm f.
    free groin f.
    free iliac bone crest f.
    free microvascular f.
    free posterior interos-
      seous f.
    free sensate f.
    free sequential f.
    free temporal fascial f.
    free temporoparietal fas-
      cial f.
    free toe-to-finger hemi-
      pulp f.
    free toe-to-fingertip neuro-
      vascular f.
    free TRAM f.
    free transverse rectus ab-
      dominis musculocuta-
      neous f.
    free vascularized f.
    French f.
    French sliding f.
    Fricke f.
    frontal bone f.
    frontogaleal f.
    full-thickness f.
    full-thickness f. loss
    fusiform f.
    fusiform island f.
    galea frontalis f.
    galea occipital f.
    galea periosteal f.
    gastrocnemius f.
    gate f.
    gauntlet f.
    geometric nasal f.
    Gillies f.

flap *(continued)*
  Gillies fan f.
  Gillies up-and-down f.
  glabellar bilobed f.
  glabellar rotation f.
  gluteal f.
  gluteal thigh f.
  gluteus maximus f.
  gluteus maximus/musculo-
    cutaneous f.
  gluteus maximus/myocuta-
    neous f.
  gracilis f.
  gracilis muscle f.
  gracilis musculocuta-
    neous f.
  great toe wraparound f.
  groin f.
  hand f.
  hemitongue f.
  hinged f.
  horizontal bipedicle der-
    mal f.
  horseshoe-shaped skin f.
  Hueston spiral f.
  Hughes f.
  ideal f.
  iliac crest free f.
  iliac crest osseous f.
  iliac crest osteocuta-
    neous f.
  iliac crest osteomuscular f.
  iliac osteocutaneous f.
  immediate f.
  inchworm f.
  Indian f.
  Indian forehead f.
  inferior gluteal f.
  innervated free f.
  innervated platysma f.
  insensate f.
  instep island f.
  interdigitated muscle f.
  interdigitating zigzag skin f.
  internal oblique osteomus-
    cular f.
  interpolated f.
  interpolation f.

flap *(continued)*
  intraoral f.
  island f.
  Island adipofascial f. in
    Achilles tendon resurfac-
    ing
  island fasciocutaneous f.
  Istanbul f. for phallic recon-
    struction
  Italian f.
  jejunal free f.
  jejunum free f.
  jump f.
  jumping man f.
  Juri f.
  Karapandzic f.
  Kazanjian f.
  Kazanjian midline fore-
    head f.
  kite f.
  Koerner f.
  Kutler lateral V-Y advance-
    ment f.
  laparoscopically harvest-
    ed f.
  lateral arm f.
  lateral cutaneous thigh f.
  lateral distally based fas-
    ciocutaneous f.
  lateral intercostal f.
  lateral supramalleolar f.
  lateral thigh f.
  lateral thigh free f.
  lateral transverse thigh f.
    (LTTF)
  lateral trapezius f.
  lateral upper arm f.
  latissimus dorsi f.
  latissimus dorsi muscle f.
  latissimus dorsi musculo-
    cutaneous f.
  latissimus dorsi myocuta-
    neous f. (LDMCF)
  latissimus dorsi/scapular
    bone f.
  latissimus fasciocutaneous
    turnover f.
  latissimus muscle f.

flap *(continued)*

Leibinger E-Z f.
lifeboat f.
Limberg local transposition f.
Limberg-type cutaneous f.
lingual f.
lingual mucoperiosteal f.
lingual tongue f.
Linton f.
lip-lip f.
lip switch f.
Littler f.
Littler neurovascular island f.
local f.
local rotation f.
lower trapezius f.
lumbar periosteal turnover f.
lumbosacral back f.
McCraw gracilis myocutaneous f.
f. maceration
McGregor forehead f.
Malaga f.
Maltese cross–patterned f.
masseter muscle f.
medial cutaneous thigh f.
medial distally based fasciocutaneous f.
medial forearm f.
medial plantar sensory f.
medial upper arm f.
median forehead f.
melolabial f.
mental V-Y island advancement island f.
mesiolabial bilobed transposition f.
microvascular free posterior interosseous f.
midface avulsion f.
midline forehead f.
Millard f.
Moberg volar advancement f.
modified Singapore f.
Monks-Esser island f.

flap *(continued)*

Morrison toe f.
mucochondrocutaneous f.
mucoperichondrial f.
mucoperiosteal periodontal f.
mucoperiosteal sliding f.
mucosal periodontal f.
mucosal prelaminated f.
muscle f.
muscle-periosteal f.
musculocutaneous f.
musculofascial f.
Mustardé lateral cheek rotation f.
Mustardé rotation-advancement f.
"mutton chop" f.
myocutaneous f.
myodermal f.
myofascial f.
myomucosal f.
Nahai-Mathes fasciocutaneous f. *(types A–C)*
Nahai tensor fasciae latae f.
nape of neck f.
nasolabial f.
nasolabial rotation f.
Nassif parascapular f.
Nataf lateral f.
neck f.
neurocutaneous f.
neurosensorial free medial plantar f.
neurosensory f.
neurovascular free f.
neurovascular infrahyoid island f. for tongue reconstruction
neurovascular island f.
oblique f. in mucogingival surgery
Ochsenbein-Luebke f.
omental f.
omental transposition f.
omocervical f.
open f.
opening f.
Orticochea f.

flap *(continued)*
  osseous f.
  osteocutaneous fillet f.
  osteocutaneous scapular f.
  osteomyocutaneous f.
  over-and-out cheek f.
  Pac-Man f. for closure of
    pressure sores
  palatal island f.
  palatal mucoperiosteal f.
  palmar f.
  palmar advancement f.
  palmaris longus compos-
    ite f.
  paramedian forehead f.
  parascapular f.
  parieto-occipital f.
  parrot beak f.
  partial-thickness f.
  pectoralis major f.
  pectoralis major myocuta-
    neous f.
  pectoralis minor f.
  pectoralis myocutaneous f.
  pectoralis myofascial f.
  pedicle f.
  pedicled galeal frontalis f.
  pedicled latissimus f.
  pedicled mucosa f.
  pedicled myocutaneous f.
  pedicled pericranial f.
  pedicled tibial bone f.
  penile f.
  perforator-based f.
  perichondrial f.
  pericranial f.
  perineal artery axial f.
  periosteal f.
  peroneus brevis f.
  peroneus longus f.
  pharyngeal f.
  platysma f.
  platysma myocutaneous f.
  posterior auricular f.
  posterior skin f.
  quadrapod f.
  quadrilobed f.
  radial forearm f.

flap *(continued)*
  radial forearm osteocuta-
    neous f.
  raised skin f.
  RAM (rectus abdominis
    musculocutaneous) f.
  RAM (rectus abdominis
    myocutaneous) f.
  random f.
  random fasciocutaneous f.
  random pattern f.
  random-pattern, palmar-
    based f.
  random temporoparietal
    fascial f.
  rectus abdominis f.
  rectus abdominis free f.
    (RAFF)
  rectus abdominis musculo-
    cutaneous (RAM) f.
  rectus abdominis myocuta-
    neous (RAM) f.
  rectus femoris f.
  rectus femoris fasciocuta-
    neous f.
  rectus femoris musculocu-
    taneous f.
  rectus turnover f.
  reflected skin f.
  regional f.
  retroauricular free f.
  retrograde-flow f.
  retrograde perfused fascio-
    cutaneous f.
  reversed digital artery f.
  reversed dorsal digital f.
  reversed extensor digito-
    rum muscle island f.
  reversed fasciosubcuta-
    neous f.
  reverse digital artery f.
  reverse digital artery is-
    land f.
  reversed island f's for fore-
    foot reconstruction
  reverse dorsal digital is-
    land f.
  reversed pedicle f.
  reverse flow island f.

flap *(continued)*
    reverse Karapandzic f.
    reverse medial arm f.
    reverse muscle f.
    reverse U-f.
    reverse ulnar hypothenar f.
      finger reconstruction
    rhomboid f.
    rhomboid transposition f.
    rope f.
    rotation f.
    rotation-advancement f.
    Rubens f.
    Rubens free f. for breast re-
      construction
    S-f.
    sandwich f.
    sandwich epicranial f.
    sartorius f.
    scalping f.
    scalping f. of Converse
    scalp sickle f.
    scapula free f.
    scapular f.
    scapular island f.
    scapular osteocutaneous f.
    Scarpa adipofascial f.
    scored alar mucocartilagi-
      nous f.
    second toe wraparound f.
    semilunar f.
    sensate f.
    sensate cutaneous f.
    sensate medial plantar
      free f.
    septal intranasal lining f.
    sequential free f's
    serratus anterior f.
    serratus anterior muscle f.
    shaped glandular f.
    shaped random pattern f.
    shoulder f.
    shutter f.
    sickle f.
    simultaneous free f's
    single-pedicle f.
    skate f.
    skin f.
    sliding f.

flap *(continued)*
    SMAS-platysma f.
    soleus f.
    spiral f.
    split-thickness f.
    steeple f.
    Stein-Abbe lip f.
    Stein-Kazanjian lower lip f.
    Stenstrom foot f.
    sternocleidomastoid f.
    sternocleidomastoid mus-
      culocutaneous f.
    sternocleidomastoid my-
      ocutaneous f.
    subcapsular f.
    subcutaneous laterodigital
      reverse f.
    subcutaneous pedicled f.
    subcutaneous turnover f.
    subgaleal f.
    submental artery f.
    submental island f.
    submentonian dermo-fatty f.
    subscapular f.
    subscapular system free f.
    superficial brachial f.
    superior gluteal f.
    superiorly based Dardour
      lateral f.
    superiorly based Nataf
      lateral f.
    supraperiosteal f.
    sural artery f.
    sural island f. for foot and
      ankle reconstruction
    switch f.
    Tagliacozzi f.
    Tait f.
    tarsoconjunctival f.
    temporal fascial f.
    temporalis f.
    temporal island pedicle
      scalp f.
    temporalis muscle f.
    temporal muscle and fas-
      cia f.
    temporoparietal fascia f.
      (TPFF)

flap *(continued)*
    temporoparietal fascial f. (TPFF)
    temporoparieto-occipital f.
    temporoparieto-occipital rotation f.
    tensor fasciae latae f.
    thenar f.
    thigh f.
    thoracoacromial f.
    thoracodorsal fascia f.
    three-paddle tensor fasciae latae free f.
    tibialis anterior (anticus) f.
    toe fillet f.
    toe pulp neurosensory f.
    toe-to-thumb f.
    TRAM f.
    transposition f.
    transverse abdominal island f.
    transverse myocutaneous f.
    transverse rectus abdominis musculocutaneous (TRAM) f.
    transverse rectus abdominis myocutaneous (TRAM) f.
    transversus and rectus abdominis musculoperitoneal (TRAMP) composite f.
    trapezius muscle/myocutaneous f.
    triangular island f.
    tunneled supraclavicular island f. for head and neck reconstruction
    "turnover" f.
    U-f
    unpedicled f.
    unrepositioned f.
    U-shaped interdigitated muscle f.
    V f.
    Vasconez tensor fasciae latae f.
    vascularity f.
    vascularized calvarial f.

flap *(continued)*
    vascularized island bone f.
    vascularized tibial bone f.
    vastus lateralis f.
    venous f.
    vermilion Abbe f.
    vertical bipedicle f.
    visor f.
    volar tissue f.
    vomer f.
    von Brun f.
    von Langenbeck bipedicle mucoperiosteal f.
    von Langenbeck palatal f.
    von Langenbeck pedicle f.
    V-Y f.
    V-Y advancement f.
    V-Y island f.
    V-Y mucosal f.
    V-Y transposition f.
    waltzed f.
    Washio f.
    web space f.
    Webster f.
    Weir pattern skin f.
    Wookey f.
    Wookey neck f.
    wraparound f.
    Y f.
    Zimany f.
    Zitelli bilobed nasal f.
    Zovickian f.

flare
    red f.
    wheal and f.

flared-W excision

flaring
    alar f.
    f. apex
    labial f.
    overzealous f.
    reverse f.

flashlamp
    f.-excited long-pulse alexandrite laser
    f.-excited pulsed dye laser
    filtered f.

flashlamp *(continued)*
- f. pulsed dye (FLPD) laser
- f.-pumped pulsed dye laser (FPPDL) 510 nm
- f.-pumped pulsed dye laser (FPPDL) 585 nm
- tunable f.-excited pulsed dye laser

flat
- f. condyloma
- f. wart

flat-bladed nasal speculum

flatness
- malar f.

flaw
- perioral f.

Fleischmann
- F. bursa
- F. hygroma

fleur-de-lis
- f.-de-l. abdominoplasty
- f.-de-l. breast reconstruction pattern
- f.-de-l. flap
- f.-de-l. forehead flap
- f.-de-l. shape
- f.-de-l.–shaped skin paddle

flexible
- f. fiberoptic
- f. laminar bone strip

Flexicon material

flexion
- f. contracture
- f. crease
- f.-extension reflex
- palmar f.
- plantar f.
- f. reflex
- f. skin lines
- wrist f.

flexor
- f. carpi radialis tendon
- f. carpi ulnaris flap
- f. carpi ulnaris muscle
- f. carpi ulnaris tendon

flexor *(continued)*
- f. digitorum brevis muscle
- f. digitorum longus muscle
- f. digitorum profundus (FDP) muscle
- f. digitorum profundus (FDP) tendon
- f. digitorum superficialis (FDS) muscle
- f. digitorum superficialis (FDS) tendon
- f. hallucis longus muscle
- f. pollicis longus (FPL) muscle
- f. pollicis longus substitution maneuver
- f. pollicis longus (FPL) tendon
- f. retinaculum
- ruptured f. tendon
- f. sheath
- f. tendon adhesion
- f. tendon grafting
- f. tendon laceration
- f. tendon repair
- f. tendon sheath

flexorplasty
- Steindler f.

flexure
- basicranial f.

Flexzan
- F. dressing
- F. foam wound dressing
- F. topical wound dressing

floating
- f. cartilage
- f. distal phalanx
- f. premaxilla
- f. thumb

floor
- f. of mouth (FOM)
- nasal f.
- f. of orbit

flora
- mouth f.

florid
- f. cutaneous papillomatosis

florid *(continued)*
    f. osseous dysplasia
flow
    antegrade blood f.
    mucociliary f.
    venous f.
Flower bone
Flowers
    F. implant
    F. mandibular glove
FLPD
    flashlamp pulsed dye
        FLPD laser
flu
    yuppie f.
fluid
    cerebrospinal f. (CSF)
    intercellular f.
    sanguineous f.
    serous f.
    temporomandibular joint
        synovial f.
fluorescein
    f. endoscopy
    f. instillation test
fluorescent antinuclear antibody test (FANA)
flutter
    alar f.
FMA
    Frankfort mandibular angle
FMI
    fixed mandibular implant
FMIA
    Frankfort mandibular incisor angle
FN
    facial nerve
FNA
    fine-needle aspiration
FNAB
    fine-needle aspiration biopsy

FNAC
    fine-needle aspiration cytology
foam
    CarraSmart f.
    fibrin f.
focal
    f. dermal hypoplasia
    f. epithelial hyperplasia
    f. inflammation
    f. keratosis
    f. osseous dysplasia
    f. tenderness
focalizing signs
Foerster
    F. capsulotomy knife
    F. surgical support brassiere
Fogarty catheter
foil
    mat f.
fold
    alar f's
    anterior mallear f.
    antihelical f.
    aryepiglottic f.
    aryepiglottic f. of Collier
    asymmetric f's of eyes
    axillary f.
    breast f's
    conjunctival f.
    Dennie infraorbital f.
    Dennie-Morgan infraorbital f.
    epicanthal f.
    eponychial f.
    fimbriated f.
    glossoepiglottic f.
    glossopalatine f.
    gluteal f.
    Hasner f.
    helical f.
    incudal f.
    inframammary f. (IMF)
    intercartilaginous f.
    interossicular f.

fold *(continued)*
    labiomental f.
    laryngeal f.
    lateral glossoepiglottic f.
    lateral mallear f.
    lateral nasal f.
    lateral umbilical f.
    malar f.
    mammary f.
    medial incudal f.
    medial umbilical f.
    median glossoepiglottic f.
    median thyrohyoid f.
    middle umbilical f.
    Morgan f.
    mucobuccal f.
    mucolabial f.
    mucosobuccal f.
    nail f.
    nasojugal f.
    nasolabial f. (NLF)
    obturatoria stapedis f.
    opercular f.
    palatine f.
    palatopharyngeal f.
    palpebronasal f.
    pharyngoepiglottic f.
    pretarsal f.
    pterygomandibular f.
    redundant upper lid skin f's
    retrotarsal f.
    rugal f's
    salpingopalatine f.
    salpingopharyngeal f.
    semilunar f.
    semilunar conjunctival f.
    sublingual f.
    tarsal f.
    thyrohyoid f.
    triangular f.
    villous f.
    white dural f.

Foley
    F. catheter
    F. operation

foliate
    f. papilla

folium *pl.* folia
    lingual f.

follicle
    hair f.
    lingual f.
    lingual lymph f.
    lymphatic f.
    lymphatic f. of tongue

follicular
    f. abscess
    f. carcinoma
    f. cyst
    f. epithelium
    f. formation
    f. infundibular cyst
    f. isthmus cyst
    f. keratosis
    f. odontogenic cyst
    f. thyroid carcinoma

follicularis
    alopecia f.
    keratosis f.

folliculitis
    f. cheloidalis
    f. decalvans
    keloidal f.
    f. nares perforans

Foltz valve

FOM
    floor of mouth

Fomon
    F. dorsal scissors
    double-pronged F. hook
    F. face-lift scissors
    F. graft augmentation
    F. lower lateral scissors
    F. nasal hook
    F. nasal rasp
    F. nasal retractor
    F. nostril elevator
    F. nostril retractor
    F. operation
    F. saber-back scissors
    F. upper lateral scissors

Fones method

fontanel (*variant of* fontanelle)

fontanelle (*spelled also* fontanel)
  anterior f.
  anterolateral f.
  bregmatic f.
  Casser f.
  casserian f.
  cranial f's
  frontal f.
  Gerdy f.
  mastoid f.
  posterior occipital f.
  posterolateral f.
  posterotemporal f.
  quadrangular f.
  sagittal f.
  sphenoidal f.
  triangular f.

foot
  cleft f.
  diabetic f.
  f. fillet flap
  ischemic f.
  Morand f.
  neuropathic f.
  plantar f. defect
  spatula f.
  trench f.

foramen *pl.* foramina
  alveolar foramina
  anastomotic f.
  anterior condyloid foramina
  anterior ethmoidal f.
  anterior palatine f.
  f. apicis dentis
  f. of Arnold
  blind f. of frontal bone
  carotid f.
  cecal f. of frontal bone
  cecal f. of tongue
  f. cecum ossis frontalis
  conjugate f.
  cribroethmoid f.
  emissary sphenoidal f.
  ethmoidal f.
  f. of Fallopio
  Ferrein f.

foramen *(continued)*
  frontal f.
  glandular f. of tongue
  greater palatine f.
  Hyrtl f.
  incisive f.
  inferior orbital f.
  infraorbital f.
  internal zygomatic f. of Meckel
  jugular f.
  lacerated f.
  f. lacerum
  lesser palatine foramina
  lingual f.
  f. magnum
  malar f.
  f. mandibulae
  mandibular f.
  mastoid f.
  maxillary f.
  mental f.
  Morgagni f.
  multiple foramina
  nasal f.
  nasopalatine f.
  olfactory f.
  foramina for olfactory nerves
  optic f.
  f. ovale
  palatine f.
  parietal f.
  posterior condyloid f.
  posterior ethmoidal f.
  postglenoid f.
  f. rotundum
  round f.
  Scarpa f.
  sphenopalatine f.
  sphenotic f.
  f. spinosum
  Stensen f.
  stylomastoid f.
  superior maxillary f.
  supraorbital f.
  teardrop f.
  thyroid f.
  venous f.
  Vesalius f.

foramen *(continued)*
   zygomatic f.
   zygomaticofacial f.
   zygomatico-orbital f.
   zygomaticotemporal f.

Forbes esophageal speculum

force
   anterior f.
   bite f.
   distal f. (DF)
   masticatory f.
   maximum bite f.
   nerve f.

forceps
   Adson f.
   Adson-Brown f.
   Adson rongeur f.
   alligator f.
   Allison f.
   Allis tissue f.
   approximation f.
   arterial f.
   articulating paper f.
   Asch f.
   Asch nasal-straightening f.
   Asch septal f.
   atraumatic tissue f.
   atraumatic visceral f.
   axis traction f.
   Bacon rongeur f.
   ball f.
   Bauer f.
   Baumgartner f.
   Baum-Hecht tarsorrhaphy f.
   Bennett epilation f.
   Berens ptosis f.
   Berke cilia f.
   Berkeley Bioengineering ptosis f.
   Berke ptosis f.
   Berne nasal f.
   biopsy punch f.
   biopsy specimen f.
   bipolar f.
   bipolar transsphenoidal f.
   biting f.
   Blake dressing f.
   Blakesley f.

forceps *(continued)*
   Blakesley ethmoid f.
   Blakesley septal bone f.
   Blakesley septal compression f.
   Blakesley-Weil upturned ethmoid f.
   Blakesley-Wilde nasal f.
   blepharochalasis f.
   Boies cutting f.
   bone f.
   Brophy dressing f.
   Brown-Adson f.
   Brown-Adson side-grasping f.
   Bruening nasal-cutting septal f.
   bulldog f.
   Callahan fixation f.
   Callahan scleral fixation f.
   Castroviejo f.
   center-action f.
   chalazion f.
   cleft palate f.
   Cottle-Arruga cartilage f.
   Cottle-Jansen rongeur f.
   Cottle-Kazanjian f.
   Cottle-Kazanjian bone-cutting f.
   Cottle-Kazanjian nasal f.
   Cottle-Kazanjian nasal-cutting f.
   Cottle-Walsham septum-straightening f.
   Defourmental rongeur f.
   Dingman f.
   double-spoon biopsy f.
   endoscopic f.
   ethmoid punch f.
   Farnham nasal-cutting f.
   foreign body f.
   Fox cartilage f.
   Freer septal f.
   Fry nasal f.
   galea f.
   Gillies dissecting f.
   Gillies tissue f.
   Goldman-Kazanjian nasal f.
   Grazer blepharoplasty f.
   Hajek-Koffler sphenoidal f.

forceps *(continued)*
 Hajek sphenoid punch f.
 Halsted curved mosquito f.
 Halsted hemostatic mos-
   quito f.
 harelip f.
 Hartmann-Gruenwald nasal-
   cutting f.
 Hartmann nasal-cutting f.
 Hartmann nasal-dressing f.
 Hartmann-Noyes nasal-
   dressing f.
 hemostatic f.
 Hinderer cartilage f.
 Hudson rongeur f.
 Hunt f.
 Hurd septal bone-cutting f.
 Hurd septum-cutting f.
 Jackson approximation f.
 Jackson broad staple f.
 Jackson button f.
 Jackson conventional for-
   eign body f.
 Jackson cross-action f.
 Jackson cylindrical object f.
 Jackson double-prong f.
 Jackson dull rotation f.
 Jackson flexible upper lobe
   bronchus f.
 Jackson globular object f.
 Jackson papilloma f.
 Jackson ring jaw globular
   object f.
 Jackson sharp-pointed ro-
   tation f.
 Jansen-Middleton punch f.
 Kahler f.
 Kazanjian f.
 Kelly f.
 Kerrison f.
 Kinder Design pedo f.
 Kleinert-Kutz bone-cut-
   ting f.
 LaLonde extra fine skin
   hook f.
 LaLonde skin hook f.
 LaRoe undermining f.
 Löwenberg f.
 lower anterior f.
 McGivney f.

forceps *(continued)*
 mandibular f.
 Matthew f.
 maxillary f.
 Mead f.
 mosquito f.
 O'Brien fixation f.
 O'Brien tissue f.
 oral rongeur f.
 Radial Jaw biopsy f.
 Rowe disimpacting f.
 Schanzioni craniotomy f.
 Semken dressing f.
 Semken-Taylor f.
 Semken tissue f.
 septal ridge f.
 serrated f.
 serrefine f.
 Snellen f.
 S&T Lalonde hook f.
 Storz nasopharyngeal biop-
   sy f.
 subglottic f.
 suction f.
 Takahashi ethmoidal f.
 Takahashi nasal f.
 Tessier disimpaction de-
   vice f.
 tissue f.
 upper universal f.
 upturned f.
 upward bent f.
 Walsham f.
 Watson duckbill f.
 West nasal-dressing f.
 Wilde ethmoid f.
 Wilde septal f.
 Wolfe eye f.
 Yankauer ethmoid-cutting f.

Fordyce
 angiokeratoma of F.
 F. disease
 F. granules
 F. spots

forehead
 f. animation
 f. asymmetry
 broad f.
 convex f.

forehead *(continued)*
  f. convexity
  f. elevation and fixation
    with percutaneous mi-
    croscrews
  f. flap
  f. lifting
  Olympian f.
  f. positioner
  f. reconstruction
  f. wrinkling

forehead-brow complex

forehead lift
  bicoronal f. l.
  biplanar f. l.
  endoscopic f. l.
  endoscopic subperiosteal
    f. l.
  modified anterior hairline
    f. l.
  transblepharoplasty f. l.

forehead-nose position

foreheadplasty
  male f.
  open f.

foreign
  f. body
  f. body aspiration
  f. body extraction
  f. body forceps
  f. body giant cell
  f. body granuloma
  f. body reaction
  f. body removal
  f. body rhinitis

forked
  f. flap
  f. tongue
  f. uvula

form
  arch f.
  disseminated f. Albright
    syndrome
  occlusal f.
  retention f.
  spherical f. of occlusion

formation
  callus f.
  crater f.
  cutaneous capillary f.
  cystic f.
  dentinoid f.
  fistula f.
  follicular f.
  hematoma f.
  heterotopic bone f.
  keloid f.
  scar f.
  seroma f.

Formatray mandibular splint

forme fruste

formula
  Callaway f.
  rule of nines f. for percent-
    age of body surface
    burned

fornix *pl.* fornices
  f. conjunctivae
  f. conjunctivae inferior
  f. conjunctivae superior
  f. pharyngis
  f. sacci lacrimalis

Forschheimer spots

fossa *pl.* fossae
  adipose fossae
  antecubital f.
  anterior cranial f.
  f. of anthelix
  articular f. of mandible
  articular f. of temporal
    bone
  axillary f.
  Bichat f.
  canine f.
  central f.
  conchal f.
  condyloid f.
  digastric f.
  distal f. (DF)
  distal triangular f. (DTF)
  elliptical scaphoid f.
  floccular f.

fossa *(continued)*
    fusiform f.
    Gerdy hyoid f.
    glandular f. of frontal bone
    glenoid f.
    glenoid f. of temporal bone
    incisive f.
    incisive f. of maxilla
    infratemporal f.
    innominate f.
    innominate f. of auricle
    jugular f.
    lacrimal f.
    f. of lacrimal gland
    f. of lacrimal sac
    lateral bulbar f.
    lingual f. (LF)
    Malgaigne f.
    mandibular f.
    mastoid f.
    maxillary f.
    Merkel f.
    mesiolingual f. (MLF)
    middle cranial f.
    nasal f.
    f. navicularis auriculae
    oral f.
    piriform f.
    posterior cranial f.
    pterygoid f.
    pterygomaxillary f.
    pterygopalatine f.
    radius f.
    retromandibular f.
    retromolar f.
    Rosenmüller f.
    saccular f.
    scaphoid f.
    sphenomaxillary f.
    subarcuate f.
    sublingual f.
    submandibular f.
    submaxillary f.
    supraclavicular f.
    supramastoid f.
    supratonsillar f.
    temporal f.
    temporal-pterygomaxil-
      lary f.

fossa *(continued)*
    temporomandibular joint f.
    triangular f.
    f. triangularis auriculae
    zygomatic f.

fossula *pl.* fossulae

four-flap
    f.-f. cleft palate repair
    f.-f. palatoplasty
    f.-f. Webster-Bernard tech-
      nique
    f.-f. Z-plasty

four-pronged liposuction can-
    nula

four-tailed bandage

fovea *pl.* foveae
    f. of condyloid process
    f. ethmoidalis
    f. nuchae
    oblong f. of arytenoid carti-
      lage
    pterygoid f.
    sublingual f.
    submandibular f.

foveate

foveated

Fox
    F. aluminum eye shield
    F. blepharoplasty
    F. cartilage forceps
    F. dermal curet
    F. scissors

FPL
    flexor pollicis longus
      FPL muscle
      FPL tendon

FPPDL
    flashlamp-pumped pulsed
      dye laser
      FPPDL 510 nm
      FPPDL 585 nm

fracture
    alveolar process f.
    anterior f.

fracture *(continued)*
    anterior cranial fossa f.
    atrophic f.
    avulsion f.
    Barton f.
    basal skull f.
    Bennett f.
    bilateral condylar f.
    blow-in f.
    blow-out f.
    blow-out f. of orbital floor
    boxer's f.
    buckling f. of the phalanx
    capitate f.
    carpal f.
    chauffeur's f.
    circumferential f.
    closed diaphyseal f.
    closed skull f.
    Colles f.
    comminuted f.
    compound f.
    condylar process f.
    cortical f.
    craniofacial disjunction f.
    f. with cross union
    f. with delayed union
    dentoalveolar f.
    depressed f.
    f. dislocation
    displaced f.
    displaced malar f.
    displaced zygomatic f.
    donor radius f.
    epiphyseal f.
    extraarticular f.
    facial f.
    fat f.
    fissured f.
    frontal sinus f.
    frontoorbitonasoeth-
      moidal f.
    glabellar f.
    greenstick f.
    greenstick Le Fort f.
    Guérin f.
    gutter f.
    hangman's f.
    hickory-stick f.

fracture *(continued)*
    f. of hook of the hamate
    horizontal maxillary f.
    horizontal oblique f.
    Hutchinson f.
    hyoid bone f.
    impacted f.
    impure blow-out f.
    infraorbital f.
    intracapsular f.
    intraorbital f.
    laryngeal cartilage f.
    Le Fort I f.
    Le Fort II f.
    Le Fort III f.
    lower frontal bone f.
    malar f.
    malar complex f.
    f. with malunion
    mandibular body f.
    mandibular condyle f.
    mandibular ramus f.
    mandibular symphysis f.
    marginal ridge f.
    maxillary f.
    maxillofacial f.
    medial orbital wall f.
    mesiodistal f.
    metacarpal head f.
    metacarpal neck f.
    metacarpal shaft f.
    midface f.
    midfacial f.
    nasal f.
    nasal-septal f.
    nasoethmoidal f.
    nasoethmoidal-orbital f.
    naso-ethmoid-orbital f.
    nasoorbitoethmoid (NOE) f.
    noncomminuted f.
    f. with nonunion
    occult scaphoid f.
    open f.
    orbital f.
    orbital blow-in f.
    orbital blow-out f.
    orbital floor f.
    orbital roof f.
    palatal alveolar f.

fracture *(continued)*
    palate f.
    pancraniomaxillofacial f.
    panfacial f.
    parasymphyseal f.
    petrous pyramid f.
    phalangeal f.
    pisiform f.
    posterior f.
    prosthetic f.
    pure blow-out f.
    pyramidal f.
    radial styloid f.
    reverse Barton f.
    reverse Bennett f.
    f. at the rhinion
    Rolando f.
    scaphoid f.
    segmental f.
    septal f.
    simple skull f.
    single f.
    Smith f.
    spiral f.
    spontaneous f.
    stellate f.
    subcondylar greenstick f.
      of the mandible
    subcondylar f. of the mandible
    f. of superior orbital fissure
    supraorbital f.
    symphyseal f.
    telescoping septal f.
    temporal bone f.
    transverse f.
    transverse facial f.
    transverse maxillary f.
    trapezial f.
    traumatic f.
    trimalar f.
    tripod f.
    triquetral f.
    undisplaced f.
    unilateral condylar f.
    unstable f.
    unstable zygomatic complex f.
    vertical f.

fracture *(continued)*
    vertical oblique pattern f.
    Volkmann f.
    Y-shaped f.
    zygoma f.
    zygomatic arch f.
    zygomatic body f.
    zygomatic complex f.
    zygomatic maxillary complex f.
    zygomaticomaxillary f.
    zygomatico-orbital f.

fracture appliance
    arch bar facial f. a.
    craniofacial f. a.
    Erich facial f. a.
    facial f. a.
    Joseph septal f. a.
    Roger Anderson facial f. a.
    Winter facial f. a.

fragment
    condylar f.

frame
    arch bars f.
    halo head f.
    implant f.
    implant superstructure f.
    Young f.

framework
    implant f.
    osteocartilaginous f.

Franceschetti
    F. syndrome
    F.-Jadassohn syndrome

Frank sign

Franke
    F. syndrome
    F. triad

Frankfort
    F. horizontal line
    F. horizontal plane
    F. mandibular angle (FMA)
    F. mandibular incisor angle (FMIA)
    F. mandibular plane

Frankfort *(continued)*
 F. mandibular plane angle

Fraser syndrome

Frazier
 F. skin hook
 F.-Adson osteoplastic flap
  clamp

Frechet extended scalp reduction

freckle
 Hutchinson f.
 melanotic f.
 melanotic f. of Hutchinson

freckled

Fredricks mammary prosthesis

free
 f. anterolateral thigh flap
 f. arterialized venous forearm flap
 f. autogenous corticocancellous iliac bone graft
 f. autogenous pearl fat graft
 f. bone flap
 f. bone reconstruction
 f. composite flap
 f. composite graft
 f. cutaneous lateral arm flap
 f. cutaneous nerve graft
 f. dermal-fat graft (FDFG)
 f. expanded flap
 f. fascial flap
 f. fasciocutaneous flap
 f. fillet extremity flap for reconstruction
 f. flap
 f. flap for burn scar revision
 f. flap procedure
 f. flap reconstruction
 f. forearm flap
 f. gracilis muscle reconstruction
 f. groin flap
 f. iliac bone crest flap
 f. mandibular movement

free *(continued)*
 f. margin of eyelid
 f. microvascular flap
 f. muscle graft
 f. omental flap transfer
 f. posterior interosseous flap
 f. sensate flap
 f. sequential flap
 f. skin graft
 f. temporal fascial flap
 f. temporoparietal fascial flap
 f. tissue transfer (FTT)
 f. tissue transfer of muscle
 f. tissue transfer reconstruction
 f. toe-to-finger hemipulp flap
 f. toe-to-fingertip neurovascular flap
 f. TRAM flap
 f. transplantation of nipple
 f. transverse rectus abdominis musculocutaneous flap
 f. vascularized flap

Freeman
 F. cookie cutter areola marker
 F. face-lift retractor
 F. punctum plug
 F. rhytidectomy scissors
 F. transorbital leukotome
 F.-Sheldon syndrome

Freer
 F. bone chisel
 F. dissector
 F. lacrimal chisel
 F. nasal chisel
 F. nasal gouge
 F. nasal knife
 F. nasal spatula
 F. nasoseptal elevator
 F. septal elevator
 F. septal forceps
 F. single-ended elevator

Freer *(continued)*
 F. skin hook
 F. skin retractor
 F. submucous retractor
 F.-Ingal nasal knife
 F.-Ingal submucous knife

freeze-dried
 f.-d. allograft
 f.-d. bone allograft
 f.-d. demineralized bone
  (FDDB)

French
 F. flap
 F. method
 F. sliding flap

French-line
 F.-l. abdominoplasty
 F.-l. method

frenectomy

frenoplasty

frenotomy

frenulum *pl.* frenula
 f. epiglottidis
 f. of inferior lip
 f. labii inferioris
 f. labii superioris
 f. linguae
 lingual f.
 f. of lower lip
 f. of superior lip
 f. of tongue
 f. of upper lip

frenum *pl.* frena, frenums
 labial f.
 lingual f.
 f. of tongue

Frenzel maneuver

frequency
 defined f.

fresh autologous deepidermalized dermis

friable
 f. mucosa

friable *(continued)*
 f. tissue
 f. vessel

Fricke flap

Friedenwald-Guyton operation

Friedreich ataxia

frog face

Frolova primary palatoplasty

Froment sign

frontal
 f. artery
 f. bone
 f. bone advancement
 f. bone advancement with
  strip craniectomy
 f. bone flap
 f. bone resorption
 f. bossing
 f. branch
 f. craniotomy
 f. fontanelle
 f. furrow
 f. irrigation
 f. lift
 f. lobe
 f. nerve
 f. ostium
 f. plagiocephaly
 f. plane
 f. process
 f. process of maxilla
 f. projection
 f. recess
 f. region
 f. resorption
 f. sinus
 f. sinus cannula
 f. sinus curet
 f. sinus fracture
 f. sinus growth
 f. sinus mucocele
 f. sinus septoplasty
 f. suture
 f. view
 f. zygomatic suture line

frontalis
  alopecia liminaris f.
  f. hyperactivity
  f. muscle
  f. muscle paralysis
  f. nerve
  f. sling procedure
  f. suspension

fronting
  palatal f.

frontocaudal

frontocranial
  f. remodeling

frontoethmoidal
  f. sphenoidectomy
  f. suture

frontogaleal flap

frontoglabellar wrinkle

frontolacrimal suture

frontolateral laryngectomy

frontomalar suture

frontomaxillary suture

frontonasal
  f. duct
  f. dysplasia
  f. process
  f. suture

fronto-occipital

fronto-orbital
  f. advancement
  f. remodeling
  f. rim

frontoparietal suture

frontotemporal
  f. craniotomy incision

frontozygomatic (FZ)
  f. suture line

Frost
  modified F. method

Frost (continued)
  modified F. suture
  F. operation
  F. stitch
  F. suture

frostbite
  deep f.
  superficial f.

Frosted Flex earmold material

frown
  corrugator f.

frown line
  glabellar f. l.
  vertical glabellar f. l's

Fry nasal forceps

FTSG
  full-thickness skin graft

FTT
  free tissue transfer

fulguration

fullness
  supratip f.

full-thickness
  f.-t. burn
  f.-t. defect
  f.-t. flap
  f.-t. flap loss
  f.-t. skin graft (FTSG)

fulminant

function
  barrier f.
  mathetic f. of language
  occlusal f.
  speech-motor f.
  velopharyngeal f.

fungating
  f. lesion
  f. mass
  f. sore
  f. tumor
  f. wound

fungoid

funicular graft

funnel chest

furca
    denuded f.

furcal

furcation
    denuded f.

Furlow
    F. closure
    F. double Z-plasty
    F. double-opposing Z-plasty
    F. double-opposing Z-plasty
      palatoplasty
    F. double-reversing Z-plasty
    F. procedure

furnace
    muffle f.

Furniss otoplasty

furrow
    digital f.
    frontal f.
    gluteal f.
    mentolabial f.

furrow *(continued)*
    nasal-labial f.
    orbital-palpebral f.
    palpebral f.
    sagittal f.
    transverse f.

furuncle

furunculosis

fusiform
    f. deformity
    f. excision
    f. flap
    f. fossa
    f. island flap
    f. plication
    f. scar
    f. skin revision
    f. swelling

fusion
    radiocarpal f.
    scaphocapitate f.
    scaphoid-capitate f.
    small joint f.
    thumb f.

FZ
    frontozygomatic

Gabarro
  G. graft
  G. operation
  G. retractor

GABEB
  generalized atrophic be-
    nign epidermolysis bul-
    losa

gag
  Crowe-Davis mouth g.
  Davis-Crowe mouth g.
  Dingman mouth g.
  Dingman-Denhardt
    mouth g.
  Dott-Kilner mouth g.
  Dott mouth g.
  Kilner mouth g.
  Kilner-Doughty mouth g.
  Millard mouth g.
  Molt mouth g.
  mouth g.

Gaillard
  G. operation
  G.-Arlt sutures

gait
  antalgic g.
  ataxic g.
  calcaneal g.
  cerebellar g.
  lurching g.
  spastic g.

galactoplania

galactorrhea

galactostasis

galea
  g. aponeurosis plication
  aponeurotic g.
  g. aponeurotica
  g. forceps
  g. frontalis
  g. frontalis advancement
  g. frontalis flap
  g.-frontalis-occipitalis re-
    lease

galea *(continued)*
  lateral g. aponeurotica
  g. occipital flap
  g. periosteal flap

galeaplasty

Galen
  G. anastomosis
  G. bandage
  G. nerve
  G. ventricle

galeoperiosteum

Gallaudet
  fascia of G.

galli
  crista g.

gamekeeper's thumb

ganglion *pl.* ganglia
  acousticofacial g.
  Acrel g.
  Andersch g.
  Arnold g.
  Blandin g.
  g. block
  Bochdalek g.
  cephalic g.
  cervical g.
  cervicothoracic g.
  ciliary g.
  Cloquet g.
  compound g.
  g. cyst
  diffuse g.
  Ehrenritter g.
  extirpation of g.
  g. extracraniale
  false g.
  Gasser g.
  gasserian g.
  geniculate g.
  g. hook
  hypoglossal g.
  inferior g. of glossopharyn-
    geal nerve
  inferior g. of vagus

ganglion *(continued)*
    jugular g. of glossopharyn-
      geal nerve
    Küttner g.
    Langley g.
    lesser g. of Meckel
    lower g. of glossopharyn-
      geal nerve
    Meckel g.
    Meissner g.
    motor roots of submandi-
      bular g.
    g. of Müller
    olfactory g.
    otic g.
    petrosal g.
    primary g.
    pterygopalatine g.
    recurrent g.
    Schacher g.
    g. scissors
    semilunar g.
    simple g.
    sphenomaxillary g.
    sphenopalatine g.
    stellate g.
    submandibular g.
    submaxillary g.
    superior g. of glossopha-
      ryngeal nerve
    sympathetic g.
    synovial g.
    thyroid g.
    trigeminal g.
    upper g.
    Valentin g.
    wrist g.
ganglionectomy
    gasserian g.
    wrist g.
ganglioneurofibroma
ganglioneuroma
ganglionic blocking agent
gangrene
    arteriosclerotic g.
    circumscribed g.
    cold g.

gangrene *(continued)*
    cutaneous g.
    decubital g.
    disseminated g.
    dry g.
    emphysematous g.
    gas g.
    hospital g.
    hot g.
    humid g.
    inflammatory g.
    mammary g.
    Meleney g.
    mephitic g.
    oral g.
    Pott g.
    pressure g.
    primary g.
    progressive g.
    progressive bacterial
      synergistic g.
    senile g.
    spontaneous g. of newborn
    static g.
    symmetric g.
    traumatic g.
    venous g.
    wet g.
gangrenous
    g. rhinitis
    g. stomatitis
Gantzer muscle
gap
    mean residual g. (MRG)
    nerve g.
    scapholunate g.
gaping
    g. wound
    g. wound edges
Garceau
    G. cheilotomy
    G. tendon technique
Garcin syndrome
gargoylism
garment
    Canfield facial plastics g.

garment *(continued)*
    compression g.
    crotchless compression g.
    elasticized compressive
        face g.
    graduated compression g's
    inelastic compression g.
    Jobst compression g.
    Marena by LySonix com-
        pression g.
    tumescent liposuction g.
        (TLG)

Garré
    G. disease
    G. osteomyelitis

Garretson bandage

gas
    argon g.
    arterial blood g.
    g. gangrene
    g. laser

Gasser ganglion

gasserian
    g. ganglion
    g. ganglion hook
    g. ganglionectomy

gastrocnemius
    g. flap
    g. muscle

gastroschisis

gate
    g. flap

gauge
    bone screw depth g.
    calibrated depth g.
    machinist's g.
    manual dermatome thick-
        ness g.

gauntlet flap

gauze
    absorbable g.
    Adaptic g.
    adhesive g.

gauze *(continued)*
    Cover-Roll adhesive g.
    impregnated g.
    Kerlix g.
    Kling g.
    nonstick g.
    g. pad
    paraffin g.
    paraffin-impregnated g.
    petrolatum g.
    Surgicel g.
    tantalum g.
    Telfa g.
    Vaseline-coated g.
    Xeroform g.

G-CSF
    granulocyte colony-stimu-
        lating factor

Gegenbaur
    ethmoidal sulcus of G.

gel
    adapalene g.
    all-trans retinoic acid
        aqueous g.
    autologous platelet g.
    autotransfusor-prepared
        platelet g.
    Benzac AC G.
    calcium alginate g.
    Cann-Ease moisturizing na-
        sal g.
    Carrington dermal
        wound g.
    Dermaflex G.
    Differin G.
    fibrin g.
    fibrin matrix g.
    g.-filled implant
    Hylaform viscoelastic g.
    hydrophilic g.
    platelet g.
    polyacrylamide g.
    g.-saline mammary implant
    silicone g.
    silicone g. implant
    SoloSite nonsterile hydro-
        gel

gelatin
  absorbable g.
  g. compression boot
  phenolized g. compound
  g.-resorcin-formalin tissue
    glue
  g. sponge

Gelfoam
  G. cookie
  G. packing
  G. pad
  G. pledget
  wire-G. prosthesis

Gell and Coombs classification

Gelocast Unna boot

GelShapes scar management
  system

gender reassignment

generalized
  g. atrophic benign epider-
    molysis bullosa (GABEB)
  g. osteoarthritis (GOA)

generator
  VNUS radiofrequency g.

genial
  g. advancement plate
  g. hypertrophy
  g. tubercle

geniculate
  g. ganglion
  medial g.

geniculum
  g. of facial canal
  g. of facial nerve

geniocheiloplasty

genioglossus muscle

geniohyoglossus

genioplasty
  advancement g.
  alloplastic augmentation g.

genioplasty (continued)
  augmentation g.
  centering g.
  jumping g.
  lengthening g.
  osseous g.
  reduction g.
  reduction-advancement g.
  sliding g.
  staged g.

genitalia
  ambiguous external g.

genitoplasty

genodermatology

genodermatosis

Gentell
  G. alginate wound dressing
  G. foam wound dressing

GentleLASE Plus

GentlePeel skin exfoliation system

genu pl. genua
  carotid g.
  g. of facial canal
  external g. of facial nerve

Georgiade breast prosthesis

geometric nasal flap

Gerdy
  G. fibers
  G. fontanelle
  G. hyoid fossa

Gerhardt sign

Geristore repair material

Gerlach tonsil

German
  G. measles
  G. method

geroderma

geromorphism
  cutaneous g.

Gerzog nasal speculum

GHRF
    growth hormone–releasing
    factor

Giampapa
    G. suture
    G. suturing technique

Giannestras step-down proce-
    dure

Gianotti-Crosti syndrome

giant
    g. congenital nevus
    g. finger
    g. pigmented nevus

giant cell
    g. c. arteritis
    g. c. fibroma
    g. c. granuloma
    g. c. lesion

Gianturco
    G. expanding metallic stent
    G.-Rösch Z-stent

gibbous deformity

gibbus deformity

Gibson
    G. bandage
    G. principle

Giedion syndrome

Gifford retractor

gigantism
    acromegalic g.
    cerebral g.
    eunuchoid g.
    hyperpituitary g.

gigantomastia

gigantosoma

Gigli
    G. saw
    G. wire saw

Gilbert stage shoulder abduc-
    tion

Gilchrist disease

Gillies
    G. approach
    G. bone hook
    G. cocked hat procedure
    G. construction of replace-
        ment thumb
    dermoepidermal G. stitch
    G. dissecting forceps
    G. ectropion graft
    G. elevation procedure
    G. fan flap
    G. flap
    G. graft
    G. hook
    G. horizontal dermal suture
    G. implant
    G. incision
    G. nasal hook
    G. needle holder
    G. operation
    G. scissors
    G. skin hook
    G. tissue forceps
    G. up-and-down flap
    G. zygomatic elevator
    G. zygomatic hook
    G.-Converse skin hook
    G.-Dingman tenaculum
        hook
    G.-Fry operation
    G.-Kilner operation
    G.-Millard technique
    G.-Sheehan needle holder

Gilmer
    G. splint
    G. wiring

gingiva
    labial g.
    lingual g.
    marginal g.

gingival embrasure

gingivectomy
    Ochsenbein g.

gingivitis
  leukemic hyperplastic g.
  marginal g.
  menstruation g.

gingivoglossitis

gingivolabial

gingivo-osseous

gingivoperiosteoplasty
  bilateral g.

gingivoplasty

gingivostomatitis
  membranous g.
  necrotizing ulcerative g.

girdle
  compression g.
  Lipo-Medi g.
  Lipopanty g.
  male compression g.

Giuffrlda-Ruggieri stigma

glabella

glabellar
  g. bilobed flap
  g. crease
  g. frown line
  g. laxity
  g. line
  g. region
  g. rotation flap
  g. wrinkle

glabrous

gland
  accessory g.
  acinar g.
  admaxillary g.
  alveolar g.
  anterior lingual g.
  apical g.
  apocrine g.
  areolar g.
  arytenoid g's
  axillary g's
  Bauhin g's

gland *(continued)*
  Baumgarten g's
  Blandin g's
  Blandin and Nuhn g's
  Bowman g's
  brachial g.
  Bruch g's
  buccal g's
  cardiac g's of esophagus
  cervical g's
  cheek g's
  Ciaccio g's
  ciliary g's
  Cobelli g's
  coil g.
  compound g.
  Ebner g's
  eccrine g.
  endocrine g's
  esophageal g's
  external salivary g.
  genal g's
  Gley g's
  glossopalatine g's
  gustatory g's
  Harder g's
  harderian g's
  Haver g's
  Henle g's
  hibernating g.
  holocrine g.
  internal salivary g.
  intraepithelial g's
  intramuscular g's of tongue
  Knoll g's
  labial g's
  labial minor salivary g.
  lacrimal g.
  lactiferous g.
  laryngeal g's
  lingual g.
  Luschka g.
  lymph g.
  major salivary g's
  malar g's
  mammary g.
  mandibular g.
  Manz g.
  maxillary g.

gland *(continued)*
    meibomian g.
    merocrine g.
    milk g.
    minor salivary g's
    molar g's
    Moll g's
    Montgomery g's
    g's of mouth
    mucoparous g.
    mucous g.
    nasal g's
    Nuhn g's
    oil g's
    palatal g.
    palatine g's
    palpebral g's
    parathyroid g.
    parotid g.
    pectoral g's
    Peyer g's
    pharyngeal g's
    pileous g.
    Poirier g's
    prehyoid g.
    racemose g.
    Rivinus g.
    salivary g.
    sebaceous g.
    sentinel g.
    Serres g's
    seromucous g.
    serous g.
    Stahr g.
    sublingual g.
    sublingual salivary g.
    submandibular g.
    submandibular salivary g.
    submaxillary g.
    submaxillary salivary g.
    superior lacrimal g.
    superior parathyroid g.
    superior thyroid g.
    suprahyoid g.
    Suzanne g.
    synovial g.
    tarsal g.
    tarsoconjunctival g's
    thyroid g.

gland *(continued)*
    tubular g.
    von Ebner g's
    Waldeyer g's
    Weber g's
    Wölfler g.
    Wolfring g's
    Zeiss g's

glandilemma

glandula *pl.* glandulae

glandular
    g. atrophy
    g. carcinoma
    g. hypertrophy
    g. hypospadias
    g. neoplasm
    g. odontogenic cyst

glandularis
    cheilitis g.

glanduloplasty *(variant of* glanuloplasty)

glanuloplasty
    meatoplasty and g.
    (MAGPI)

glaserian fissure

Glasgow Coma Scale

Gley glands

glide
    acentric g.
    mandibular g.

glioma
    ganglionic g.
    nasal g.
    peripheral g.
    g. sarcomatosum

glioneuroma

gliosarcoma

globe
    g. dystopia
    ocular g.
    proptotic g.
    g. retropulsion

globulin
    immune g.
    intramuscular immune g.
    intravenous immune g.

Glogau
    G. classification for pho-
        toaging (groups I–IV)
    G. system of skin evalua-
        tion

glomangioma

glomangiosis

glomus
    g. jugulare
    g. tumor

glossa

glossagra

glossanthrax

glossectomy
    partial g.
    subtotal g.
    total g.

glossitis
    g. areata exfoliativa
    atrophic g.
    benign migratory g.
    Clarke-Fournier g.
    g. desiccans
    Hunter g.
    idiopathic g.
    median rhomboid g.
    g. migrans
    Moeller g.
    rhomboid g.

glossocele

glossodynia
    g. exfoliativa

glossoepiglottic
    g. fold

glossohyal

glossoncus

glossopalatine

glossopexy

glossopharyngeal

glossoplasty

glossorrhaphy

glossosteresis

glossotomy
    labiomandibular g.
    median labiomandibular g.
    midline sagittal g.

glottal

glottic
    g. carcinoma
    g. closure
    g. larynx
    g. prosthesis
    g. spasm
    g. squamous cell carci-
        noma
    g. stenosis

glottis pl. glottides

glottitis

glove
    Biogel g.
    Biogel Diagnostic surgical
        g's
    Biogel M surgical g's
    Biogel Neotech surgical g's
    Biogel Reveal/Indicator sur-
        gical g's
    Biogel Super-Sensitive sur-
        gical g's
    Flowers mandibular g.
    Nouvisage Deep-Hydra-
        tion g.
    utility g.

gloving
    double g.

glucose 6-phosphate dehydro-
    genase

glue
    CoSeal fibrin g.
    CoStasis fibrin g.

glue *(continued)*
    cyanoacrylate g.
    fibrin g.
    fibrin g. adhesive
    fibrin g. polymer
    hydroxyapatite fibrin g.
    Tisseel fibrin g.
    tissue g.

gluteal
    g. bonnet
    g. cleft
    g. fascia
    g. flap
    g. thigh flap

gluteus
    g. maximus
    g. maximus flap
    g. maximus/musculo-
      cutaneous flap
    g. maximus/myocutaneous
      flap
    g. minimus

glycolic
    g. acid
    g. skin peel

glycosialorrhea

Gly Derm
    G. D. alpha hydroxy acid
    G. D. glycolic acid

GM
    gingival margin

gnathalgia

gnathic

gnathion

gnathitis

gnathodynamometer
    bimeter g.

gnathodynia

gnathography

gnathoplasty

gnathoschisis

gnathostomatics

GOA
    generalized osteoarthritis

Goddio disposable cannula

Godtfredsen syndrome

Godwin tumor

Goeminne syndrome

Goethe
    suture of G.

goiter
    multinodular g.

gold
    mat g.
    MF-Y g.

Goldenhar syndrome

Goldman
    G. cartilage punch
    G. curet
    G. nasal tip reconstruction
    G. septal elevator
    G. septal scissors
    G.-Fox knife
    G.-Fox wound débridement
      scissors
    G.-Kazanjian nasal forceps
    G.-Kazanjian rongeur

Goldner modification

Goldscheider disease

Goldstein retractor

Golgi
    G. corpuscles
    G.-Mazzoni corpuscles

Goltz syndrome

gomphosis

gonadal
    mixed g. dysgenesis
    pure g. dysgenesis

gonial angle

goniocraniometry

gonion

Gonzalez specialized dissecting cannula

Gooch retractor

Goode nasal splint

Gore
G. Resolut regenerative tissue membrane
G. subcutaneous augmentation material (S.A.M.)
G. suture passer

Gore-Tex
G.-T. alloplastic material
G.-T. augmentation material (GTAM)
G.-T. augmentation membrane (GTAM)
G.-T. closure
G.-T. DUALMESH biomaterial
G.-T. graft
G.-T. lip augmentation
G.-T. membrane
G.-T. mesh
G.-T. MYCROMESH biomaterial
G.-T. nasal implant
G.-T. periodontal material
G.-T. regenerative material
G.-T. S.A.M. facial implant
G.-T. soft-tissue patch
G.-T. strips
G.-T. suture
G.-T. tube

Gorlin
G. cyst
G. syndrome
G.-Chaudhry-Moss syndrome

Gorney
G. dissector
G. face-lift scissors
G. rhytidectomy scissors
G. septal scissors

Gorney (continued)
G. septal suction elevator
G. turbinate scissors

Goshgarian transpalatal bar

Gosset
spiral band of G.

Gothic arch

Gottlieb epithelial attachment

gouge
Freer nasal g.
X-Acto g.

Gougerot-Sjögren syndrome

Goulian
G. blade
G. knife
G. mammaplasty
G. mastopexy
G. procedure to harvest skin graft

goundou

gracilis
g. flap
g. muscle
g. muscle flap
g. musculocutaneous flap
g. myocutaneous vaginal reconstruction

graciloplasty
double dynamic g.
dynamic g.
dynamic urethral g.
electrostimulated g.
single dynamic g.
stimulated g.
unstimulated g.

grade
Baker g.
Brackmann g.
House-Brackmann g. (I–VI)
Kaplan-Feinstein comorbidity g.
Meurmann external ear anomaly g.

grading
  insufficient jaw g.
  jaw g.
  mean rejection g. (MRG)

Gradle
  G. eyelid retractor
  G. scissors

Graefe spot

graft
  acellular muscle g.
  accordion g.
  activated g.
  adipodermal g.
  alar batten g.
  AlloDerm acellular dermal g.
  AlloDerm cellular dermal g.
  AlloDerm onlay g.
  AlloDerm processed tissue g.
  AlloDerm universal dermal tissue g.
  allogeneic g.
  allogeneic keratinocyte g.
  AlloMatrix injectable putty bone g. substitute
  alloplastic g.
  alveolar bone g.
  alveolar cleft g.
  amnion g.
  anastomosed g.
  animal g.
  Apligraf (graftskin) g.
  augmentation g.
  auricular cartilage g.
  auricular composite g.
  autodermic g.
  autoepidermic g.
  autogeneic g.
  autogenous g.
  autogenous bone g.
  autogenous cartilage g.
  autogenous corticocancellous g.
  autogenous fat g.
  autogenous nerve g.
  autologous g.

graft (continued)
  autologous fat g.
  autologous iliac crest bone g.
  autologous rib bone g.
  autoplastic g.
  avascular g.
  Baker composite g.
  B-B g.
  Biobrane glove g.
  Biobrane/HF substitute skin g.
  BioGran resorbable synthetic bone g.
  BioGran synthetic g.
  BIO-OSS bone filler g.
  Blair-Brown g.
  Blair-Brown skin g.
  bolus tie-over g.
  bone g.
  bone g. substitute
  bovine heterograft
  Braun g.
  Braun skin g.
  Braun-Wangensteen g.
  brephoplastic g.
  buccal mucosa g.
  buccal mucosal g.
  buccal mucosa g. for urethra reconstruction
  B-W g.
  cable g.
  cadaveric g.
  calvarial bone g.
  cancellous bone g.
  cancellous cellular bone g.
  cantilever g.
  cantilevered bone g.
  Capset bone g. barrier
  cartilage g.
  cartilaginous g.
  cartilaginous autologous thin septal g.
  carved cartilage g.
  cavum conchal cartilage g.
  chessboard g.
  chip g.
  chondromucosal g.
  collagen g.

graft *(continued)*
    Collagraft bone g. matrix
    composite g.
    composite auricular g.
    composite biodegradable
      skin g.
    composite inlay antral and
      nasal bone g.
    compound g.
    conchal cartilage g.
    conchal cartilage–ethmoid
      bone g.
    connective tissue g.
    convex cartilage g.
    cortical bone g.
    corticocancellous g.
    corticocancellous block g.
    costal cartilage g.
    costochondral g. (CCG)
    Cotton cartilage g.
    Cotton cartilage g. to crico-
      laryngeal area
    cranial bone g.
    cross-facial nerve g.
    crossover g.
    crushed cartilage g.
    cultured epithelial auto
      graft
    cultured mucosal g.
    cutis g.
    cymba conchal cartilage g.
    Davis g.
    defatted skin g.
    delayed g.
    Dembone g.
    demineralized bone g.
    dermal g.
    dermal fat g.
    Dermamesh g. expander
    dermis-fat g.
    dermofat g.
    diced cartilage g.
    dorsal onlay g.
    double-barreled fibular
      bone g.
    double-end g.
    double papilla g.
    double papilla pedicle g.
    Douglas g.

graft *(continued)*
    Douglas mesh skin g.
    Dragstedt g.
    DualMesh biomaterial g.
    earlobe composite g.
    epidermic g.
    Esser g.
    facial skin g.
    fascia g.
    fascia-fat composite g.
    fascia lata g.
    fascicular g.
    fat g.
    fat cell g.
    fibular onlay strut g.
    filler g.
    free g.
    free autogenous cortico-
      cancellous iliac bone g.
    free autogenous pearl fat g.
    free bone g.
    free composite g.
    free cutaneous nerve g.
    free dermal-fat g. (FDFG)
    free fat g.
    free muscle g.
    free non-vascularized com-
      posite nail g.
    free skin g.
    full-thickness skin g. (FTSG)
    funicular g.
    Gabarro g.
    gauntlet g.
    Gillies g.
    Gillies ectropion g.
    good g. take
    Gore-Tex g.
    Grafton DBM bone g.
    gull-wing concha compos-
      ite g.
    hair-bearing g.
    hair replacement g.
    hard palate mucosa g.
    g. harvesting
    Hedrocel bone substitute
      material g.
    heterodermic g.
    heterogenous g.

graft *(continued)*
  heterologous g.
  heteroplastic g.
  heterospecific g.
  heterotopic g.
  heterotrophic bone g.
  homologous g.
  homoplastic g.
  hydroxyapatite block g.
  hyperplastic g.
  iliac crest bone g.
  implantation g.
  infusion g.
  inlay g.
  inlay bone g.
  in situ tricortical iliac crest
    block bone g.
  intercalary bone g.
  interspecific g.
  island g.
  isogeneic g.
  isologous g.
  isoplastic g.
  jump g.
  Kebab g.
  Kiel g.
  Kimura cartilage g.
  Konig g.
  Krause g.
  Krause-Wolfe g.
  lateral pedicle g.
  LifeCell AlloDerm acellular
    dermal g.
  linear g.
  lyophilized dura g.
  McIndoe inlay g.
  McIndoe skin g.
  Mangoldt epithelial g.
  mattressed onlay g.
  Meek island sandwich g.
  mesh g.
  meshed g.
  meshed split-thickness
    skin g.
  metatarsal free vasculari-
    zed g.
  microvascular g.
  mucoperiosteal periodon-
    tal g.

graft *(continued)*
  mucosal g.
  mucosal periodontal g.
  multi-layered g.
  muscular g.
  nerve g.
  neuromuscular pedicle g.
  nonvascularized bone g.
    (NVBG)
  nonvascularized fibular
    strut g.
  Ollier g.
  Ollier-Thiersch g.
  omental skin g.
  onlay g.
  onlay bone g.
  onlay tip g.
  oral mucosa g.
  orthotopic g.
  orthotopic bone g.
  osseous g.
  OsteoGen bone g.
  osteoperiosteal g.
  overlay cantilever bone g.
  Padgett mesh skin g.
  papilla g.
  papillary pedicle g.
  Papineau g.
  Papineau cancellous g.
  partial-thickness g.
  patch g.
  pedicle g.
  pedicled cartilage g.
  pedicled skin g.
  pelvic peritoneal g.
  perichondrocutaneous g.
  PerioGlas synthetic bone g.
  periosteal g.
  Phemister g.
  pinch g.
  polytetrafluoroethylene
    membrane g.
  porcine g.
  postage-stamp skin g.
  postauricular g.
  primary bone g.
  primary skin g.
  ProOsteon 500 bone im-
    plant g.

graft *(continued)*
   punch g.
   rectangular cartilage g.
   g. resorption
   revascularized bone g.
   reverse-flow vascularized
    bone g.
   Reverdin g.
   Reverdin epidermal free g.
   Reverdin skin g.
   rib costochondral dorsal
    onlay g.
   Robinson vein g.
   rolled g.
   rope g.
   rotational flap g.
   sagittal cartilage g.
   saphenous vein interposi-
    tion g.
   scapula crest pedicled
    bone g.
   Seddon nerve g.
   seed g.
   segmental g.
   g. sensation
   sentinel skin paddle g.
   septal cartilage g.
   septal chondromucosal g.
   sequential g.
   sheet g.
   shield-type g.
   sieve g.
   skate g.
   skin g.
   sleeve g.
   slice g.
   sliding inlay bone g.
   Solvang g.
   split calvarial g.
   split-skin g.
   split-thickness g.
   split-thickness skin g.
    (STSG)
   sponge g.
   spreader g.
   Stent g.
   straight tubular g.
   strut g.
   subdermal g.

graft *(continued)*
   subepithelial connective
    tissue g.
   sural nerve cable g.
   sutured-in-place, shield-
    shaped tip g.
   swaging g.
   syngeneic g.
   synthetic bone g.
   Tait g.
   Tanner-Vandeput g.
   tantalum mesh g.
   Teflon g.
   temporalis fascia g.
   tendon g.
   thick-split g.
   Thiersch g.
   Thiersch medium-split
    free g.
   Thiersch thin-split free g.
   thin-split g.
   tip g.
   Transcyte skin substitute g.
   transposition of g.
   T-shaped g.
   tube g.
   tunnel g
   twin-barreled fibular g.
   umbrella g.
   undemineralized bone g.
   underlayer cantilever
    bone g.
   unmeshed split-thickness
    skin g.
   valise handle g.
   Van Millingen g.
   vascularized g.
   vascularized bone g. (VBG)
   vascularized metaphyseal
    bone g.
   vascularized scapular
    bone g.
   vascularized tendon g.
   Verdan g.
   white g.
   Wolfe g.
   Wolfe-Krause g.
   XenoDerm g.
   xenogeneic g.

graft *(continued)*
　　xenograft
　　Y g.
　　zooplastic g.

Graftac
　　G. absorbable skin tack
　　G.-S skin stapler

GraftAssist vein and graft
　holder

GraftCyte
　　G. gauze wound dressing
　　G. hydrating mist
　　G. moist dressing
　　G. post-surgical shampoo

grafting
　　alveolar g.
　　areolar g.
　　autogenous g.
　　bone g.
　　cartilage g.
　　cranial bone g.
　　dermal g.
　　dermis-fat g.
　　fascial g.
　　flap g.
　　flexor tendon g.
　　hair g.
　　Mangoldt epithelial g.
　　mucosal g.
　　nipple g.
　　one-stage g.
　　onlay bone g.
　　osseous g.
　　simultaneous g.
　　skin g.
　　two-step g.

Grafton DBM bone graft

Graftpatch

Graftskin

graft-versus-host (GVH)
　　g.-v.-h. disease *(grades 1–4)*
　　g.-v.-h. reaction

Gram cannula

granular
　　g. bed

granular *(continued)*
　　g. cell layer
　　g. degeneration
　　g. layer
　　g. reticulum

granulation
　　exuberant g's
　　red g.
　　Reilly g's
　　g. tissue

granule
　　Birbeck g.
　　DynaGraft g.
　　Fordyce g's
　　lamellar g.
　　Langerhans cell g.
　　Langley g's
　　membrane-coating g.
　　mucigen g.
　　ProOsteon Implant 500 g.

granulocyte colony-stimulating
　factor (G-CSF)

granuloma
　　actinic g.
　　g. annulare
　　caseating g.
　　central giant cell g.
　　eosinophilic g.
　　epithelial g.
　　g. faciale
　　foreign body g.
　　g. gangrenescens
　　giant cell g.
　　g. gluteale infantum
　　histiocytic g.
　　Langerhans cell eosinophil-
　　　ic g.
　　laryngeal g.
　　lethal midline g.
　　lipophagic g.
　　malignant g.
　　midline lethal g.
　　midline malignant reticu-
　　　losis g.
　　necrotizing g.
　　pyogenic g.
　　sarcoidal g.

granuloma *(continued)*
    silica g.
    silicone g.
    swimming pool g.
    g. telangiectaticum
    ulcerated g.

granulomatosa
    cheilitis g.
    Miescher cheilitis g.

granulomatosis
    Langerhans cell g.
    Wegener g.

granulomatous
    g. angiitis
    g. cheilitis
    g. dermal infiltrate
    g. disease
    g. inflammatory reaction
    g. mastitis
    g. rosacea
    g. sialadenitis
    g. slack skin
    g. tenosynovitis
    g. tissue

granulosum
    stratum g.

grasp
    modified pen g.

gray line of upper eyelid

Grayson ligament

Grazer
    G. abdominoplasty
    G. blepharoplasty forceps

great
    g. auricular nerve
    g. toe implant
    g. toe transplant
    g. toe wraparound flap

greater
    g. alar cartilage
    g. palatine artery
    g. palatine canal
    g. palatine foramen
    g. palatine nerve

greater *(continued)*
    g. palatine sulcus of maxilla
    g. petrosal nerve
    g. superficial petrosal
    nerve
    g. wing of sphenoid
    g. zygomatic muscle

Green lid clamp

greenstick fracture

Greig
    G. cephalopolysyndactyly
    syndrome
    G. syndrome

Griesinger
    G. sign
    G. symptom

Groenholm lid retractor

groin flap

groove
    ala-facial g.
    alar facial g.
    alveolobuccal g.
    alveololabial g.
    alveolollingual g.
    anterior auricular g.
    anterior palatine g.
    basilar g. of occipital bone
    basilar g. of sphenoid bone
    cavernous g. of sphenoid
    bone
    costal g.
    g. of crus of the helix
    distal oblique g. (DOG)
    ethmoidal g.
    gingivobuccal g.
    gingivolabial g.
    gingivolingual g.
    greater palatine g.
    hamular g.
    inframalar g.
    infraorbital g.
    infraorbital g. of maxilla
    intermandibular g.
    labial g.
    labiomental g.
    lacrimal g.

groove *(continued)*
    lacrimal g. of maxilla
    g. of lacrimal bone
    laryngotracheal g.
    lingual g. (LG)
    lingual developmental g.
     (LDG)
    linguogingival g.
    mastoid g.
    median g. of tongue
    mesiobuccal developmen-
     tal g. (MBDG)
    mesiolingual g. (MLG)
    mesiolingual developmen-
     tal g. (MLDG)
    mylohyoid g.
    mylohyoid g. of inferior
     maxillary bone
    nail g.
    g. of nail matrix
    g. for nasal nerve
    nasofacial g.
    nasolabial g.
    nasolacrimal g.
    nasomaxillary g.
    nasopalatine g.
    nasopharyngeal g.
    olfactory g.
    palatine g.
    palatine g. of maxilla
    palatine g. of palatine bone
    palatomaxillary g.
    palatomaxillary g. of pala-
     tine bone
    palatovaginal g.
    paraglenoid g.
    pharyngeal g's
    posterior auricular g.
    preauricular g.
    pterygopalatine g.
    g. for radial nerve
    sinus g.
    skin g's
    transverse nasal g.
    Verga lacrimal g.
    vomeral g.
    vomerine g.

Grossan nasal irrigator tip

Grosse-Kempf interlocking nail

ground-glass
    g.-g. appearance
    g.-g. lesion
    g.-g. pattern

growth
    asymmetric maxillomandi-
     bular g.
    basicranial sagittal g.
    axonal g.
    cartilaginous g.
    chondromatous g.
    condylar g.
    cranial g.
    facial g.
    frontal sinus g.
    hamartomatous g.
    g. hormone–releasing fac-
     tor (GHRF)
    g. retardation

growth factor
    autologous g. f. (AGF)
    basic fibroblastic g. f.
     (bFGF)
    epidermal g. f. (EGF)
    fibroblast g. f. (FGF)
    human fibroblast g. f.-1
     (FGF-1)
    insulin-like g. f.
    nerve g. f. (NGF)
    platelet-derived g. f. (PDGF)
    recombinant human insu-
     lin-like g. f. (rhIGF)
    transforming g. f. (TGF)
    transforming g. f. beta
     (TGF-β)
    vascular endothelial g. f.
     (VEGF)

Gruber
    petrosphenooccipital su-
     ture of G.

Gruver method

gryphosis

grypposis

GTAM
    Gore-Tex augmentation material
    Gore-Tex augmentation membrane

guard
    mouth g.

gubernaculum dentis

Guérin fracture

Guibor Silastic tube

guidance
    endoscopic g.

guide
    adjustable anterior g.
    condylar g.
    Cooper nasal ganglia g.
    Cottle bone g.
    Cottle cartilage g.
    Cottle knife g.
    Cottle knife g. and retractor
    custom drill g.
    Joseph saw g.
    Kazanjian g.
    microdrilling g.
    nasal cartilage g.

guided
    g. bone regeneration
    g. tissue regeneration

Guidi
    G. canal
    canal of G.

gull-wing incision

gummatous necrosis

Gunning splint

gusher
    labyrinthine g.

gustatory
    g. lacrimation
    g. rhinorrhea

Gustilo
    G. fracture score
    G. scoring for open fractures (*types II, IIIA, IIIB, IIIC*)
    G.-Anderson classification

Guthrie skin hook

guttural duct

Guyon
    G. canal
    G. canal release
    G. canal syndrome

GVH
    graft-versus-host
        graft-versus-host disease
        graft-versus-host reaction

gynecomastia
    surgical classification of g. (*grades 1, 2A, 2B, 3*)

gynoplasty

gyrus
    angular g.

H
H-flap incision

HA
hydroxyapatite

Haagensen staging of breast carcinoma

Haber syndrome

Haelan tape

Haemogram blood loss monitor

Hagedorn
H. cheiloplasty
H. needle holder
H. suture needle
H.-Le Mesurier method of cleft lip repair

Hagerty operation

Hahnenkratt lingual bar

Haid Universal bone plate system

Haines-Zancolli test

hair
h. bulb
burrowing h.
h. collar sign
cuticle of h.
exclamation point h.
h. follicle
h. grafting
laser h. removal
laser h. transplantation
h. transplantation
h. transplant punch
vellus h.

hair-bearing
h.-b. area
h.-b. graft
h.-b. reconstruction

hairline
h. incision

hairy
h. mole

hairy (continued)
h. nevus

Hajdu-Cheney syndrome

Hajek
H. elevator
H. lip retractor
H. retractor
H. septal chisel
H. sphenoid punch forceps
H.-Ballenger septal dissector
H.-Ballenger septal elevator
H.-Koffler sphenoidal forceps
H.-Koffler sphenoidal punch
H.-Koffler sphenoidal rongeur
H.-Skillern sphenoidal punch
H.-Tieck nasal speculum

Hall
H. dermatome
H. mandibular implant system
H. mastoid bur
H. surgical drill

Halle
H. ethmoidal curet
H. nasal elevator
H. nasal speculum
H. septal elevator
H. septal needle
H. sinus curet
H.-Tieck nasal speculum

Haller
H. ansa
H. circle
H. plexus

Hallermann
H.-Streiff syndrome
H.-Streiff-François syndrome

Hallpike maneuver

halo
  h. blue nevus
  h. deformity
  h. head frame
  h.-Ilizarov distraction in-
    strumentation
  h. melanoma
  h. nevus
  h. test for cerebrospinal
    fluid (CSF) leak
  h. test for cerebrospinal
    fluid (CSF) rhinorrhea

Halsted
  H. curved mosquito for-
    ceps
  H. hemostatic mosquito
    forceps
  H. law
  H. mattress sutures
  H. mosquito hemostat
  H. radical mastectomy
  H. suture

hamartoma
  angiomatous lymphoid h.
  Becker hair h.
  facial h.
  hairy h.
  neuromuscular h.

hamartomatous lesion

hamate
  body of the h.
  h. bone
  hook of the h.
  pole of the h.

Hamilton bandage

hammer
  h. finger
  h. nose
  Quisling intranasal h.

Hammock bandage

hammock ligament

hamular
  h. notch
  h. process

hamulus
  h. of ethmoid bone
  frontal h.
  h. frontalis
  h. of hamate bone
  lacrimal h.
  h. lacrimalis
  h. ossis hamati
  pterygoid h.
  h. pterygoideus

hand
  accoucheur's h.
  ape h.
  benediction h.
  claw h.
  cleft h.
  congenital h. duplication
  crab h.
  dead h.
  drop h.
  frozen h.
  h. flap
  intrinsic minus h.
  h. ischemia
  Krukenberg h.
  lobster-claw h.
  metacarpal h.
  mirror h.
  mitten h.
  monkey h.
  Myobock artificial h.
  opera-glass h.
  phantom h.
  preacher's h.
  skeleton h.
  spade h.
  split h.
  spoon-shaped h.
  trench h.
  trident h.
  ulnar claw h.
  ulnar club h.
  windblown h.

Handages

hand cock-up
  h. c.-u. sling
  h. c.-u. splint

handicapped
   multiply h.

Handisol phototherapy device

handle
   Bard-Parker knife h.
   Cottle knife h.
   Cottle modified knife h.
   Cottle protected knife h.
   Klein Delrin Luer-Lok h.
   love h's
   h. of malleus
   measurement control h.
   rotatable transsphenoidal
      knife h.
   scaphoid spoon h.
   Universal h. with nasal-cut-
      ting tips

handpiece
   Chill Tip cooling h.
   collimated beam h. for la-
      ser surgery
   Dermacerator h.
   Dermastat dermatology h.
   Hexascan computerized
      dermatology h.
   large diameter h.
   M4 safety h.
   Micro oral surgery h.
   Micro-Pen h.
   micropigmentation h.
   Microstat h.
   Permark micropigmenta-
      tion h.
   Platinum 5000 micropig-
      mentation h.
   Revolution micropigmenta-
      tion h.
   Sapphire 2000 micropig-
      mentation h.

Hand-Schüller-Christian disease

hanging
   h. columella
   h. panniculus
   h. skin

hangman's fracture

Hanhart syndrome

Hanna classification of head
   and neck defects (classes A,
   B, C)

Hannover canal

Hapex bioactive material

Hapsburg
   H. jaw
   H. lip

hard
   h. calculus
   h. cleft palate
   h. palate
   h. subcutaneous node
   h. tissue
   h. tissue replacement
      (HTR)
   h. ulcer

Harder glands

hardness
   Mohs h.

hard-soft palate junction

Hardy
   H. lip retractor
   H. sellar punch

harelip
   acquired h.
   double h.
   h. forceps
   median h.
   h. needle
   single h.
   h. suture

harlequin
   h. deformity
   h. orbit

harmony
   facial h.
   functional occlusal h.
   occlusal h.

Hartel technique

Hartmann
H. nasal conchotome
H. nasal-cutting forceps
H. nasal-dressing forceps
H. nasal speculum
H.-Gruenwald nasal-cutting
forceps
H.-Noyes nasal-dressing for-
ceps

harvest
bone h.
double rectus h.
endoscope-assisted rectus
abdominis muscle flap h.
endoscopic h.
endoscopically-assisted h.
free gracilis muscle h.
graft h.
in situ graft h.
open method h.
tissue h.

harvested
h. fat
laparoscopically h. flap

harvesting
bone graft h. technique
in situ graft h.
open h. technique
h. skin

Haslinger retractor

Hasner
H. fold
H. valve

Haver glands

haversian
h. canals
h. lamella
h. spaces
h. system

Haws type brachydactyly

Haynes-Griffin mandibular
splint

HBIG
hepatitis B immunoglobulin

HBO
hyperbaric oxygen
HBO-induced angioge-
nesis

head
bulldog h.
condylar h.
condyle h.
h. of condyloid process of
mandible
fibular h.
hourglass h.
h. of malleus
little h. of mandible
mandibular h.
oblique h.
pointed h.
saddle h.
steeple h.
tower h.
transverse h.

headache
migraine h.
muscle contraction h.
muscle tension h.
ocular h.

healing
h. biopsy incision
delayed wound h.
h. by first intention
h. by granulation
h. by second intention
wound h.

heart and hand syndrome

Heath
H. operation
H. suture scissors
H. wire-cutting scissors

Heberden rheumatism

Heck disease

Hedrocel bone substitute material graft

Heidenhain
H. crescents

Heidenhain *(continued)*
    H. law

height
    alveolar h.
    anterior facial h. (AFH)
    buccopalatal h.
    eyebrow h.
    facial h.
    h. of mandibular ramus
    mental h.
    nasal h.
    orbital h.
    h. of palate
    philtral h.
    posterior facial h.
    vertical bony h.
    vertical facial h.

Heimlich maneuver

Heiss retractor

Hejdu-Cheney syndrome

helical
    h. crease
    h. crus
    h. fold
    h. rim
    h. surgery

helicis
    cauda h.
    crus h.
    musculus h. major
    musculus h. minor
    spina h.
    sulcus cruris h.

helium-neon (He-Ne) laser

helix *pl.* helices
    auricular h.
    h. of ear

helmet
    molding h.
    h. therapy

HEMA
    2-hydroxyethyl methacry-
    late

hemangiectasia

hemangiectasis

hemangiectatic hypertrophy

hemangioendothelioma
    kaposiform h.
    malignant h.
    spindle cell h.
    h. tuberosum multiplex

hemangiofibroma

hemangioma *pl.* hemangiomas,
  hemangiomata
    adnexal h.
    ameloblastic h.
    arteriovenous h.
    h. birthmark
    capillary h.
    cavernous h.
    central h.
    cervicofacial h.
    cherry h.
    choroidal h.
    circumscribed choroidal h.
      (CCH)
    congenital h.
    congenital subglottic h.
    craniofacial h.
    deep h.
    epithelioid h.
    esophageal h.
    facial h.
    hypertrophic h.
    intramuscular h.
    involuting flat h.
    laryngeal h.
    lumbar h.
    mixed h.
    h. planum extensum
    sclerosing h.
    scrotal h.
    senile h.
    h. simplex
    spider h.
    strawberry h.
    subcutaneous h.
    subglottic h.

hemangioma *(continued)*
   superficial h.
   synovial h.
   verrucous h.

hemangiomatosis
   Osler h.
   Parkes-Weber h.
   thrombocytopenic h.

hemangiopericytoma
   benign h.
   borderline malignant h.
   congenital h.
   malignant h.

hemangiosarcoma

hematapostema

hematocephalus

hematoma
   h. auris
   epiglottic h.
   h. evacuation
   expanding h.
   face-lift h.
   fibrosed h.
   orbital h.
   postoperative h.
   rectus sheath h.
   retrobulbar h.
   septal h.
   spectacle h.
   sublingual h.
   submental h.
   subungual h.

hemiacrosomia

hemiageusia

hemiarthroplasty

hemiatrophy
   facial h.
   facial h. of Romberg
   lingual h.
   progressive lingual h.
   Romberg h.

hemiclavicular line

hemicraniosis

hemidystrophy

hemiectromelia

hemifacial
   h. atrophy
   h. hypertrophy
   h. microsomia
   h. spasm

hemigigantism

hemiglossal

hemiglossectomy

hemignathia

hemihyperplasia

hemihypertrophy
   facial h.

hemihypoplasia

hemilaryngectomy

hemilingual

hemimacroglossia

hemimandible

hemimandibulectomy

hemimaxillectomy
   radical h.

hemimelia

hemipagus

hemiparesis

hemiplegia
   facial h.
   faciobrachial h.
   faciolingual h.

hemisection

hemiseptum of interalveolar
   bone

hemithorax

hemithyroidectomy

hemitongue flap

hemodynamics
  venous h.

hemolysis
  autoimmune h.

hemoptysis
  massive h.

hemorrhage
  arterial h.
  capillary h.
  laryngeal h.
  nasal h.
  petechial h.
  punctate h.
  retrobulbar h.
  splinter h.
  submucosal h.
  venous h.

hemorrhagic
  h. cyst
  h. pyoderma gangrenosum
  h. telangiectasia

hemosialemesis

hemostasis
  h. scalp clip

hemostat
  Allis h.
  Avitene microfibrillar collagen h.
  bulldog h.
  Carmault h.
  curved mosquito h.
  Dean tonsil h.
  fine-tipped mosquito h.
  Halsted mosquito h.
  Hemotene absorbable collagen h.
  Instat collagen absorbable h.
  Instat MCH microfibrillar collagen h.
  Kelly h.
  microfibrillar collagen h.
  mosquito h.
  straight mosquito h.

hemostatic
  h. agent
  h. clip
  h. collodion
  h. forceps
  h. material
  h. suture

Hemotene absorbable collagen hemostat

Hemovac
  H. drain
  H. suction tube

He-Ne
  helium-neon
    He-Ne laser

Henderson lag screw

Henke
  H. space
  H.-Stille conchotome

Henle
  H. glands
  H. spine

Hennebert reflex

henpuye

Hensen's duct

hepatitis
  h. B immunoglobulin (HBIG)
  serum h. (SH)
  viral h.

heptadactyly

Herbert
  H. alphanumeric classification system for scaphoid fractures (*types A1, A2, B1–4, C, D1, D2*)
  H. screw
  H.-Whipple screw

hereditary
  h. bone dysplasia

hereditary *(continued)*
 h. hemorrhagic telangiectasia

hermaphrodite

hermaphroditism
 bilateral h.
 h. with excess
 false h.
 spurious h.
 synchronous h.
 transverse h.
 unilateral h.

hernia
 abdominal wall h.
 h. defect
 diaphragmatic h.
 incisional h.
 intermuscular h.
 muscle h.
 parastomal h.
 TRAM flap h.
 umbilical h.
 ventral h.

herniated fat pad

herpes
 h. desquamans
 h. digitalis
 h. facialis
 h. genitalis
 h. labialis
 h. mentalis
 h. simplex
 h. simplex virus
 h. virus
 h. zoster
 h. zoster virus

herpetic
 h. paronychia
 h. ulcer
 h. whitlow

herpetiform

Hess
 H. eyelid operation
 H. ptosis operation

heterodermic
 h. graft

heterogeneous

heterogenesis

heterogenetic

heterogenic

heterogenote

heterogenous
 h. graft

heterograft
 bovine h.
 h. implant
 h. prosthesis

heterologous
 h. graft
 h. material
 h. tissue

hetero-osteoplasty

heteroplasia
 osseous h.

heteroplastic graft

heteroplasty

heterosexual

heterotopic
 h. bone formation
 h. ossification
 h. transplantation

heterotransplantation

heterotrophic

Hexascan
 H. computerized dermatology handpiece
 krypton laser with H.
 H. mode
 Nd:YAG laser with H.
 tunable dye laser with H.

Heyer-Schulte
 H.-S. breast implant

Heyer-Schulte *(continued)*
 H.-S. breast prosthesis
 H.-S. chin prosthesis
 H.-S. malar prosthesis
 H.-S. mammary prosthesis
 H.-S. rhinoplasty implant
 H.-S. subcutaneous tissue
  expander
 H.-S. testicular prosthesis
 H.-S. tissue expander

Heyman nasal scissors

Heyring sign

H-flap incision

HGM Spectrum K1 krypton yellow and green laser

hiatus
 h. of canal for greater petrosal nerve
 h. of canal for lesser petrosal nerve
 esophageal h.
 h. ethmoidalis
 h. of facial canal
 fallopian h.
 h. of fallopian canal
 maxillary h.
 semilunar h.

Hickman catheter

hidradenitis
 h. axillaris of Verneuil
 axillary h.
 eccrine h.
 h. suppurativa

hidradenoma
 clear cell h.
 cystic h.
 h. eruptivum
 nodular h.
 papillary h.
 solid h.

hidrocystoma

Hierst perineoplasty

Highet and Sander modified criteria of MacKinnon and Dellon for sensory recovery following nerve repair

Highet and Sander modified criteria of Zachary and Holmes for sensory recovery following nerve repair

high-flow
 h.-f. arterial malformation
 h.-f. arterial stenosis
 h.-f. arteriovenous fistula
 h.-f. arteriovenous malformation

high lateral tension abdominoplasty

Highmore antrum

Hilger facial nerve stimulator

Hillis retractor

hillock
 auricular h.

Hilton
 laryngeal saccule of H.
 H. sac

Hinderer
 H. cartilage forceps
 H. malar prosthesis
 H. lower nasal base implant

hindfoot ulcer

hinged
 h. flap
 h. great toe replacement prosthesis

Hinsberg operation

hippocratic
 h. fingers
 h. wreath

hip rotationplasty

Hirschfield method

hirsutism
    Apert h.

His line

histiocyte

histiocytic
    h. cytophagic panniculitis
    h. granuloma
    h. response

histiocytoma
    angiomatoid fibrous h.
        (AFH)
    benign fibrous h.
    cutaneous fibrous h.
    lipoid h.
    malignant fibrous h. (MFH)

histiocytomatosis

histiocytosis
    acute disseminated h. X
    benign cephalic h.
    juvenile xanthogranulo-
        ma h.
    Langerhans cell h.
    malignant h.
    nodular h.
    skin-limited h.

histochromatosis

histocompatibility

histocompatible

histoincompatibility

histopathologic

histophysiology

historrhexis

HMTV
    human mammary tumor vi-
        rus

hockey-stick incision

hoe
    monangle h.

Hoen retractor

Hoffman
    H. external fixation device
    H. external fixation system
    H. external fixator
    H. transfixion pin
    H. and Mohr procedure

Hogan and Converse graft aug-
    mentation

Holdaway
    H. line
    H. ratio

holder
    Dale Foley catheter h.
    Dale tracheostomy tube h.
    GraftAssist vein and
        graft h.
    Lewy laryngoscope h.
    lion jaw bone h.
    Margraf beam aligning
        film h.
    Young rubber dam h.

hole
    bur h.

Holinger anterior commissure
    laryngoscope

Hollister medial adhesive band-
    age

hollow
    cheek h's
    Sebileau h.

holmium
    h. laser
    h.:YAG laser

holoprosencephalic malforma-
    tion

holoprosencephaly

Holt-Oram
    H.-O. atriodigital dysplasia
    H.-O. syndrome

Holzheimer retractor

homeotransplant

homogeneous

homogenous

homograft

homologous

homoplastic

homoplasty

homotransplantation

honeycomb appearance

hooding

hook
  Blair palate h.
  blunt dissecting h.
  Carroll skin h.
  cleft palate sharp h.
  Converse hinged skin h.
  Cottle double h.
  Cottle-Joseph h.
  Cottle nasal h.
  Cottle skin h.
  Cottle tenaculum h.
  Crile nerve h.
  delicate skin h.
  DePuy nerve h.
  Dingman zygoma h.
  double-pronged Cottle h.
  double-pronged Fomon h.
  embrasure h.
  Fomon nasal h.
  Frazier skin h.
  Freer skin h.
  gasserian ganglion h.
  Gillies h.
  Gillies bone h.
  Gillies-Converse skin h.
  Gillies-Dingman tenaculum h.
  Gillies nasal h.
  Gillies skin h.
  Gillies zygomatic h.
  Guthrie skin h.
  h. of the hamate
  hinged skin h.
  House tragus h.
  Humby h.

hook (continued)
  Jameson muscle h.
  Jarit palate h.
  jaw h.
  Johnson skin h.
  Joseph nasal h.
  Joseph sharp skin h.
  Joseph single-prong h.
  Joseph skin h.
  Joseph tenaculum h.
  Kilner sharp h.
  Kilner skin h.
  Kleinert-Kutz skin h.
  Lange plastic surgery h.
  long palate h.
  Meyerding skin h.
  Meyerding skin h. and retractor
  Miltex tenaculum h.
  Moe alar h.
  Nova jaw h.
  O'Connor tenotomy h.
  palate pusher h.
  Schnitman skin h.
  Scoville curved nerve h.
  skin graft h.
  Sluder sphenoidal h.
  Smith lid-retracting h.
  Stevens h.
  Tyrrell skin h.
  Universal nerve h.
  Volkmann bone h.
  zygoma h.
  Zylik-Joseph h.

Hopf
  acrokeratosis verruciformis of H.
  H. disease
  H. keratosis

Hopkins
  H. endoscopy telescope
  H. rod endoscope
  H. II rod lens

hordeolum
  acute h.

horizontal
  h. bipedicle dermal flap

horizontal *(continued)*
    h. growth phase
    h. lid laxity
    h. mattress suture
    h. maxillary fracture
    h. osteotomy
    h. plate of palatine bone
    h. projection
    h. resorption
    h.-shaped skin paddle

horizontovertical laryngectomy

hormone
    adrenocorticotropic h.
      (ACTH)
    recombinant human
      growth h. (rhGH)
    melanocyte-stimulating h.

horn
    cicatricial h.
    cutaneous h.
    greater h. of hyoid bone
    inferior h. of thyroid carti-
      lage
    lateral h. of hyoid bone
    lesser h.
    lesser h. of hyoid bone
    mucosal h.
    sebaceous h.
    warty h.

Horner
    H. muscle
    H. syndrome

hornified epithelium

horseshoe
    h. abscess
    h. Le Fort I osteotomy
    h.-shaped skin flap
    h. tear

Horton arteritis

hose
    delivery h.

Hoskins-Westcott tenotomy
    scissors

host
    surrogate h.

Hotchkiss operation

hound-dog facies

hourglass nasal deformity

House
    H. grade facial palsy
    H. tragus hook
    H.-Brackmann classification
    H.-Brackmann classification
      for facial nerve function
    H.-Brackmann facial weak-
      ness scale
    H.-Brackmann grade (I–VI)
    H.-Brackmann scoring
    H.-Brackmann system

Howe silver precipitation
    method

HTR
    hard tissue replacement
    HTR-MFI implant

Huber technique

Hudson
    H. cranial bur
    H. rongeur forceps

Hueston
    H. finger amputation
    H. flap procedure
    H. spiral flap

Hueter
    H. maneuver
    H. perineal dressing

Huger diamond-back nasal scis-
    sors

Hughes
    H. eye reconstruction
    H. eyelid operation
    H. flap

human
    h. fibroblast growth factor-
      1 (FGF-1)
    h. mammary tumor virus
      (HMTV)
    h. tissue collagen matrix

Humby
    H. alar cartilage relocation
    H. hook
    H. knife

Hummelsheim operation

Hummer microdebrider

hump
    buffalo h.
    dowager h.
    nasal h.

Hunstad system for tumescent
    anesthesia

Hunt
    H. atrophy
    H. clamp
    H. forceps
    H. neuralgia
    H. syndrome

Hunter
    H. glossitis
    H. line
    mucopolysaccharidosis
        type II H. (MPS-II)
    H. syndrome
    H.-Schreger line

Hurd
    H. dissector
    H. pillar retractor
    H. septal bone-cutting for-
        ceps
    H. septal elevator
    H. septum-cutting forceps

Hurler
    mucopolysaccharidosis
        type I H. (MPS-IH)
    H. syndrome
    mucopolysaccharidosis
        type I H.-Scheie (MPS-IHS)
    H.-Scheie syndrome

Hürthle
    H. adenoma
    H. cell
    H. cell tumor

Huschke
    H. cartilage

Huschke *(continued)*
    H. valve

Husk rongeur

Hutchinson
    H. crescentic notch
    H. facies
    H. fracture
    H. freckle
    melanotic freckle of H.
    H. sign
    H.-Gilford disease
    H.-Gilford progeria
    H.-Gilford syndrome

Huxley
    H. layer
    H. membrane
    H. sheath

hyaline
    h. articular cartilage
    h. basement membrane
    h. cartilage
    h. degeneration

hyCURE
    h. hydrolyzed protein pow-
        der and exudate absorber
    h. collagen hemostatic
        wound dressing

Hydrasorb foam wound dress-
    ing

hydraulic dissection

Hydrocal cast material

hydrocele
    cervical h.

hydrochloric acid

hydrocolloid dressing

HydroDerm transparent dress-
    ing

Hydroflex
    H. penile implant
    H. penile implant rod
    H. penile prosthesis

hydrogel
    Carrasyn h.

hydrogel *(continued)*
  h. dressing
  SoloSite nonsterile h.

Hydro-Jel alginate

Hydron burn bandage

hydrophilic
  h. gel
  h. polymer dressing
  h. semipermeable absorbent polyurethane foam dressing

hydrops
  labyrinthine h.

HydroSKIN

hydroxyapatite (HA)
  h. adhesive
  h. block graft
  h. fibrin glue
  h. implant material
  nonresorbable h.
  porous h.

11-hydroxysteroid dehydrogenase

HyFil hydrogel dressing

hygiene
  mouth h.

hygroma
  cervical h.
  h. colli cysticum
  cystic h.
  Fleischmann h.

hygromatous

Hylaform viscoelastic gel

Hylasine

Hynes pharyngoplasty

hyoepiglottic ligament

hyoglossal
  h. membrane
  h. muscle

hyoid
  h. arch

hyoid *(continued)*
  h. bone
  h. branchial arch
  h. cartilage
  low-set h.
  mandibular plane to h.
  h. myotomy

hyperactive
  h. glabellar muscle

hyperactivity
  frontalis h.

hyperbaric
  h. chamber
  h. oxygen (HBO)
  h. oxygen–induced angiogenesis

hyperdactyly

hyperdivergent
  h. facial pattern
  h. patient
  h. skeletal pattern

hyperemia
  reactive h.
  rebound h.

hyperesthesia
  cervical h.
  laryngeal h.

hypereuryopia

hyperfunctional
  h. facial line
  h. glabellar line

Hypergel wound dressing

hyperkeratosis
  h. congenita
  epidermolytic h.
  h. figurata centrifuga atrophica
  h. follicularis
  h. penetrans
  subungual h.

hyperkeratotic epidermis

hyperkinesis
  mimetic h.

hypermastia

hypermelanosis
　linear and whorled nevoid h.
　nevoid h.

hypermobility
　temporomandibular joint h.

hyperostosis
　ankylosing h.
　h. corticalis deformans
　h. corticalis generalisata
　h. cranii
　diffuse idiopathic skeletal h.
　generalized cortical h.
　infantile cortical h.
　reactive h.
　subpontic h.

hyperparathyroidism
　primary h.

hyperparotidism

hyperperfusion
　h. injury

hyperphalangism

hyperpigmentation
　centrofacial h..
　cutaneous h.
　postpeel h.
　postsclerotherapy h.

hyperplasia
　adenomatous h.
　angiolymphoid h. with eosinophilia
　atypical melanocytic h.
　basal cell h.
　benign h.
　condylar h.
　congenital sebaceous h.
　coronoid h.
　cystic h.
　ductal h.
　fibrous h.
　focal epithelial h.
　hemimandibular h.
　idiopathic gingival h.

hyperplasia (continued)
　inferior pole h.
　inflammatory fibrous h.
　inflammatory papillary h.
　medication-induced h.
　neoplastic h.
　papillary h.
　parotid lymph node h.
　pseudocarcinomatous h.
　pseudoepitheliomatous h.
　sebaceous h.
　senile sebaceous h.
　tissue h.
　verrucous h.

hyperplastic
　h. epidermis
　h. epithelial lesion
　h. graft
　h. lesion
　h. mucosa

hypersensitivity
　anaphylactic h.
　delayed h.
　immediate h.

hypertelorism
　canthal h.
　orbital h.
　Munro classification of orbital h.
　pseudo-orbital h.

hypertension
　ambulatory venous h.
　postoperative h.
　venous h.

hyperthermia
　h. of anesthesia
　malignant h.

hypertonia
　lip h.

hypertrichosis

hypertrophic
　h. burn scar
　h. cicatrix
　h. hemangioma
　h. osteoarthropathy

hypertrophic *(continued)*
   h. port-wine stain
   h. rosacea
   h. scar
   h. scarring

hypertrophied

hypertrophy
   bilateral masseteric h.
   breast h.
   fat h.
   fatty h.
   fibrovascular h.
   genial h.
   glandular h.
   hemangiectatic h.
   hemifacial h.
   labial h.
   limb h.
   masseteric h.
   masseter muscle h.
   mixed h.
   skeletal h.
   submucosal gland h.
   unilateral h.
   unilateral facial h.
   virginal h.

hypesthesia
   bilateral h.

hyphema
   anterior chamber h.

hypocondylar

hypodactyly

hypoderm

hypodermatomy

hypodermoclysis

hypoesthesia

hypogenesis

hypoglossal
   h. canal
   h. ganglion
   h. nerve
   h. paralysis
   h. plexus

hypoglossal-facial neuroanastomosis

hypoglossia
   h.-hypodactylia syndrome
   h.-hypodactyly syndrome

hypoglottis

hypognathous

hypomastia

hypomelanosis
   congenital circumscribed h.
   idiopathic guttate h.

hyponychium

hyponychon

hypoperfusion

hypophalangism

hypopharyngeal
   h. carcinoma
   h. eminence
   h. lipoma
   h. squamous cell carcinoma

hypopharynx

hypophysis
   pharyngeal h.

hypopigmentation
   cutaneous h.
   postinflammatory h.
   postpeel h.

hypopigmented
   h. macular eruption

hypoplasia
   breast h.
   condylar h.
   focal dermal h.
   lingual h.
   malar h.
   mandibular h.
   mandibular condylar h.

hypoplasia *(continued)*
  maxillary h.
  maxillary-zygomatic h.
  midface h.
  midfacial h.
  soft tissue h.
  thenar muscle h.
  thumb h.
  zygomaticomaxillary h.

hypoplastic
  h. mandible
  h. tuberous breast
  h. urethra

hyposiagonarthritis

hyposomia

hypospadias
  balanic h.
  female h.
  glandular h.
  mid-penile h.
  penile h.
  penoscrotal h.
  perineal h.
  pseudovaginal h.

hypostasis

hypotelorism
  ocular h.
  orbital h.

hypotension
  orthostatic h.

hypotension *(continued)*
  vascular h.

hypothenar
  h. eminence
  h. hammer syndrome
  h. septum
  h. space

hypothyroidism
  iatrogenic h.

hypotonicity

hypoxemia
  arterial h.

hypsibrachycephalic

hypsicephalic

hypsicephaly

hypsiconchous

hypsistaphylia

hypsistenocephalic

hypsocephalous

Hyrtl
  H. anastomosis
  H. foramen
  H. loop

hysterotrachelectomy

hysterotracheloplasty

Hy-Tape surgical tape

IAN
    inferior alveolar nerve

iatrogenic
    i. cholesteatoma
    i. deformity
    i. disease
    i. hypothyroidism
    i. nasal stenosis
    i. perforation
    i. trauma

IBSL
    internal branch of superior
      laryngeal
        IBSL nerve

ICA
    internal carotid artery

ictus laryngis

I&D
    incision and drainage

IDC
    interdigitating dendritic
      cell

ideal
    i. flap
    i. occlusion

idioglossia

idioglottic

idiolalia

idiolect

idiopathic
    i. bone cavity
    i. enlargement
    i. facial paralysis
    i. fibromatosis
    i. gingival hyperplasia
    i. guttate hypomelanosis
    i. multiple hemorrhagic sar-
      coma

IgA
    immunoglobulin A

IgE
    immunoglobulin E

3i implant

ileocystoplasty

ileus

iliac
    i. crest
    i. crest bone graft
    i. crest free flap
    i. crest osseous flap
    i. crest osteocutaneous flap
    i. crest osteomuscular flap
    i. osteocutaneous flap

iliocostalis
    i. dorsi muscle
    i. lumborum muscle

iliohypogastric
    i. nerve
    i. neuralgia

ilioinguinal
    i. nerve
    i. neuralgia

iliotibial
    i. band
    i. tract

ilium microvascular transfer

Ilizarov
    halo-I. distraction instru-
      mentation
    I. internal fixation
    I. procedure
    I. technique

illocution

Illouz
    I. aspirative lipoplasty
    I. cannula
    I. liposuction technique
    I. modified tip
    reserve fat of I.
    I. standard tip

ILP
    intralesional laser photoco-
      agulation

ILVEN
    inflammatory linear verru-
    cous epidermal nevus

image
    x-ray i.

imaging
    magnetic resonance i.
        (MRI)
    magnetic source i. (MSI)
    MedMorph III patient vi-
        deo i.

imbalance
    occlusal i.
    orofacial muscle i.

imbricate

imbrication
    i. lines of von Ebner
    platysmal i.

IMCOR implant

IMF
    inframammary fold
    intermaxillary fixation

imipenem and cilastatin

immediate
    i. echolalia
    i. extension technique
    i. flap
    i. hypersensitivity

Immediate Load implant

immobility
    ciliary i.

immobilizer
    sternal-occipital-mandibu-
        lar i. (SOMI)

immotile cilia syndrome

immune
    i. adherence
    i. complex
    i. deficiency
    i. globulin
    intramuscular i. globulin

immune *(continued)*
    intravenous i. globulin
    i. modulation
    i. response
    i. system

immunity
    active i.
    adaptive i.
    cell-mediated i.
    humoral i.
    innate i.
    passive i.
    tumor-specific transplanta-
        tion i. (TSTI)

immunization

immunobiology

immunocompetent
    i. cell
    i. site
    i. squamous cell cancer
        model

immunocytochemical

immunocytochemistry

immunodeficiency
    severe combined i. (SCID)

immunoelectrophoresis

immunofluorescence
    direct i.

immunogenicity

immunoglobulin
    i. A (IgA)
    i. E (IgE)
    hepatitis B i. (HBIG)
    salivary i.
    secretory i.

immunohistochemical study

immunohistochemistry

immunologic memory

immunology

immunomodulation

immunoperoxidase stain

immunoprophylaxis

immunoradiometric analysis
(IRMA)

immunoreactivity

immunosuppressant

immunosuppression
drug-induced i.
iatrogenic i.

immunosuppressive
i. agent
i. therapy

immunosurveillance

immunotherapy

IMPA
incisal mandibular plane
angle

impact
i. injury

impaction
Le Fort I i.
mesioangular i.

impairment
motor i.
sensory i.

impalement injury

implant
adjustable breast i.
adjustable saline breast i.
alar-columella i.
alloplastic i.
alloplastic facial i.
anatomical Tobin malar
prosthetic i.
anterior subperiosteal i.
arthroplastic i.
articulated chin i.
autologous i.
bag-gel i.
Becker i.
bilumen i.
bilumen mammary i.
Binder i.

implant *(continued)*
Binder submalar i.
Biocell anatomical recon-
structive mammary i.
Biocell RTV i.
Biocell smooth surface i.
Biocell textured i.
Biocell textured shell surface i.
Biocell textured surface i.
BioCurve saline-filled
breast i.
BioDIMENSIONAL saline-
filled i.
bioresorbable i.
Bio-Vent i.
bivalve nasal splint i.
blade endosteal i.
blade-form i.
Blair-Brown i.
Brånemark i.
Brånemark osseointegra-
tion i.
breast i.
Brink PeriPyriform i.
i. button
calcification of breast i.
ceramic endosteal i.
i. cervix
cheek i.
chin i.
collagen i.
columellar i.
complete-arch blade endosteal i.
complete subperiosteal i.
Contigen Bard collagen i.
Contour Profile Natural saline breast i.
Crete-Manche i.
Cronin i.
Cronin mammary i.
cylinder-type i.
Dacron-backed i.
i. deflation
double lumen i.
D-shaped i.
dual-chambered i.
i. elastomer shell

implant *(continued)*
    endodontic endosseous i.
    endodontic endosteal i.
    Endopore i.
    endosseous blade i.
    endosseous hydroxyapatite
      (HA) i.
    endosseous vent i.
    endosteal i.
    endosseous i.
    ePTFE (expanded polytet-
      rafluoroethylene) i.
    esthetic Taylor mandibular
      angle i.
    expanded polytetrafluoro-
      ethylene (ePTFE) i.
    expansible infrastructure
      endosteal i.
    fabricated i.
    facial i.
    facial alloplastic i.
    Fibrel gelatin matrix i.
    fixed mandibular i. (FMI)
    i. fixture
    Flowers i.
    i. frame
    i. framework
    free-standing i.
    gel-filled i.
    gel-saline mammary i.
    Gillies i.
    Gore-Tex nasal i.
    Gore-Tex S.A.M. facial i.
    great toe i.
    i. gingival sulcus
    gold eyelid i.
    helicoid endosseous i.
    helicoid endosteal i.
    heterograft i.
    hex i.
    hexlock i.
    Heyer-Schulte breast i.
    Heyer-Schulte rhinoplasty i.
    Hinderer lower nasal
      base i.
    histoclasia i.
    HTR-MFI i.
    hybrid-type i.
    Hydroflex penile i.

implant *(continued)*
    hydroxyapatite-coated i.
    3i i.
    IMCOR i.
    Immediate Load i.
    Implantech Binder i.
    Implantech facial i.
    Implantech Flowers i.
    Implantech Mittelman i.
    Implantech Terino i.
    Imtec premounted thread-
      ed i.
    IMZ i.
    inflatable i.
    inflated i.
    i. infrastructure
    integral i.
    intracochlear i.
    intramuscular gluteal i.
    intraosseous i.
    intraperiosteal i.
    ITI-Bonefit endosseous i.
    ITI type-F endosseous i.
    LaminOss i.
    large-pore polyethylene i.
    Lifecore Restore wide dia-
      meter i.
    Linkow blade i.
    liposuction fat fillant i.
    Luhr i.
    468 McGhan Biocell ana-
      tomical breast i.
    Maestro i.
    magnetic i.
    i. malposition
    mammary i.
    MedDev gold eyelid i.
    Medpor facial i.
    Medpor malar i.
    Medpor reconstructive i.
    Medpor surgical i.
    Meme i.
    Mentor 1600 i.
    Mentor breast i.
    Mentor H/S Siltex i.
    mesostructure i.
    i. mesostructure
    i. metal
    metallic i.

implant *(continued)*
    Mettelman prejowl chin i.
    Micro-Lok i.
    Micro-Vent i.
    Micro-Vent2 i.
    Mini-Matic i.
    Mittelman i.
    3M mammary i.
    i. model
    monostructure i.
    mucosal i.
    multichannel cochlear i.
    i. neck
    needle endosseous i.
    needle endosteal i.
    Nobelpharma i.
    nonautologous i.
    Novagold mammary i.
    Nucleus 22 cochlear i.
    Nucleus multichannel coch-
        lear i.
    Octa-Hex i.
    oral i.
    osseointegrated cylinder i.
    osseointegrated oral i.
    Osseotite dental i.
    Osseotite two-stage proce-
        dure i.
    Osteo i.
    osteointegrated dental i.
    Osteoplate i.
    Paragon i.
    perigingival i.
    Periotest i.
    permucosal endosteal i.
    pin i.
    pin endosseous i.
    platinum eyelid i.
    polytetrafluoroethylene i.
    polyurethane-coated sili-
        cone breast i.
    Porex i.
    porous polyethylene i.
    post i.
    i. post
    Proplast i.
    Proplast-Teflon disk i.
    prosthetic i.
    PTFE-containing i.

implant *(continued)*
    Radovan breast i.
    ramus blade i.
    ramus endosteal i.
    RBM i.
    i.-related complications
        (IRC)
    Replace system tapered i.
    i. restoration
    Restore bone i.
    Restore RBM i.
    rhinoplasty i.
    saline breast i.
    S.A.M. facial i.
    Sargon i.
    i. screw
    screw-type i.
    Screw-Vent i.
    self-tapping screw-type i.
    i. shelf
    Silastic i.
    Silastic chin i.
    Silastic finger i.
    Silastic penile i.
    Silastic rhinoplasty i.
    Silastic silicone rubber i.
    Silastic subdermal i.
    Silastic testicular i.
    Silastic toe i.
    silicone-filled i.
    silicone-filled mammary i.
    silicone gel i.
    silicone gel breast i.
    silicone gel–filled breast i.
        (SGBI)
    silicone gel–filled mam-
        mary i. (SGMI)
    silicone nasal strut i.
    silicone textured mam-
        mary i.
    Siltex mammary i.
    single-chambered saline i.
    single-channel cochlear i.
    single-stage screw i.
    i. site dilator
    Small-Carrion Silastic rod
        for penile i.
    Smith orbital floor i.
    SoftForm facial i.

implant *(continued)*
    solid silicone buttock i.
    Spectra-System i.
    spiral endosseous i.
    spiral endosteal i.
    STAR*LOCK multi-purpose submergible threaded i.
    STAR*LOCK Press-Fit cylinder i.
    stock i.
    Straith chin i.
    Straith nasal i.
    i. structure
    subdermal i.
    submucosal i.
    submuscular i.
    subpectoral i.
    subperiosteal i.
    subperiosteal i. one-phase technique
    i. substructure interspace
    i. substructure strut
    superficial i.
    i. superstructure attachment
    i. superstructure connector
    i. superstructure frame
    i. superstructure neck
    Supramid mesh i.
    supraperiosteal i.
    i. surgical splint
    i. surgical splint superstructure
    Surgitek Flexi-Flate II penile i.
    Surgitek mammary i.
    synthetic i.
    i. system
    teardrop-shaped breast i.
    Teflon i.
    Teflon mesh i.
    Teflon orbital floor i.
    i. template
    Terino i.
    Terino anatomical chin i.
    textured saline breast i.
    TG Osseotite single-stage procedure i.

implant *(continued)*
    thick-walled Dacron-backed i.
    TiMesh patient-configured titanium craniomaxillofacial i.
    titanium-sprayed IMZ i.
    TMI i.
    transmandibular i. (TMI)
    transosseous i.
    transosteal i.
    triplant i.
    triple lumen i.
    Twist MTX i.
    Twist Ti i.
    two-piece i.
    universal subperiosteal i.
    vent i.
    vent-plate i.
    Vitek interpositional i.
    Zest i.
    Zyderm collagen i.
    Zyplast i.

implantation
    i. graft
    muscle i.
    Sewell internal mammary i.
    subcutaneous i.
    subpectoral-subserratus muscle i.
    vascular bundle i.
    vascular bundle i. into bone

implant-bearing surface

implant-bone interface

implant-borne prosthesis

Implantech
    I. Binder implant
    I. facial implant
    I. Flowers implant
    I. Mittelman implant
    I. SE-100 smoke aspiration tip
    I. Terino implant

implant/flap reconstruction

Implant Innovations titanium screw

implantodontics

implantodontist

implantodontology

implantologist

implantology
oral i.

Implant Support Systems titanium screw

impression
cleft palate i.
mandibular i.
maxillary i.
modeling plastic i.

impulse
nerve i.

Imtec
I. BioBarrier membrane
I. premounted threaded implant

IMZ
IMZ implant
IMZ implant system
titanium-sprayed IMZ implant
IMZ-type restoration

inchworm flap

incisal
i. angle
i. embrasure
i. mandibular plane angle (IMPA)

incision
access i.
alar i.
angular i.
anterior hairline i.
apron U-shaped i.
areolar i.

incision *(continued)*
back cut i.
bicoronal i.
bikini i.
blepharoplasty i.
Caldwell-Luc i.
chevron i.
circumareolar i.
collar i.
Conley i.
counter i.
contoured pretragal i.
coronal i.
crevicular i.
cross-hatch i.
cross-tunneling i.
crow's foot i.
crucial i.
cruciate i.
curved longitudinal i.
curvilinear i.
donor i.
i. and drainage (I&D)
elliptical i.
endaural mastoid i.
endonasal i.
external bevel i.
external paralateronasal skin i.
Fergusson i.
frontotemporal craniotomy i.
Gillies i.
gull-wing i.
hairline i.
healing biopsy i.
H-flap i.
hockey-stick i.
inferior conjunctival fornix i.
inframammary i.
inner bevel i.
intercartilaginous i.
internal bevel i.
intra-areolar i.
intraoral i.
inverse bevel i.
inverted bevel i.

incision *(continued)*
    inverted-U i.
    Killian i.
    Kocher i.
    labicolumellar crease i.
    lip-splitting i.
    lower lip–splitting i.
    low-flying bird i.
    MacFee i.
    marginal i.
    Martin i.
    Meisterschnitt i.
    Mercedes i.
    modified Weber-Fergus-
       son i.
    palmar i.
    periareolar i.
    preauricular i.
    releasing i.
    relief i.
    Rethi i.
    retroauricular i.
    retrotragal i.
    Risdon extraoral i.
    Risdon pretragal i.
    Skoog i. in palmar fasciec-
       tomy
    stepladder i.
    Steri-Stripped i.
    subciliary i.
    sublabial i.
    submammary i.
    submental i.
    supraciliary i.
    supraumbilical i.
    T-i.
    three-armed stellate i.
    transfixation i.
    U-shaped i.
    vertical elliptical i.
    volar transverse i.
    Wise breast i.
    wound i. and suction
    W-shaped i.
    xiphoid to os pubis i.
    xiphoid to umbilicus i.
    Y i.
    Y-shaped i.

incisional
    i. biopsy
    i. pain

incision-halving technique

incisionless otoplasty

incisive foramen

incisolabial

incisolingual

incisoproximal

incisura
    i. Santorini

incisor
    mandibular i.
    maxillary i.

incisure
    sagittal i.

inclination
    lateral condylar i.
    lingual i.

inclusion
    i. cyst
    i. disease

incompetence
    lip i.
    palatal i.
    valvular i.
    velopharyngeal i. (VPI)

incompetency *(variant of* in-
    competence)

incompetent upper lip

incomplete
    i. cleft
    i. cleft of earlobe
    i. cleft palate
    i. facial paralysis
    i. medialization
    i. paralysis
    i. recruitment
    i. syndactyly

inconsistent velopharyngeal closure

incontinence
  neuropathic i.

incontinentia pigmenti

incorporated tissue

incremental
  i. appositional pattern
  i. instrumentation
  i. line
  i. lines of cementum
  i. lines of von Ebner
  i. therapy

incudal
  i. fold
  i. ligament

incudectomy

incudomalleolar mass

incudostapedial joint

incus
  eroded i.
  i. interposition

index *pl.* indexes, indices
  alveolar i.
  apnea-hypopnea i. (AHI)
  articulation i.
  body mass i. (BMI)
  Broders i. (*grades 1–4*)
  cephalic i.
  Dean fluorosis i.
  debris i.
  Facial Disability I. (FDI)
  i. finger
  i. finger pollicization
  i. finger polydactyly
  gnathic i.
  Marginal Line Calculus I. (MLCI)
  maxilloalveolar i.
  Mohs i.
  moiré topography i.
  palatal i.

index *(continued)*
  palatal height i.
  palatine i.
  palatomaxillary i.
  Sciatic Function I.

Indian
  I. flap
  I. forehead flap
  I. method
  I. operation
  I. rhinoplasty

India rubber skin

induration
  brawny i.

inelastic
  i. lower eyelid

infancy
  melanotic neuroectodermal tumor of i.
  sternocleidomastoid (SCM) tumor of i.

infantile
  i. apertognathia
  i. aphasia
  i. fibrosarcoma
  i. perseveration

infarction
  myocardial i.

infection
  bacterial i.
  candidal i.
  fulminant invasive i.
  fungal i.
  indolent invasive i.
  invasive fungal i.
  middle ear i.
  mycobacterial i.
  mycobacterial nodal i.
  necrotizing myofascial fungal i.
  necrotizing soft tissue i. (NSTI)
  nonopportunistic i.
  nosocomial i.

infection *(continued)*
    opportunistic i.
    orbital i.
    periorbital i.
    pneumococcal i.
    recurrent i.
    run-around i.
    secondary i.
    subcutaneous necrotizing i.
    subeschar i.
    upper respiratory tract i.
    Vincent i.
    viral i.
    wound i.

infective endocarditis

inferior
    i. alveolar nerve (IAN)
    i. alveolar nerve block
    i. alveolar nerve fascicle
    i. alveolar neurovascular bundle
    arcus dentalis i.
    i. cantholysis
    chorditis vocalis i.
    i. colliculus
    i. concha
    i. conjunctival fornix incision
    i. constrictor pharyngeal muscle
    i. crus of lateral canthal tendon
    i. deep cervical node
    i. dental arch
    i. dental thrombosis
    i. ethmoidal concha
    i. extensor retinaculum
    i. gluteal flap
    i. laryngeal artery
    i. laryngeal nerve
    i. laryngotomy
    i. lip
    i. lip of pons
    i. longitudinal muscle of tongue
    i. malposition
    i. marginotomy
    i. maxillary bone

inferior *(continued)*
    i. meatal antrostomy
    i. meatus
    i. nasal concha
    i. nasal nerve
    i. oblique muscle
    i. orbital fissure
    i. orbital foramen
    i. pedicle
    i. petrosal sinus
    i. pharyngeal constrictor
    i. pole peritonsillar abscess
    i. rectus muscle
    i. retinacular lateral canthoplasty
    i. retrognathia
    i. surface
    i. surface of tongue
    i. teeth
    i. thyroid artery
    i. thyroid vein
    i. turbinate
    i. turbinate bone
    i. turbinate concha
    i. tympanic artery
    i. vestibular nucleus

infiltrate
    granulomatous dermal i.
    multifocal lymphocytic i.

infiltrating carcinoma

infiltration
    leukocyte i.
    leukocytic i.
    superwet preoperative subcutaneous i.

infiltrative
    i. fasciitis
    i. local anesthesia

infiltrator
    Klein i.

inflammation
    acute i.
    central zone i.
    chronic i.
    fibrinous i.
    focal i.

inflammation *(continued)*
  granulomatous i.
  purulent i.
  sanguineous i.
  serous i.
  subacute i.
  suppurative i.
  ulcerative i.

inflammatory
  i. cell
  i. cyst
  i. disease
  i. edema
  i. fibrous hyperplasia
  i. lesion
  i. linear verrucous epidermal nevus (ILVEN)
  i. oncotaxis
  i. papillary hyperplasia
  i. papillomatosis
  i. process
  i. response
  i. zone

inflatable implant

inflation
  CT-guided balloon i.

infolded

infolding
  basal i.

infra
  vide i.

infra-areolar scar

infra-auricular mass

infrabony
  i. pocket
  i. pocket curettage

infrabrow scar

infrabulge
  i. clasp

infracartilaginous

infraciliary line

infraclusion

infracrestal pocket

infraglottic
  i. squamous cell carcinoma

infrahyoid
  i. artery
  i. muscle
  i. strap muscle

infralabyrinthine
  i. air cell
  i. approach

inframalar groove

inframammary
  i. crease
  i. distance
  i. fold (IMF)
  i. incision
  i. scar

inframandibular

inframaxillary

inframaxillism

infraocclusion

infraorbital
  i. artery
  i. block
  i. fissure
  i. foramen
  i. margin
  i. nerve
  i. nerve block
  i. plate
  i. region
  i. ridge of maxilla
  i. rim
  i. space
  i. space abscess
  i. sulcus of maxilla
  i. tear trough

infraspinatus muscle

infrastructure
  implant i.

infratemporal
  i. fossa

infratemporal *(continued)*
    i. fossa approach
    i. space
    i. surface of maxilla
    i. wall

infratrochlear nerve

infundibular cell

infundibulotomy

infundibulum
    ethmoidal i.

infusion
    colloid i.
    crystalloid i.
    i. graft

infusion/infiltration cannula

Ingals nasal speculum

ingrowth
    bone i.
    bony i.
    fibrovascular i.
    squamous i.
    squamous epithelial i.

inherent extensibility of skin

injection
    bolus i.
    collagen i.
    fat i.
    intralesional i.
    intralesional steroid i.
    intramuscular i.
    mental block i.
    Microfil i.
    nasopalatine i.
    sclerosing i.
    serial scar i's
    silicone i.
    Zyderm collagen i.

injector
    Dermo-Jet i.
    Dermo-Jet high pressure i.

injury
    acute phase of burn i.
    avulsion i.
    avulsion flap i.

injury *(continued)*
    axonotmetic i.
    basement membrane
      zone i.
    blunt carotid i. (BCI)
    closed brachial plexus i.
    closed degloving i.
    closed head i. (CHI)
    clothesline i.
    cold i.
    contrecoup i.
    cotton roll i.
    cribriform plate i.
    crush i.
    degloving i.
    dentinoblastic i.
    dural venous sinus i.
    extra-axial i.
    fingertip i.
    greater arc i. of the carpus
    hyperperfusion i.
    impact i.
    impalement i.
    lesser arc i. of the carpus
    maxillofacial i.
    nerve crush i.
    neurotmetic i.
    obstetric brachial plexus i.
    radial mutilation i.
    radiation i.
    reperfusion i.
    ring avulsion i.
    Sunderland classification
      for nerve i's *(grades I–V)*
    thermal i.
    through-and-through avul-
      sion i.
    traumatic i.
    zone of i.

inlay
    composite i.
    epithelial i.

inner
    i. bevel incision
    i. ear
    i. fibrous layer

innervated
    i. free flap

innervated *(continued)*
    i. platysma flap

innervation
    reciprocal i.

innominate
    i. artery
    i. fascia
    i. line

Innovation implant system

inosculation

insane finger

insensate flap

insert
    intramucosal i.
    mucosal i.

insertion
    endoscopic-assisted facial
        implant i.
    i. loss
    myringotomy and grom-
        met i.
    path of i

in situ
    carcinoma in s.
    melanoma in s. (MIS)

inspissate

inspissatum
    cerumen i.

instability
    atlantoaxial i.
    carpal i.
    dorsal intercalated segmen-
        tal i. (DISI)
    dynamic i. of wrist
    lunotriquetral i.
    perilunar i.
    progressive perilunar i.
        (stages I–IV)
    scapholunate i.
    static i. of wrist
    volar intercalated segmen-
        tal i. (VISI)

installation

Insta-Mold silicone ear impres-
    sion material

Instat
    I. collagen absorbable he-
        mostat
    I. MCH microfibrillar colla-
        gen hemostat

instep island flap

instillation
    intravesical i.

instrument
    ASSI nasal and sinus i's
    binocular i.
    B.I.P. biopsy i.
    Daniel EndoForehead i.
    ESI Lite-Pipe fiberoptic i.
    ESI Lite-Pipe plastic sur-
        gery i.
    Exprin DQI biopsy i.
    Farrior flap exposure i's
    gnathologic i.
    handcutting i.
    intracanal i.
    Isse endo brow i.
    Kapp surgical i.
    McCall i.
    M4 Kerr Safety Hedstrom i.
    NOVA DPM 9003 skin tes-
        ting i.
    Obwegeser orthognathic
        surgery i.
    Rosenberg gynecomastia
        dissection i.
    Tessier craniofacial i.
    Vilex plastic surgery i.

instrumentation
    Baxter V. Mueller laparos-
        copic i.
    craniofacial i.
    EndoMax endoscopic i.
    halo-Ilizarov distraction i.
    incremental i.
    insufficient i.
    Midas Rex i.
    minimal i.

insufficiency
    abdominal wall i.
    arterial i. of lower extremities
    palatal i.
    superficial valvular i.
    velar i.
    velopharyngeal i. (VPI)
    venous i.

insufficient
    i. instrumentation
    i. jaw grading
    i. lip support

insulin-like growth factor

intact canal wall technique

intaglio view

Integra
    I. artificial skin
    I. tissue expander

integral
    i. implant
    i. intraoral bilateral posterior mesostructure

integration
    prosthetic i.

integrative
    i. mastoplasty

integrity
    marginal i. of amalgam
    skin i.

intensity
    electrosurgical current i.

interalveolar
    i. bone crater
    i. distance
    i. space

interameloblast

interarch
    i. distance

interarticular disk of temporomandibular joint

interarytenoid
    i. muscle
    i. notch

intercalated
    i. defect
    i. duct
    i. duct lumen
    i. joint

intercalation

intercartilaginous
    i. fold
    i. incision

intercellular
    i. bridge
    i. canaliculus
    i. fenestration
    i. fluid
    i. layer
    i. matrix process
    i. space
    i. substance

intercostal
    i. artery
    i. nerve
    i. vessel

intercostalis
    i. externus muscle
    i. internus muscle

intercricothyrotomy

intercuspation
    maximum i.

interdental embrasure

interdigitate

interdigitated muscle flap

interdigitating
    i. dendritic cell (IDC)
    i. zigzag skin flap

interendognathic suture

interface
    implant-bone i.
    metal i.

interface *(continued)*
   structural i.

interfacial
   i. surface tension

interference
   occlusal i.

interfragmentary wiring

intergluteal
   i. cleft
   i. sulcus

interincisal
   i. angle
   i. distance
   i. opening

interlobular duct

intermaxillary fixation (IMF)

intermediate
   i. fascia
   i. fiber
   i. layer
   i. nerve
   i. plexus
   i. restoration
   i. restorative material
     (IRM)
   i. string
   i. suture
   i. tendon
   i. zone

intermedium
   stratum i.

intermetatarsal ligament

internal
   i. bevel incision
   i. branch of the superior la-
     ryngeal (IBSL) nerve
   i. carotid artery (ICA)
   i. defatting
   i. derangement (ID)
   i. elastic membrane
   i. ethmoidectomy
   i. jugular vein
   i. juncture
     astopexy

internal *(continued)*
   i. maxillary artery
   i. oblique aponeurosis
   i. oblique osteomuscular
     flap
   i. occipital ridge
   i. traction

internum
   osteum i.

interodontoblastic collagen fibril

interorbital space

interosseous
   i. wire
   i. wiring

interossicular fold

interphalangeal (IP)
   distal i. (DIP)
   i. joint
   proximal i. (PIP)

interplacodal area

interpolated flap

interpolation flap

interposing fascia

interposition
   colonic i.
   incus i.
   jejunal i.
   temperoparietal facial
     flap i.

interpositional gap arthroplasty

interradicular
   i. abscess
   i. alveoloplasty
   i. artery
   i. fiber
   i. lesion
   i. osseous defect
   i. septum
   i. space

intersection
   tendinous i.

interseptal osteoclasia

interspace
  implant substructure i.

interspecific graft

intertriginous area

intestinal vaginoplasty

intima
  tunica i.

intimal dehiscence

intolerance
  cold i. after fingertip injury

intra-alveolar
  i. pocket
  i. root

intra-areolar incision

intrabony
  i. defect
  i. lesion
  i. pocket

intracapsular
  i. fracture
  i. rupture
  i. temporomandibular joint
    arthroplasty
  i. tumor removal

intracartilaginous

intracavitary anesthesia

intraconal fat

intracorporeal lithotripsy

intracranial
  i. tumor

intracuticular running sutures

intradermal
  i. nevus
  i. sutures

intraepithelial
  i. carcinoma
  i. dyskeratosis

intraepithelial *(continued)*
  i. excementosis

intrafascicular suture

intrajugular
  i. process of temporal bone

intralabyrinthine fistula

intralesional
  i. injection
  i. laser photocoagulation
    (ILP)
  i. triamcinolone

intraligamentary anesthesia

intralingual
  i. cyst of foregut origin

intralobular duct

intramastoid abscess

intramedullary
  i. fixation
  i. pin

intramembranous

intramuscular
  i. glands of tongue
  i. gluteal implant
  i. hemangioma
  i. injection

intraoperative
  i. skin expansion
  i. spatial confirmation
  i. tumor staging

intraoral
  i. antrostomy
  i. approach
  i. cyst
  i. flap
  i. incision
  i. Kaposi sarcoma
  i. lining deficiency
  i. meloplasty
  i. mucosal defect

intraosseous
  i. ameloblastoma
  i. carcinoma

intraosseous *(continued)*
  i. cyst
  i. ganglion cyst
  i. implant
  i. lesion

intraparotideal metastasis

intraparotid mesenchymal tumor

intraperiosteal implant

intraseptal alveoloplasty

intravelar veloplasty

introitus
  neovaginal i.

intrusion
  maxillary i.

invaginate

invagination
  epithelial i.
  eyelid i.
  Oehlers type 3 dens i.
  skin envelope i.
  i. of umbilicus

invaginatus
  dens i.

invasion
  laryngotracheal i.

invasive
  i. fungal infection
  i. fungal infection of tempo-
    ral bone
  i. keratitis
  i. lobular carcinoma

inventory
  MacArthur Communicative
    Development I's

inverse
  i. bevel incision

inversion
  nipple i.
  penile skin i.

inverted
  i. bevel incision

inverted *(continued)*
  i. ductal papilloma
  i.-L osteotomy
  i. schneiderian papilloma
  i.-T scar
  i.-T skin excision
  i.-U incision

inverting papilloma

inviscation

in vitro–grown palatal mucosa
  sheet

involvement
  regional node i.
  skin i.

IP
    interphalangeal
      IP joint

IRC
    implant-related complica-
      tions

IRMA
    immunoradiometric assay

irradiation
  elective neck i.

irregularity
  contour i's

irrigation
  antibiotic i.
  bacitracin i.
  frontal i.
  saline i.
  sinus i.
  tendon sheath i.

irritability
  electric i.
  myotatic i.

ischemia
  hand i.
  wound i.

ischemic
  i. necrosis
  i. neuropathy

ischemic *(continued)*
i. ulatrophy

island
i. adipofascial flap in Achilles tendon resurfacing
attached i.
cartilage i.
epimyoepithelial i.
i. fasciocutaneous flap
i. flap
i. frontalis muscle transfer
myoepithelial cell i.
septocutaneous i.
septofasciocutaneous i.
skin i.
teres major skin i.

isogenic graft

isognathus

isograft

Isolagen human collagen

isolation
carotid i.

isologous graft

Isomet
I. low speed saw
I. Plus precision saw

isotransplantation

Israel nasal rasp

Isse endo brow instrument

Istanbul flap for phallic reconstruction

isthmus
thyroid i.

Italian
I. flap
I. method
I. operation
I. rhinoplasty

iter
i. dentis
i. dentium

ITI
ITI-Bonefit endosseous implant
ITI type-F endosseous implant

Ito nevus

Ivy
I. rongeur
I. wire

Jackson
J. anterior commissure la-
ryngoscope
J. appliance
J. approximation forceps
J. broad staple forceps
J. button forceps
J. conventional foreign
body forceps
J. crib
J. cross-action forceps
J. cylindrical object forceps
J. double-prong forceps
J. dull rotation forceps
J. esophagoscope
J. flexible upper lobe bron-
chus forceps
J. globular object forceps
J. laryngoscope
J. papilloma forceps
J. ring jaw globular object
forceps
J. sharp-pointed rotation
forceps
J. steel-stem woven filiform
bougie
J. syndrome
J. triangular brass dilator
J.-Pratt drain

Jacobson
J. cartilage
J. nerve
J. organ
J. plexus
J. reflex

Jacob ulcer

Jacquart angle

Jaeger
J. bone plate
J. lid plate
J. retractor

Jaffe
J. eyelid speculum
J. retractor

Jahss
J. maneuver
J. position

Jako laryngoscope

Jameson
J. face-lift scissors
J. muscle hook

Janeway spot

Jannetta retractor

Jansen
J. operation
J. retractor
J.-Gifford retractor
J.-Middleton punch forceps

Japan Facial Score

Jarit palate hook

jaw
bird-beak j.
j. bone
j. brace
cleft j.
Cox regression analysis of
partially edentulous j.
crackling j.
j. grading
Hapsburg j.
j. hook
lumpy j.
j. movement
multiple exostoses of j.
parrot j.
progonoma of j.
j. protrusion
j. radiograph
ramus of j.
receding lower j.
j. reflex
j. relation
j. relation record
j. repositioning
j. separation
j. stabilization
upper j.
wide j.

jawline

jaw-to-jaw
  j.-t.-j. position
  j.-t.-j. relation

jaw-winking
  j.-w. phenomenon

J/cm²
  joules per square centimeter

JedMed TRI-GEM microscope

jejunal
  j. free flap
  j. interposition

jejunoplasty

jejunum free flap

Jena method

Jessner
  J. solution
  J. solution peel

Jobst
  J. compression garment
  J. stockings

Johnson
  J. cheek retractor
  J. skin hook

Johnston method

joint
  Ackerman bar j.
  j. arthrodesis
  axial rotation j.
  ball and socket j.
  bar j.
  butt j.
  capitolunate j.
  capsule of temporomandibular j.
  carpometacarpal (CMC) j.
  Charcot j.
  j. contracture
  cranial suture j.
  cricoarytenoid j.
  cricothyroid j.
  distal interphalangeal (DIP) j.

joint *(continued)*
  frozen knee j.
  incudostapedial j.
  intercalated j.
  interphalangeal (IP) j.
  Lisfranc j.
  lunotriquetral j.
  metacarpophalangeal (MCP) j.
  metatarsal j.
  metatarsophalangeal (MTP) j.
  midcarpal j.
  pisotriquetral j.
  proximal interphalangeal (PIP) j.
  radiocarpal j.
  radiolunate j.
  rotation j.
  saddle j.
  scaphoid-trapezium-trapezoid (STT) j.
  scaphotrapeziotrapezoid (STT) j.
  j. sepsis
  septic j.
  single sleeve bar j.
  socket j.
  j. space
  Steiger j.
  sternoclavicular j.
  temporomandibular j. (TMJ)
  triscaphe j.
  ulnocarpal j.

Joint-Jack finger splint

Jones nasal splint

Joseph
  J. clamp
  J. knife
  J. nasal hook
  J. nasal rasp
  J. nasal scissors
  J. nasal splint
  J. periosteal elevator
  J. rhinoplasty
  J. saw
  J. saw guide
  J. septal fracture appliance

Joseph *(continued)*
    J. septal splint
    J. serrated scissors
    J. sharp skin hook
    J. single-prong hook
    J. skin hook
    J. tenaculum
    J. tenaculum hook
    J.-Maltz saw

joule
    j. counter

jowl
    j. fat
    neck j.
    j. reduction lipectomy

jugal bone

jughandle
    j. view
    j. roentgenogram

jugomasseteric mutilation

jugomaxillary point

jugular
    j. bulb
    j. bulb decompression
    j. chain lymph node
    j. foramen
    j. foramen syndrome
    j. fossa
    j. lymph node
    j. vein
    j. venography

jugulare
    glomus j.

jugulodigastric
    j. node
    j. region

jugulo-omohyoid node

jugum *pl.* juga
    juga alveolaria mandibulae
    juga alveolaria maxillae

jump flap

jumping
    j. genioplasty
    j. man flap

junction
    alar-facial j.
    chondroethmoidal j.
    dentoepithelial j.
    dentogingival j.
    gap j.
    hard-soft palate j.
    impermeable j.
    intermediate j.
    mucocutaneous j.
    mucogingival j. (MGJ)
    neuromuscular j.
    nexus-type j.
    pontomedullary j.
    squamocolumnar j.
    sternoclavicular j.
    vermilion-skin j.

junctional
    j. complex
    j. epithelium
    j. nevus

juncture
    internal j.

Juri
    J. II, III degree of male pattern baldness
    J. flap

jut
    columellar j. of nose

juxta-articular ankylosis

juxtabrow skin

juxtacapillary receptor

juxtacortical
    j. chondroma
    j. osteogenic sarcoma

Kadon primer

Kahler forceps

kallikrein

Kallmann syndrome

Kanavel cock-up splint

Kanner syndrome

Kaplan-Feinstein comorbidity
grade

Kaposi
pseudo-K. sarcoma
K. sarcoma
K. sarcoma of mastoid
K. varicelliform eruption

kappacism

Kappa test

Kapp surgical instrument

Karamar-Mailatt tarsorrhaphy
clamp

Karapandzic
K. flap
K. method
reverse K. flap
K. technique

Karman cannula

Karoli effect

Kartagener
K. syndrome
K. triad

Kasabach
K.-Merritt phenomenon
K.-Merritt syndrome

Kawamoto technique

Kawasaki disease

Kaye
K. face-lift scissors
K. minimal-incision anterior
approach

Kazangia
K. and Converse facial fracture classification
K. and Converse mandibu-
lar fracture classification

Kazanjian
K. flap
K. forceps
K. guide
K. midline forehead flap
K. nasal cutting scissors
K. nasal splint
K. operation
K. splint
K. T-bar
T-bar of K.
K. vestibuloplasty
K. vestibuloplasty tech-
nique
K. vestibulotomy

K cell

Kebab graft

keel
Montgomery laryngeal k.

Keel tip

Keith needle

Keizer retractor

Kelly
K. forceps
K. hemostat

keloid
earlobe k.
k. formation
k. scar
k. tumor

Kennedy bar

keratinization
intracellular k.

keratinized
k. epithelium
k. tissue

keratinizing
  k. epithelial odontogenic cyst
  k. epithelial odontogenic tumor
  k. squamous cell carcinoma

keratinocyte
  cultured autologous k.

keratitis
  exposure k.
  invasive k.
  xerotic k.

keratoacanthoma
  Ferguson-Smith k.
  nodulo-vegetating k.
  solitary k.
  subungual k. (SUKA)

keratocoagulation

keratoconjunctivitis
  bacterial k.

keratocyst
  odontogenic k.

keratocyte

keratoderma
  k. blennorrhagica
  k. climactericum
  senile k.

keratolysis

keratolytic agent

keratoma
  senile k.

keratopachyderma

keratopathy

keratoplasty
  Sourdille k.

keratosis pl. keratoses
  actinic k.
  k. blennorrhagica
  k. climactericum

keratosis (continued)
  focal k.
  follicular k.
  k. follicularis
  Hopf k.
  k. labialis
  k. obliterans
  k. obturans
  papillary k.
  seborrheic k.
  senile k.
  solar k.

keratotic papilloma

kerion
  tinea k.

Kerlix
  K. gauze
  K. gauze bandage

Kernahan and Elsahy striped Y classification for cleft lip and palate

kernicterus

Kerr
  K. Permplastic material
  K. Traycon material

Kerrison
  K. forceps
  K. rongeur

Kesselring
  K. aspirative lipoplasty
  K. curette technique

ketamine

ketoacidosis

ketoconazole

ketoprofen

Khan-Jaeger clamp

Kiel
  K. graft
  modified K. mastopexy

Kienböck disease

kieselguhr

Kiesselbach
  K. area
  K. plexus
  K. triangle

Killian
  K. dehiscence
  K. frontoethmoidectomy
    procedure
  K. incision
  K. nasal speculum
  K. operation
  K.-Halle nasal speculum
  K.-Lynch suspension laryn-
    goscope

Kilner
  K. mouth gag
  K. sharp hook
  K. skin hook
  K.-Doughty mouth gag

Kimura cartilage graft

Kinder Design pedo forceps

King operation

Kingsley
  reverse K. splint
  K. splint

kinking
  pedicle k.

Kinzie method

Kirby retractor

Kirkland knife

Kirschner
  K. pin fixation
  K. wire (K-wire)
  K. wire splint

Kisch reflex

kiss
  angel's k.

kit
  ACE bone screw tacking k.
  McGhan fill k.
  micro-bicinchoninic acid
    protein assay k.

kit (continued)
  Straith nasal splint k.

Kitano and Okada method

kite flap

Kiwisch bandage

kleeblattschädel
  k. anomaly
  k. craniosynostosis
  k. syndrome

Klein
  K. cannula
  K. cannula tip
  K. Delrin Luer-Lok handle
  K. 1-hole infiltrator tip
  K. infiltration needle
  K. infiltrator
  K. multihole infiltrator tip
  K. pump

Kleinert
  K. dynamic traction splint
  K.-Kutz bone-cutting for-
    ceps
  K.-Kutz skin hook
  K.-Kutz tenotomy scissors
  K.-Ragnell retractor

Kleinman test

Kleinsasser anterior commissure laryngoscope

Klinefelter syndrome

Kling
  K. gauze
  K. gauze bandage

Klippel-Trénaunay syndrome

Klumpke palsy

Knapp lacrimal sac retractor

knee salvage

knife pl. knives
  Agnew canaliculus k.
  Alexander otoplasty k.
  Austin k.
  Ballenger cartilage k.

knife *(continued)*
- Ballenger nose k.
- Berens ptosis k.
- bistoury k.
- Blair k.
- Blair-Brown k.
- Blair-Brown skin graft k.
- Blair cleft palate k.
- Bodenham-Blair skin graft k.
- Bodenham-Humby skin graft k.
- Brophy k.
- Brophy bistoury k.
- Brophy cleft palate k.
- Brown-Blair skin graft k.
- Brown cleft palate k.
- Buck k.
- Caltagirone skin graft k.
- cautery k.
- chalazion k.
- cleft palate k.
- Cobbett skin graft k.
- Cottle k.
- Cottle nasal k.
- Cronin palate k.
- diathermy k.
- k.-edged finishing line
- electronic k.
- endotherm k.
- Farrior otoplasty k.
- Farrior septal cartilage stripper k.
- Fergusson k.
- finishing k.
- Foerster capsulotomy k.
- free-hand k.
- Freer-Ingal nasal k.
- Freer-Ingal submucous k.
- Freer nasal k.
- gamma k.
- gold k.
- Goldman-Fox k.
- Goulian k.
- Humby k.
- interdental k.
- Joseph k.
- Kirkland k.
- Merrifield k.

knife *(continued)*
- Monahan-Lewis k.
- myringotomy k.
- Orban k.
- periodontal k.
- Reese ptosis k.
- Rehne skin graft k.
- serrated k.
- Sharpoint microsurgical k.
- sickle k.
- straight tympanoplasty k.
- Thiersch skin graft k.
- tympanoplasty k.
- Virchow skin graft k.
- Watson skin grafting k.
- Webster skin graft k.

Knight
- K. nasal scissors
- K. and North classification of malar fractures *(groups I–VI)*

Knoll glands

Kocher incision

Koerner flap

kojic acid

Kole procedure

Konig graft

Koplik spots

Körner septum

Korsakoff disease

Krause
- K. corpuscle
- K. graft
- K. method
- transverse suture of K.
- K. valve
- K.-Wolfe graft

Krönlein orbitotomy

Krukenberg
- K. hand
- modified K. procedure
- K. procedure

KTP/Nd:YAG XP surgical laser
 system

KTP/YAG laser

Kuhnt-Szymanowski
  K.-S. ectropion repair pro-
   cedure
  K.-S. technique

Kürsteiner canals

Kutler lateral V-Y advancement
 flap

Küttner
  K. ganglion
  K. wound stretcher

K-wire
  Kirschner wire

kyphectomy

kyphos
  bony k.

kyphosis
  basilar k.

L

L
    L approach
    L-shaped skin excision

lab
    earmold l.

Laband syndrome

Labbé vein

labia

labial
    l. angle
    l. arch
    l. artery
    l. assimilation
    l. bar
    l. cavity
    l. cleft
    l. commissure
    l. curve
    l. edema
    l. embrasure
    l. filter
    l. flange
    l. flaring
    l. frenum
    l. gingiva
    l. glands
    l. hypertrophy
    l. lamina
    l. line
    l. and lingual arches
    l. minor salivary gland
    l. movement
    l. notch
    l. occlusion
    l. pad
    l. pit
    l. region
    l. splint
    l. stent
    l. sulcus
    l. surface
    l. teeth
    l. torque
    l. tubercle

labial *(continued)*
    l. vestibule
    l. wire

labial-buccal sulcus

labialis
    facies l.
    herpes l.
    keratosis l.

labialism

labialization

labicolumellar crease incision

labioalveolar

labioaxiogingival

labiocervical

labiochorea

labioclination

labiodental
    l. area
    l. sulcus

labiogeniomandibular mutila
    tion

labiogingival (LAG)

labioglossolaryngeal
    l. paralysis

labioglossopharyngeal

labiograph

labioincisal (LAI)
    l. edge (LIE)
    l. line angle

labiolingual
    l. plane
    l. splint
    l. technique

labiolingually

labiomandibular
    l. glossotomy
    l. ligament

labiomarginal sulcus

labiomaxilloseptocolumellar
    amputation

labiomental
    l. amputation
    l. fold
    l. groove

labionasal

labiopalatal amputation

labiopalatine

labioplacement

labioplasty

labioproximal

labiotenaculum

labioversion

labium
    l. inferius oris
    l. mandibulare
    l. maxillare
    l. oris
    l. superior oris

labrale
    l. inferius
    l. superioris
    l. superius

labrum *pl.* labra

labyrinth
    bony l.
    ethmoidal l.
    membranous l.
    osseous l.
    otic l.
    vestibular l.

labyrinthectomy
    chemical l.
    mechanical l.

labyrinthine
    l. angiospasm
    l. aplasia
    l. artery
    l. cryptococcosis
    l. fenestration

labyrinthine *(continued)*
    l. fistula
    l. gusher
    l. hydrops
    l. membrane
    l. nystagmus
    l. ossification
    l. righting reflex
    l. segment
    l. torticollis
    l. vertigo

labyrinthitis
    circumscribed l.
    congenital luetic l.
    diffuse serous l.
    diffuse suppurative l.
    obliterative l.
    suppurative l.
    viral l.

labyrinthotomy

lacerated
    l. foramen
    l. wound

laceration
    avulsed l.
    flexor tendon l.

lacerum
    foramen l.

lacrimal
    l. bone
    l. duct
    l. fossa
    l. gland
    l. groove of maxilla
    l. lake
    l. probe
    l. process
    l. sac
    l. sulcus of maxilla

lacrimation
    gustatory l.
    l. test

lacrimoauriculodentodigital
    (LADD)
    l. syndrome

lacteal fistula

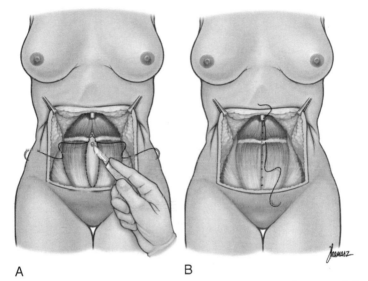

A   B

Type III, modified abdominoplasty. *A,* Longer skin incision is demarcated. Operation begins with liposuction as indicated. Umbilicus, which has dual blood supply from skin and below from muscle, can be left intact or can be detached at its base ("floating"). *B,* Musculoaponeurotic plication is then performed to extent indicated. If umbilicus is detached, it is reinserted with sutures. (From Achauer, BM, et al.: Plastic Surgery. St. Louis, Mosby, Inc., 2000.)

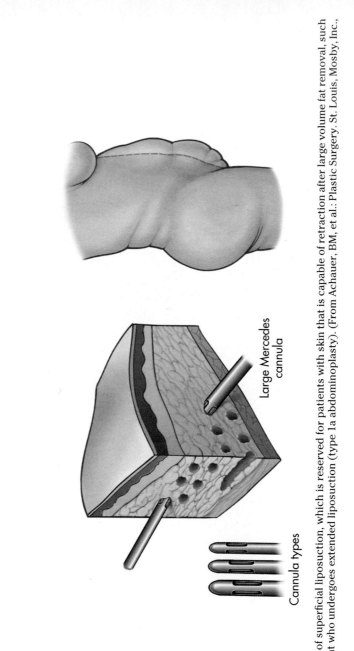

Concept of superficial liposuction, which is reserved for patients with skin that is capable of retraction after large volume fat removal, such as patient who undergoes extended liposuction (type 1a abdominoplasty). (From Achauer, BM, et al.: Plastic Surgery. St. Louis, Mosby, Inc., 2000.)

Cannula types

Large Mercedes cannula

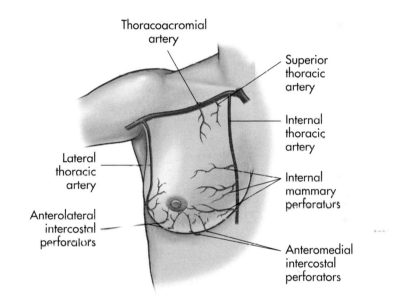

Blood supply to breast. (From Achauer, BM, et al.: Plastic Surgery. St. Louis, Mosby, Inc., 2000.)

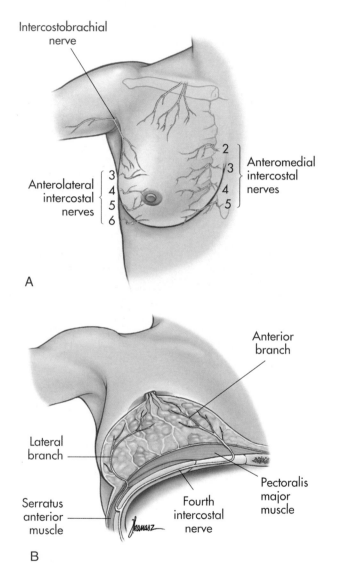

A, Innervation of breast. *B,* Innervation of NAC (nipple-areola complex). (From Achauer, BM, et al.: Plastic Surgery. St. Louis, Mosby, Inc., 2000.)

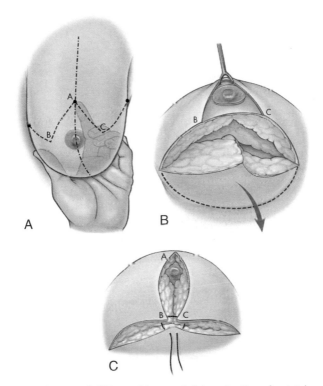

Pitanguy technique. *A,* Skin markings and determination of point A as the forward projection of IMF (inframammary fold). *B,* Deepithelialization within triangle ABC. En bloc excision of glandular tissue and skin in inverted "keel" shape from lower breast. *C,* closure of pillars is accomplished with few if any internal sutures. New areolar site is determined after partial closure of vertical limb of incision at approximately 4.5 to 5 cm from midline of IMF. (From Achauer, BM, et al.: Plastic Surgery. St. Louis, Mosby, Inc., 2000.)

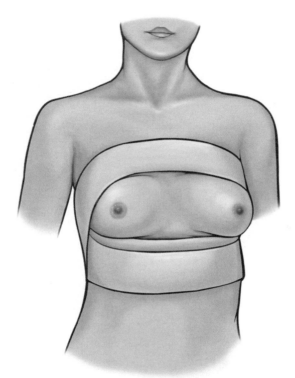

Example of elastic wrap used to maintain implant location and prevent implant migration immediately after surgery. Some wraps do not have an inframammary band, but rather simply a band over superior aspect of implant and breast. (From Achauer, BM, et al.: Plastic Surgery. St. Louis, Mosby, Inc., 2000.)

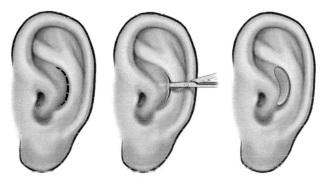

Anterior approach for harvesting ear cartilage graft. (From Achauer, BM, et al.: Plastic Surgery. St. Louis, Mosby, Inc., 2000.)

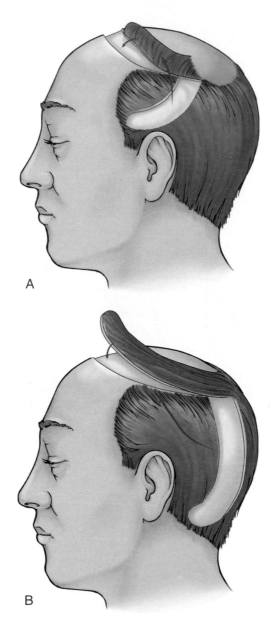

Dardour flaps. *A,* Preauricular. *B,* Postauricular. (From Achauer, BM, et al.:
Plastic Surgery. St. Louis, Mosby, Inc., 2000.)

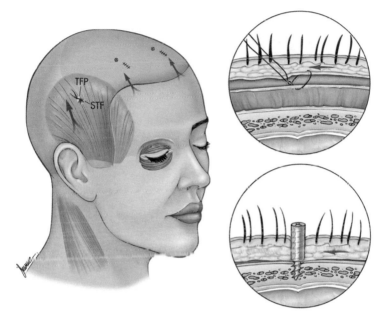

Endoforehead fixation technique. Superficial temporal fascia (STF) is anchored to temporal fascia proper (TFP) with two 3-0 PDS sutures (see inset, *top*). Frontal scalp is typically anchored with two endoscopic scalp posts (14 mm long, 4-mm stopper, 1.5-mm diameter screw portion). These posts are applied percutaneously away from frontal slit incisions and do not require skin staples for support of scalp against posts (see inset, *bottom*). (From Achauer, BM, et al.: Plastic Surgery. St. Louis, Mosby, Inc., 2000.)

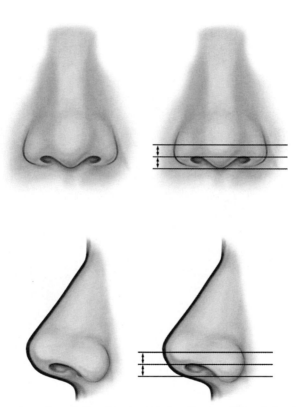

Ideal alar-columellar relationship, frontal view *(top)* and lateral view *(bottom)*.
(From Achauer, BM, et al.: Plastic Surgery. St. Louis, Mosby, Inc., 2000.)

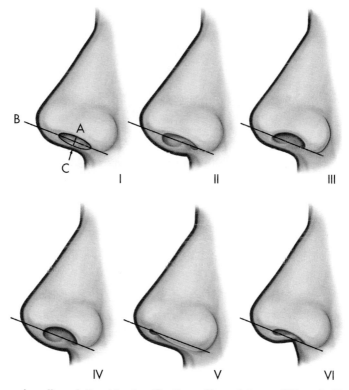

Alar-columellar relationship classifications. (From Achauer, BM, et al.: Plastic Surgery. St. Louis, Mosby, Inc., 2000.)

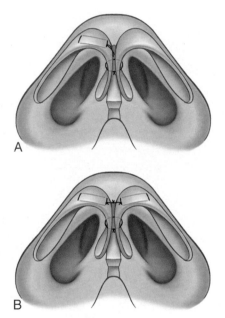

A, Transdomal suture. *B,* Joined transdomal sutures. (From Achauer, BM, et al.: Plastic Surgery. St. Louis, Mosby, Inc., 2000.)

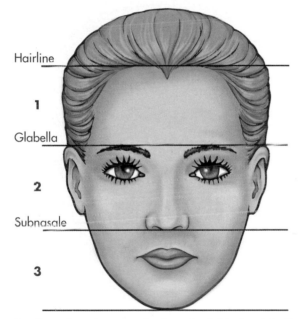

Lines passing through eyebrows and subnasale divide face into three equal zones. (From Achauer, BM, et al.: Plastic Surgery. St. Louis, Mosby, Inc., 2000.)

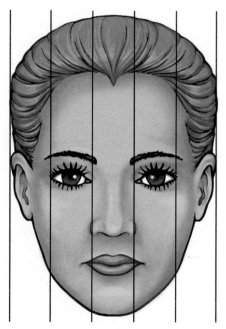

Width of upper face is 5 times that of palpebral fissure. Of five equal segments, two are occupied by eyes, one by nose, and two by temples. (From Achauer, BM, et al.: Plastic Surgery. St. Louis, Mosby, Inc., 2000.)

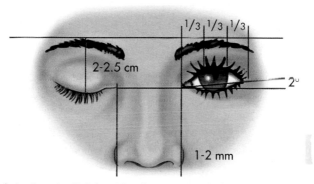

Width of alar base is slightly wider than intercanthal distance. Distance from eyelid to eyebrow and position of eyebrow arch in relation to iris are shown. (From Achauer, BM, et al.: Plastic Surgery. St. Louis, Mosby, Inc., 2000.)

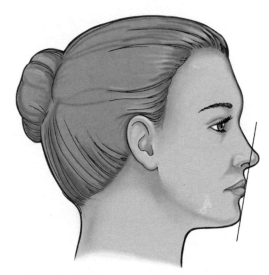

Reidel's plane of lip and chin line-up is straight line connecting most prominent portion of upper lip to lower lip. In pleasing profiles, line usually contacts most prominent portion of soft tissue chin. (From Achauer, BM, et al.: Plastic Surgery. St. Louis, Mosby, Inc., 2000.)

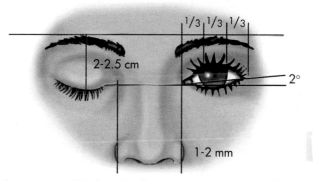

Width of alar base is slightly wider than intercanthal distance. Distance from eyelid to eyebrow and position of eyebrow arch in relation to iris are shown. (From Achauer, BM, et al.: Plastic Surgery. St. Louis, Mosby, Inc., 2000.)

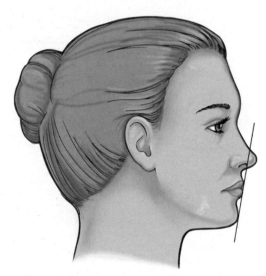

Reidel's plane of lip and chin line-up is straight line connecting most prominent portion of upper lip to lower lip. In pleasing profiles, line usually contacts most prominent portion of soft tissue chin. (From Achauer, BM, et al.: Plastic Surgery. St. Louis, Mosby, Inc., 2000.)

lactic
  l. acid
  l. dehydrogenase

LactoSorb
  L. resorbable craniomaxillofacial fixation
  L. craniofacial plate fixation system

lacuna
  absorption l.

LADD
  lacrimoauriculodentodigital
    LADD syndrome

Ladd lid clamp

LAG
  labiogingival

lag
  maturational l.
  l. screw
  l. screw fixation

lagophthalmos
  paretic l.

LaGrange scissors

lag screw
  l. s. fixation
  l. s. technique of interfragmentary compression

Lahey
  L. clamp
  L. tenaculum

LAI
  labioincisal

Laimer-Haeckerman area

lake
  lacrimal l.
  venous l.

Lakeside nasal scissors

LaLonde
  L. extra fine skin hook forceps
  L. skin hook forceps

lambdoid
  l. suture
  l. synostosis deformity
  l. synostotic plagiocephaly

Lambert-Eaton myasthenic syndrome

Lambone
  L. demineralized laminar bone
  L. freeze-dried bone

lamella
  cornoid l.
  haversian l.

lamina
  basal l.
  basal l. of ciliary body
  dentogingival l.
  l. dura
  l. dura–like appearance
  labial l.
  l. medialis
  palatine l.
  palatine l. of maxilla
  l. papyracea
  l. profunda
  l. propria
  vestibular l.

lamina-bud stage

laminagraph

laminagraphy
  cephalometric l.

laminar
  l. bone
  l. fat

LaminOss implant

Lamont
  L. nasal rasp
  L. saw

lamp
  mouth l.

lancet
  l. blade
  gingival l.

lancet *(continued)*
    gum l.
    Lipectron ultrasonic l.
    ultrasonic l.

lancinating

landmark
    cephalometric l.
    cranial base l.
    facial l.

Landolt eyelid reconstruction

Landry-Guillain-Barré syndrome

Landsmeer ligament

Lange
    L. plastic surgery hook
    L.-Converse nasal root ron-
    geur

Langenbeck
    L. operation
    L. palatorrhaphy
    L. with pharyngeal flap pal-
    atorrhaphy
    L. repair
    L. saw

Langer
    L. arch
    L. cleavage line
    L. line

Langerhans
    L. cells
    L. cell eosinophilic granu-
    loma
    L. cell granule
    L. cell granulomatosis
    L. cell histiocytosis
    L.-type giant cells

Langley
    L. ganglion
    L. granules

laparoscope

laparotomy pad

L approach

large-caliber nonabsorbable suture

large-cell lymphoma

large-pore polyethylene implant

LaRoe undermining forceps

Larsen syndrome

laryngeal
    l. abscess
    l. anesthesia
    l. angioleiomyoma
    l. anomaly
    l. artery
    l. atresia
    l. blastomycosis
    l. burn
    l. cancer
    l. carcinoid
    l. carcinoma
    l. cartilage
    l. cartilage fracture
    l. chondroma
    l. chondroradionecrosis
    l. chorea
    l. cleft
    l. cramp
    l. crisis
    l. diversion
    l. edema
    l. epilepsy
    external branch of the su-
    perior l. (EBSL) nerve
    l. fold
    l. framework surgery
    l. granuloma
    l. hemangioma
    l. hemorrhage
    l. hyperesthesia
    l. image biofeedback
    internal branch of the su-
    perior l. (IBSL) nerve
    l. lipoma
    l. mask
    l. mask airway (LMA)
    l. melanosis (LM)
    l. motor paralysis
    l. neoplasm

laryngeal *(continued)*
  l. nerve
  l. neuroendocrine carci-
    noma
  l. obstruction
  l. oscillation
  l. papillomatosis
  l. paraganglioma
  l. paresthesia
  l. perichondritis
  l. polyp
  l. prominence
  l. reflex
  l. release
  l. respiration
  l. saccular cyst
  l. saccule of Hilton
  l. sensory paralysis
  l. spasm
  l. stenosis
  l. stent
  l. stridor
  l. stuttering
  l. syncope
  l. syringe
  l. tension
  l. tuberculosis
  l. vein
  l. ventricle
  l. vestibule
  l. web

laryngectomy
  anterior partial l.
  frontolateral l.
  horizontovertical l.
  narrow-field l.
  near-total l.
  salvage l.
  subtotal l.
  subtotal supraglottic l.
    (SSL)
  supracricoid l.
  supraglottic l.
  total l.
  wide-field total l.

larynges *(pl.* of larynx)

laryngis
  ictus l.

laryngis *(continued)*
  myasthenia l.
  pachyderma l.
  ventriculus l.

laryngismus
  l. stridulus

laryngitic

laryngitis
  acute l.
  acute supraglottic l.
  chronic l.
  chronic hyperplastic l.
  chronic subglottic l.
  croupous l.
  hemorrhagic l.
  hyperplastic l.
  hypertrophic l.
  membranous l.
  l. sicca
  spasmodic l.
  l. stridulosa
  traumatic l.

laryngocele
  symptomatic l.

laryngofissure
  l. with tracheotomy

Laryngoflex reinforced endotracheal tube

laryngograph

laryngography

laryngology

laryngomalacia

laryngoparalysis

laryngopathy

laryngopharyngeal sensation

laryngopharyngectomy
  partial l. (PLP)
  total l. (TLP)

laryngopharyngitis

laryngopharyngoesophagec-
  tomy procedure

laryngopharynx

laryngophthisis

laryngoplasty
    sternothyroid muscle flap l.

laryngoplegia

laryngoptosis

laryngopyocele

laryngoscope
    Benjamin binocular slim-
      line l.
    Benjamin pediatric opera-
      ting l.
    Benjamin-Lindholm micro-
      suspension l.
    Dedo l.
    fiberoptic l.
    Holinger anterior commis-
      sure l.
    Jackson l.
    Jackson anterior commis-
      sure l.
    Jako l.
    Killian-Lynch suspension l.
    Kleinsasser anterior com-
      missure l.
    Lindholm operating l.
    Lynch suspension l.
    Storz-Hopkins l.
    Weerda distending opera-
      ting l.

laryngoscopic
    l. view

laryngoscopist

laryngoscopy
    direct l.
    flexible fiberoptic l.
    indirect l.
    laser l.
    microdirect l.
    suspension l.

laryngospasm

laryngospastic reflex

laryngostenosis

laryngostomy

laryngostroboscope

laryngotomy
    inferior l.
    median l.
    superior l.
    thyrohyoid l.
    transepiglottic l.

laryngotracheal
    l. diversion
    l. invasion
    l. reconstruction (LTR)
    l. stenosis
    l. trauma

laryngotracheitis

laryngotracheobronchitis

laryngotracheoesophageal cleft

larynx *pl.* larynges
    artificial l.
    chondromalacia of l.
    Cooper-Rand intraoral arti-
      ficial l.
    electrical artificial l.
    electronic artificial l.
    extrinsic muscles of l.
    glottic l.
    intrinsic muscles of l.
    neuroendocrine tumor of l.
    neurofibroma of l.
    Nu-Vois artificial l.
    pneumatic artificial l.
    supraglottic l.

Laschal scissors

LaseAway
    L. ruby laser system
    L. ruby and Q-switched Nd:
      YAG laser
    L. Smooth Touch laser

laser
    alexandrite l.
    ALEXlazr l.
    argon green l.
    argon tunable dye l.
    l.-assisted uvulopalato-
      plasty (LAUP)

laser *(continued)*
    Candela l.
    Candela pulsed dye l.
    carbon dioxide (CO_2) l.
    CB Erbium/2.94 l.
    char-free carbon dioxide l.
    CLR 2940 erbium l.
    CO_2 (carbon dioxide) l.
    CO_2 l. blepharoplasty
    CO_2 FeatherTouch Silk-
      Laser
    CO_2 SilkLaser
    l. coagulation
    Coherent argon l.
    Coherent UltraPulse l.
    Coherent UltraPulse
      5000C l.
    cold beam l.
    continuous wave l.
    continuous wave CO_2 l.
    copper vapor l.
    Cynosure l.
    Derma 20 l.
    Derma K combination l.
    diode pumped Nd:YAG l.
    l. dissection technique
    l. Doppler flowmeter
    l. Doppler flowmetry
    l. Doppler perfusion moni-
      tor
    l. endoforeheadplasty
    endoscopic brow lift with
      simultaneous carbon di-
      oxide l. resurfacing
    EpiLaser hair removal l.
    erbium CrystaLase l.
    esthetic CO_2 l.
    excimer ultraviolet l.
    l. festoon reduction
    flashlamp-excited long-
      pulse alexandrite l.
    flashlamp-excited pulsed
      dye l.
    flashlamp pulsed dye
      (FLPD) l.
    flashlamp-pumped pulsed
      dye l. (FPPDL) 510 nm
    flashlamp-pumped pulsed
      dye l. (FPPDL) 585 nm
    gas l.

laser *(continued)*
    25 Gold portable CO_2 l.
    l. hair transplant
    l. hair transplantation
    helium-neon (He-Ne) l.
    HGM Spectrum K1 krypton
      yellow and green l.
    holmium l.
    holmium:YAG l.
    l. holography
    I.L.MED l.
    l. incisional blepharoplasty
    2.5 joule Erbium resurfa-
      cing l.
    krypton l.
    krypton l. with Hexascan
    KTP l.
    KTP/532 l.
    KTP/YAG l.
    l. laryngoscopy
    LaseAway ruby and Q-
      switched Nd:YAG l.
    LaseAway Smooth Touch l.
    l. lower lid transconjuncti-
      val blepharoplasty
    Luxar NovaPulse CO_2 l.
    MedLite Q-Switched neo-
      dymium-doped yttrium-
      aluminum-garnet l.
    MedLite Q-Switched YAG l.
    l. meloplasty
    MultiLase D copper vapor l.
    NaturaLase Erbium l.
    NaturaLase Er:YAG l.
    Nd:YAG (neodymium:yt-
      trium-aluminum-garnet) l.
    Nd:YAG l. with Hexascan
    neodymium:yttrium-alumi-
      num-garnet (Nd:YAG) l.
    510-nm pigmented lesion
      dye l.
    NovaPulse l.
    NovaPulse CO_2 l.
    Paragon l.
    PBI Medical copper vapor l.
    PBI MultiLase D copper va-
      por l.
    PhotoDerm PL l.
    PhotoDerm T l.
    PhotoDerm T10 l.

laser *(continued)*
  PhotoDerm V l.
  PhotoDerm VL l.
  PhotoDerm VLS pulsed
    dye l.
  PhotoGenica LPIR with
    TKS l.
  PhotoGenica T10 l.
  PhotoGenica V l.
  PhotoGenica VLS pulsed
    dye l.
  Polytec LaseAway Q-
    switched ruby l.
  potassium titanyl phos-
    phate l.
  pulsed dye l.
  pulsed tunable dye l.
  pulsed yellow dye l.
  QS alexandrite l.
  QS neodymium:yttrium-alu-
    minum-garnet (Nd:YAG) l.
  QS ruby l.
  QS ruby/YAG l.
  Q-switched alexandrite l.
  Q-switched neodymium:
    yttrium-aluminum-garnet
    (Nd:YAG) l.
  Q-switched ruby l.
  Q-switched ruby/YAG l.
  resurfacing l.
  l. resurfacing
  ruby l.
  Sharplan l.
  Sharplan L. 710 Acuspot
  Sharplan argon l.
  Sharplan CO_2 l.
  Sharplan SilkTouch flash-
    scan surgical l.
  SharpLase Nd:YAG l.
  l. shield
  Silhouette endoscopic l.
  SilkLaser aesthetic CO_2 l.
  Silktouch l.
  Skinlight erbium:YAG (yt-
    trium-aluminum-garnet) l.
  l. skin resurfacing
  l. smoke evacuation
  SoftLight l.
  Spectrum K1 l.

laser *(continued)*
  Spectrum ruby l.
  l. stapedectomy
  l. stapedotomy
  l. stereolithography pro-
    cess
  l. surgery
  Surgica K6 l.
  Surgipulse XJ 150 CO_2 l.
  l. system
  TKS l.
  Tru-Pulse carbon dioxide l.
  Tru-Pulse CO_2 skin resur-
    facing l.
  tunable dye l.
  tunable dye l. with Hexas-
    can
  tunable flashlamp-excited
    pulsed dye l.
  two-joule erbium l.
  UltraPulse carbon dioxide l.
  UltraPulse CO_2 l.
  ultrapulsed l.
  Unilase CO_2 l.
  Vbeam pulsed dye l.
  VersaLight l.
  l. welding
  YAG (yttrium-aluminum-
    garnet) l.

laserbrasion
  UltraPulse carbon dioxide l.

Lasercare
  Elysee L.

Laserflo BPM laser Doppler
  monitor

Laserscope

Laser-Shield XII wrapped endotracheal tube

LaserSite
  L. facial mask
  L. wound dressing

Laser Trach wrapped endotracheal tube

Lasertubus

lasing

latissimus
l. dorsi breast reconstruction
l. dorsi flap
l. dorsi muscle
l. dorsi muscle flap
l. dorsi musculocutaneous
flap
l. dorsi myocutaneous flap
(LDMCF)
l. dorsi/scapular bone flap
l. dorsi segmental musculovascular pedicle
l. fasciocutaneous turnover
flap
l. muscle flap
total autogenous l. (TAL)

LATRAM
simultaneous LATRAM and
mastectomy (SLAM)

Latrobe retractor

lattice
l. fiber
l. space

LAUP
laser-assisted uvulopalatoplasty

LAV
lymphadenopathy-associ-
ated virus

LaVeen helical stripper

law
Halsted l.
Heidenhain l.
Virchow l.

laxity
aponeurotic l.
l. of cheeks
eyelid l.
fascial l.
glabellar l.
horizontal lid l.
ligamentous l.
musculofascial l.

laxity *(continued)*
orbicularis l.
skin l.
submental l.

layer
adipose l's of anterior abdominal wall
basal l.
cambrium l.
closed in anatomic l's
cornified l.
Dermanet wound contact l.
facial fascial l.
fascial l.
granular l.
granular cell l.
Huxley l.
inner fibrous l.
intercellular l.
intermediate l.
musculoaponeurotic l.
outer fibrous l.
parakeratotic l.
parietal l.
silica-carbon l.
subdermal l.
submucous l.
surface cell l.
Weil basal l.

LCS
lateral crural steal

LDMCF
latissimus dorsi myocuta-
neous flap

leak
cerebrospinal fluid l.
halo test for cerebrospinal
fluid (CSF) l.

leakage
silicone l.

leash
subcutaneous l.

Le Dentu suture

leech
medicinal l.

Le Fort
  Le F. I fracture
  Le F. I impaction
  Le F. I osteotomy
  Le F. I procedure
  Le F. I–type osteotomy
  Le F. II fracture
  Le F. II osteotomy
  Le F. II procedure
  Le F. II–type midface oste-
    otomy
  Le F. III advancement oste-
    otomy
  Le F. III craniofacial dis-
    junction
  Le F. III fracture
  Le F. III procedure
  Le F. classification of maxil-
    lary fractures (I, II, III)
  greenstick Le F. fracture
  horseshoe Le F. osteotomy
  Le F. maxillary osteotomy
  Le F. osteotomy procedure
  Le F. suture

Leibinger
  L. 3-D bone plate
  L. E-Z flap
  L. Micro Plus plate
  L. Micro Plus screw
  L. Mini-Würzburg plate
  L. Mini-Würzburg screw
  L. plating
  L. plating system
  self-tapping L. lag screw
  L. titanium Würzburg man-
    dibular reconstruction
    system
  L. Würzburg screw

leiomyoma

leiomyosarcoma
  mandibular l.

leishmaniasis
  Brazilian l.

Leitz 1600 Saw microtome

Lejour
  L. breast reduction

Lejour (continued)
  L. mammaplasty
  L. mastoplasty
  L. technique

Leksell rongeur

Lell laryngofissure saw

Le Mesurier repair

length
  anterior arch l.
  arch l.
  available arch l.
  basialveolar l.
  l. of mandible
  mandibular body l.
  maxilloalveolar l.
  muscle moment arm l.
  Nance analysis of arch l.
  palatal l.
  l. of palate
  physiognomic l.
  required arch l.
  sill l.
  upper lip l.

lengthening
  distraction l.
  levator Müller complex l.
  penile l.
  tendon l.

lens
  Hopkins II rod l.

lentigo pl. lentigines
  l. maligna melanoma
  senile l.
  l. senilis
  simple l.
  l. simplex
  solar l.

Leon
  L. cannula
  L. cobra cannula
  L. cobra tip

leonine facies

leprosy

Leri
  L.-Weill disease

Leri *(continued)*
    L.-Weill syndrome

Leser-Trélat sign

Lesgaft space

lesion
    acneiform l.
    aggressive l.
    benign epidermal pigmen-
        ted l.
    benign lymphoepithelial l.
        (BLL)
    bullous l.
    caviar l.
    circumscribed l.
    clival l.
    combined-flow l.
    cutaneous vascular l.
    cylindromatous l.
    cystic l.
    cystic lymphoepithelial
        AIDS-related l.
    epulis-like l.
    erythroplakic l.
    fibromyxomatous l.
    fibro-osseous l.
    floor-of-mouth l.
    fungating l.
    giant cell l.
    gross l.
    ground-glass l.
    hamartomatous l.
    hyperplastic l.
    hyperplastic epithelial l.
    inflammatory l.
    interradicular l.
    intrabony l.
    intraosseous l.
    lateral hemifacial l.
    lymphoepithelial l.
    melanocytic l.
    monostotic l.
    mucoepidermoid l.
    neurapraxic l.
    nonneoplastic tumorlike l.
    oromandibular l.
    osteoporotic l.
    papulosquamous l.
    papulovesicular l.
    pigmented l.

lesion *(continued)*
    precancerous l.
    primary l.
    radiolucent l.
    radiopaque l.
    reticular l.
    satellite l.
    scalene l.
    scaling l.
    scaling skin-colored l.
    secondary l.
    sessile l.
    skin l.
    skip l.
    slope-shouldered l.
    smooth l.
    smooth skin-colored l.
    soft l.
    solitary l.
    spiculated l.
    spongiotic l.
    square-shouldered l.
    Stener l.
    systemic l.
    target l.
    varicelliform l.
    variegated l's
    vasculitic l.
    Vaughan-Jackson l.
    verrucous l.
    vesicobullous l.
    vesiculobullous l.
    weeping l.
    white-spot l.

lesser
    l. horn
    l. palatine artery
    l. petrosal nerve
    l. superficial petrosal nerve
    l. wing of sphenoid

leukemia

leukemic hyperplastic gingivitis

leukocyte
    l. infiltration
    neutrophilic l.
    polymorphonuclear l.

leukocytic infiltration

leukodontia

leukoedema

leukokeratosis
l. nicotina palati

leukopenia

leukoplakia
l. buccalis
dyskeratotic l.
friction/trauma-associ-
ated l.
hairy l. (HL)
idiopathic/tobacco-associ-
ated l.
l. lingualis
nondyskeratotic l.
oral l.
oral hairy l.
speckled l.
verruciform l.
verrucous l.

leukotome
Freeman transorbital l.

Leurs nasal rasp

levator
l. anguli oris muscle
l. aponeurosis surgery
l. complex
l. costae muscle
l. dehiscence
l. disinsertion
l. glandulae thyroidea muscle
l. labii superioris alaeque
nasi muscle
l. labii superioris muscle
l.-Müller complex lengthening
l. muscle
l. muscle of angle of mouth
l. palatini muscle
l. palpebrae superioris
l. resection
l. veli palatini muscle

level
serum complement l.

Levy articulating retractor

Lewis-Tanner esophagectomy

Lewy
L. laryngoscope holder
L. suspension device

Lezinski Flex-HA PORP ossicu-
lar chain prosthesis

LF
lingual fossa

lichen
atrophic l. planus
bullous l. planus

Lichtman classification of Kienböck disease (*stages I, II, IIIA,
IIIB, IV*)

lid
l. retraction
l. retractor
scalloping of lower l.
l.-loading technique
l.-sharing technique

LIE
labioincisal edge
linguoincisal edge

lifeboat flap

LifeCell AlloDerm acellular dermal graft

Lifecore
L. cutting advance technology
L. Restore wide diameter
implant

lift
arm l.
bicoronal forehead l.
biplanar forehead l.
breast l.
brow l.
brow-forehead l.
buttocks l.
canthal l.
chin l.
corner mouth l.
coronal brow l.
deep-plane l.

lift *(continued)*
    endoforehead l.
    endoforehead-endomid-
      face l.
    endoforehead-periorbital-
      cheek l.
    endomidface l.
    endoscopically assisted
      brow l.
    endoscopic brow l.
    endoscopic brow l. with si-
      multaneous carbon diox-
      ide laser resurfacing
    endoscopic forehead l.
    endoscopic subperiosteal
      forehead l.
    endoscopic subperiosteal
      forehead and midface l.
    endoscopic subperiosteal
      midface l.
    endotemporal l.
    endotemporal-endomid-
      face l.
    eyebrow l.
    face-l. *(see* face-lift)
    facial subcutaneous l.
    FAME midface l.
    forehead l.
    frontal l.
    functional l.
    inner thigh l.
    mask l.
    midface l.
    modified anterior hairline
      forehead l.
    open coronal brow l.
    palatal l.
    scalp l.
    SMAS (superficial muscu-
      loaponeurotic system) l.
    subcutaneous temporofa-
      cial face-l.
    subcutaneous temporoma-
      lar face-l.
    subperiosteal brow l.
    subperiosteal malar
      cheek l.
    subperiosteal mid-face l.
    subperiosteal minimally in-
      vasive face-l.

lift *(continued)*
    subperiosteal minimally in-
      vasive laser endoscopic
      (SMILE) rhytidectomy
    temporomandibular endos-
      copic l.
    thigh l.
    transblepharoplasty fore-
      head l.
    transcoronal eyebrow l.

lifting
    face l.
    forehead l.

ligament
    accessory collateral l.
    alar l.
    alveolodental l.
    annular l.
    anterior mallear l.
    anterior suspensory l.
    apical dental l.
    Berry l.
    Broyle l.
    capitolunate l.
    carpometacarpal l.
    circular dental l.
    Cleland l.
    collateral l.
    Colles l.
    Cooper l's
    cricothyroid l.
    dentoalveolar l.
    dorsal radioulnar l.
    external l. of mandibular
      articulation
    external l. of temporoman-
      dibular articulation
    external l. of temporoman-
      dibular joint
    facial retaining l's
    Ferrein l.
    gingival l.
    gingivodental l.
    Grayson l.
    hammock l.
    hyoepiglottic l.
    incudal l.
    interdental l.
    intermetatarsal l.

ligament *(continued)*
- labiomandibular l.
- Landsmeer l.
- lateral l. of temporomandibular articulation
- lateral accessory l. of Henle
- lateral collateral l.
- lateral mallear l.
- lateral maxillary l.
- lateral thyrohyoid l.
- lateral TMJ l.
- Lockwood l.
- lunotriquetral l.
- lunotriquetral interosseous l. (LTIL)
- mallear l.
- maxillary l.
- median thyrohyoid l.
- nasolabial l.
- nasomandibular l.
- oblique retinacular l.
- palmar l's
- palmar beak l.
- palmar radioulnar l.
- peridental l.
- periimplant l.
- periodontal l. (PDL)
- petroclinoid l.
- posterior incudal l.
- posterior suspensory l.
- Poupart l.
- radiocarpal l.
- radioscapholunate l.
- l. reinsertion
- Sappey l.
- scapholunate l.
- scapholunate interosseous l.
- Soemmering l.
- sphenomandibular l.
- spiral l.
- stylohyoid l.
- stylomandibular l.
- superior incudal l.
- superior mallear l.
- suspensory l.
- temporomandibular l.
- thyroepiglottic l.
- thyrohyoid l.
- transseptal l.

ligament *(continued)*
- transverse l. of Landsmeer
- transverse metacarpal l.
- Treitz l.
- true collateral l.
- Valsalva l's
- volar beak l.
- volar carpal l.
- volar radiocarpal l.
- Whitnall l.
- Zinn l.
- zygomatic l.
- zygomatic osteocutaneous l.
- zygomatic retaining l's

ligamental anesthesia

ligamentous facial fence

ligate

ligation
- endoscopic band l. (EBL)
- endoscopic variceal l. (EVL)
- interdental l.
- parotid l.
- parotid duct l.
- sling l.
- surgical l.
- teeth l.
- tooth l.
- transesophageal varix l.
- transnasal l. of internal maxillary artery

ligature
- anchor with suture l.
- catgut l.
- l. cutter
- elastic l.
- grass-line l.
- l.-locking pliers
- occluding l.
- orthodontic l.
- plastic l.
- steel l.
- l. tie wire
- l.-tying pliers

ligatureless bracket

light
    Wood l.

limb
    l. bud
    complete cutaneous syn-
        dactyly of all four l's
    l. duplication
    horizontal l.
    l. hypertrophy
    l. salvage
    supernumerary l.

Limberg
    L. local transposition flap
    L.-type cutaneous flap

limb-sparing procedure

limbus
    alveolar l. of mandible
    alveolar l. of maxilla
    l. alveolaris mandibulae
    l. alveolaris maxillae

Linburg sign

Lindeman
    L. bone cutter
    L. bur

Lindholm operating laryngo-
    scope

line
    accretion l.
    alveolar point–basion l.
    alveolar point–nasal
        point l.
    alveolar point–nasion l.
    alveolobasilar l.
    alveolonasal l.
    l. angle
    anterior axillary l.
    antitension l. (ATL)
    arcuate l.
    Burton l.
    Camper l.
    canthomeatal l.
    cerebral reference l.
    cervical l. (CL)
    Clapton l.
    contour l.

line (continued)
    cross arch fulcrum l.
    demarcation l.
    developmental l.
    external oblique l.
    feathered-edge proximal
        finishing l.
    feather-edged proximal fin-
        ishing l.
    fine l.
    finish l.
    flexion skin l's
    Frankfort horizontal l.
    frontal zygomatic suture l.
    frontozygomatic suture l.
    frown l's
    gingival l.
    gingival finishing l.
    glabellar l.
    glabellar frown l.
    gray l. of upper eyelid
    gum l.
    hemiclavicular l.
    high lip l.
    high smile l.
    His l.
    Holdaway l.
    Hunter l.
    Hunter-Schreger l.
    hyperfunctional facial l.
    hyperfunctional glabellar l.
    imbrication l's of von Eb-
        ner
    incremental l.
    incremental l's of cemen-
        tum
    incremental l's of von Eb-
        ner
    infraciliary l.
    innominate l.
    knife-edged finishing l.
    labial l.
    Langer l.
    Langer cleavage l.
    lead l.
    lip l.
    load l.
    low lip l.

line *(continued)*
    marionette l.
    median l.
    mercurial l.
    methylene blue l.
    middle cranial fossa l.
    milk l.
    mucogingival l.
    mylohyoid l.
    nasion-alveolar point l.
    nasolabial l.
    neonatal l.
    oblique l.
    l. of occlusion
    Öhngren l.
    orbital l.
    Owen's l.
    Pickerill imbrication l.
    protrusive l.
    radiolucent l.
    recessional l.
    relaxed skin tension l's
     (RSTL)
    resting l.
    retentive fulcrum l.
    l's of Retzius
    reversal l.
    sagittal suture l.
    Salter incremental l's
    S-BP l.
    Schreger l's
    sinus l.
    smoker's l's
    S-N l.
    sphenofrontal suture l.
    sphenoparietal suture l.
    Spigelius l.
    squamous suture l's
    stabilizing fulcrum l.
    subcutaneous fat l's
    submammary l.
    survey l.
    Tatagiba l.
    temporal l.
    tension skin l's
    Terry l.
    Thompson l.
    vertical corrugator l.
    vertical glabellar frown l's

line *(continued)*
    von Ebner l.
    l's of von Ebner
    Webster l.
    wrinkle l's
    zygomatic suture l.

linea
    l. alba
    l. alba buccalis
    l. aspera
    l. temporalis

linear
    l. graft
    l. osteotomy
    l. scleroderma

lined flap

liner
    Ac'cents permanent
     lash l.
    Accu-Spense cavity l.
    cavity l.
    lash l.

lingua *gen. and pl.* linguae
    l. alba
    copula linguae
    l. dissecta
    l. fissurata
    l. frenata
    frenulum linguae
    l. geographica
    l. nigra
    nigrities linguae
    pityriasis linguae
    l. plicata
    tylosis linguae
    l. villosa alba
    l. villosa nigra

linguadental *(variant of* linguodental*)*

lingual
    l. alveolus
    l. angle
    l. approach

lingual *(continued)*
  l. apron
  l. arch
  l. arch-forming pliers
  l. artery
  l. attachment
  l. bone
  l. button
  l. cavity
  l. clasp
  l. cortical plate
  l. cyst
  l. developmental groove
    (LDG)
  l. dovetail
  l. duct
  l. embrasure
  l. flange
  l. flap
  l. follicle
  l. foramen
  l. fossa (LF)
  l. frenulum
  l. frenum
  l. gingiva
  l. gland
  l. groove (LG)
  l. hemiatrophy
  l. hypoplasia
  l. inclination
  l. lobe
  l. lymph follicle
  l. lymph node
  l. mandibular periosteum
  l. movement
  l. mucoperiosteal flap
  l. mucosa
  l. nerve
  l. occlusion
  l. papilla
  l. paralysis
  l. peak
  l. periosteum
  l. placement
  l. plate
  l. plexus
  l. root
  l. saliva
  l. salivary gland depression

lingual *(continued)*
  l. septum
  l. shield
  l. splint
  l. split-bone technique
  l. strap
  l. sulcus
  l. surface
  l. thyroid
  l. thyroid carcinoma
  l. tongue flap
  l. trophoneurosis
  l. wire

lingualis
  papillae linguales

lingula *pl.* lingulae
  l. of mandible
  l. mandibulae

lingulectomy

linguoalveolar
  l. area

linguoangular

linguoaxial

linguoaxiogingival

linguocervical
  l. ridge

linguoclination

linguoclusion

linguodental
  l. area

linguodistal (LD)

linguogingival
  l. fissure
  l. ridge
  l. shoulder

linguoincisal (LI)
  l. edge (LIE)
  l. line angle

linguopalatal contact

linguopapillitis

linguoplacement

linguoplasty

linguoplate
  l. major connector
  palatal l.

linguoproximal

linguopulpal (LP)

lining
  mucoperiosteal l.

Linkow blade implant

Linscheid test

Linton flap

lion jaw bone holder

lip
  l. augmentation
  bilateral cleft l. and palate
    (BCLP)
  l. biting
  l. border advancement
  l. bumper
  cleft l. (CL)
  cleft l./alveolus (CLA)
  cleft l. and palate (CLP)
  l. competency
  complete cleft l.
  l. curtain
  double l.
  l. elevator
  l. enhancement
  frenulum of superior l.
  l. furrow band
  l. habit appliance
  Hapsburg l.
  l. hypertonia
  incisive muscle of lower l.
  incisive muscle of upper l.
  l. incompetence
  incompetent upper l.
  inferior l.
  inferior l. of pons
  isolated unilateral cleft l./
    alveolus (UCLA)
  l. line
  lower l.
  median cleft l.

lip (continued)
  mucous membrane of l.
  l. paresthesia
  l. pit
  l. plumper
  l. pucker
  quadrate muscle of lower l.
  quadrate muscle of upper l.
  red zone of l.
  l. retractor
  l. rounding
  square muscle of lower l.
  square muscle of upper l.
  superior l.
  l. switch flap
  tubercle of upper l.
  unilateral cleft l.
  unilateral cleft l. and palate
  upper l.
  vermilion border of l.
  vermilion surface of l.

lipectomy
  abdominal l.
  blunt suction l.
  jowl reduction l.
  orbital l.
  suction l.
  suction-assisted l. (SAL)
  transjunctival l.
  ultrasound-assisted l.
    (UAL)

Lipectron
  L. ultrasonic lancet
  L. ultrasonic scalpel

lipexeresis

lip-lip flap

lipoaspirated material

lipoaspiration

lipoatrophy

lipoblastoma
  benign l.

lipocontour

lipocontouring
  suction-assisted l.

lipodissector
    Aspiradeps l.

lipodystrophy
    congenital generalized l.
    facial l.
    traumatic l.

lipofilling

lipogenic tumor

lipogranuloma

lipogranulomatosis
    sclerosing l.

lipohypertrophic mass

lipohypertrophy
    insulin-induced l.

lipoidosis cutis et mucosae

lipoinfiltration
    periorbital l.

lipoinjection technique

lipo layering technique

lipolysis
    suction-assisted l.

lipoma
    l. arborescens
    l. aspiration
    atypical l.
    hypopharyngeal l.
    laryngeal l.
    posttraumatic l.
    salivary l.
    spindle cell l.
    subcutaneous l.

lipomatosis
    benign symmetric l.

Lipo-Medi girdle

lipomyxoma

liponecrosis

liponecrotic pseudocyst

Lipopanty girdle

lipoplasty
    blunt suction-assisted l.
    Fischer aspirative l.
    Illouz aspirative l.
    Kesselring aspirative l.
    Schrudde aspirative l.
    Teimourian aspirative l.
    traditional l.

liporestructure

liposarcoma
    adult-type well-differentia-
        ted l.
    myxoid l.
    pleomorphic l.
    round-cell l.

liposculpture
    superficial l.
    syringe l.

liposculpturing
    ultrasonic l.

liposhaver

lipostructure

liposuction
    l.-assisted
    l. cannula
    l. divot
    extended l.
    l. fat fillant implant
    massive all layer l. (MALL)
    submental l.
    syringe-assisted l.
    l. technique
    tumescent l.
    ultrasonic l.
    ultrasound l.
    ultrasound-assisted l.
    wet technique l.

liposuctioning

liposurgery
    cervicofacial l.

Lipovacutainer canister

lip-splitting incision

lipstick sign

lip-sucking habit crib

liquefaction
    bone l.
    l. necrosis

liquefactive necrosis

Lisfranc joint

lisp
    dental l.
    frontal l.
    interdental l.
    lateral l.
    lingual l.
    nasal l.
    occluded l.
    protrusion l.
    strident l.
    substitutional l.

Lister tubercle

Lite blade

Lite-Pipe
    Millard L.-P.

lithiasis
    salivary l.

lithotomy
    l. position
    l. procedure

lithotripsy
    intracorporeal l.

Littauer
    L. dissecting scissors
    L. Junior suture scissors
    L. stitch scissors
    L. suture scissors

Little area

Littler
    L. flap
    L. neurovascular island flap
    L. suture carrying scissors

liver spot

LM
    laryngeal melanosis

LM (continued)
    light microscopy

LMA
    laryngeal mask airway

lobe
    deep parotid l.
    ear l. (variant of earlobe)
    flocculonodular l.
    frontal l.
    lingual l.
    occipital l.
    parietal l.
    parotid l.
    supplemental l.
    temporal l.
    thyroid l.

lobectomy
    deep l.
    ipsilateral total l. and con-
       tralateral subtotal l.
    thyroid l.
    total ipsilateral l.

lobular carcinoma

lobulated tongue

lobule
    ear l.
    myxoid l.
    prominent l.

local
    l. analgesia
    l. anesthesia
    l. anesthetic
    l. excision
    l. flap
    l. infiltrative anesthesia
       (LIA)
    l. nerve block
    l. rotation flap
    l. vasodilation

locally invasive congenital cellular blue nevus of scalp

locator
    apex l.

locked septal displacement

Lockwood ligament

Lombard-Boies rongeur

Longacre graft augmentation

long bone reconstruction

longitudinal
  l. cerebral fissure
  l. melanonychia
  l. muscle of tongue
  l. raphe
  l. raphe of tongue
  l. ridge of hard palate
  l. suture
  l. suture of palate

longitudinalis
  l. inferior muscle
  l. superior muscle

long-skin flap blepharoplasty

longus
  l. capitis muscle
  l. colli muscle
  palmaris l.

loop
  arterial l.
  Hyrtl l.
  venous l.

loose premaxilla

Looser zones

lop ear
  persistent l. e.

Lorenz-Rees nasal rasp

loss
  crestal bone l.
  full-thickness flap l.
  insertion l.
  nerve l.
  segmental l. of helix
  sensory l.
  vertical bone l.
  weight l.

Love
  L. nasal splint

Love (continued)
  L. nerve retractor

love handles

Löwenberg forceps

lower
  l. anterior forceps
  l. arch
  l. lateral cartilage
  l. lip
  l. lip–splitting incision
  l. trapezius flap

low-flying bird incision

low lip line

LTIL
  lunotriquetral interosseous
  ligament

LTTF
  lateral transverse thigh flap

LTR
  laryngotracheal reconstruction

lubricant
  silicone l.

Lucas alveolar curet

Luc operation

Luer-Lok
  L.-L. adapter
  Klein Delrin L.-L. handle

Luhr
  L. fixation plate
  L. implant
  L. maxillofacial fixation sys-
  tem
  L. microfixation system
  L. Vitallium micromesh
  plate
  L. Vitallium screw

Lukens
  L. collecting tube
  L. needle
  L. retractor
  L. trap

lumbar
l. drainage
l. periosteal turnover flap
l. puncture
l. roll

lumbosacral back flap

lumbrical-plus finger

lumen
acinar l.
intercalated duct l.

lumpectomy

lumpy jaw

Lund and Browder chart for
burn estimation

lunotriquetral
l. instability
l. interosseous ligament
(LTIL)
l. joint
l. ligament
l. motion
l. tear

lunate
l. bone
l. excision
l. sinus of radius
l. sinus of ulna

lupus
l. erythematosus
l. pernio
l. vulgaris

Luschka
L. bursa
L. cartilage
L. gland
L. sinus

lusoria
dysphagia l.

Luxar NovaPulse CO$_2$ laser

luxation
habitual temporomandibu-
lar joint l.

luxation *(continued)*
temporomandibular l.
traumatic l.

lymph
l. capillary
dental l.
dentinal l.
l. node
l. nodule

lymphadenectomy

lymphadenitis
mycobacterial l.
Toxoplasma l.

lymphadenoma
sebaceous l.

lymphadenopathy
infectious l.
persistent generalized l.

lymphadenopathy-associated
virus (LAV)

lymphadenosis
benign l.

lymphangiohemangioma
cavernous l.

lymphangioma
capillary l.
cavernous l.
l. circumscriptum
cystic l.
solitary simple l.
l. superficium simplex

lymphangioplasty

lymphangitis
sclerosing l.

lymphatic
afferent l.
l. capillary
l. drainage
l. fistula
l. follicle
l. follicle of tongue
l. malformation
l. massage

lymphatic *(continued)*
    l. metastasis
    l. nodule
    l. vessel

lymphaticovenous anastomosis

lymphedema

lymphocytic choriomeningitis

lymphocytoma
    benign l. cutis

lymphoepithelial
    l. cyst
    l. lesion
    l. proliferation

lymphoepithelioma
    malignant l.

lymphoma
    Burkitt l.
    Burkitt l. of nasal ala
    Castleman l.
    cutaneous T-cell l. (CTCL)
    diffuse large cell l.
    endemic Burkitt l.
    extranodal malignant l.
    extranodal non-Hodgkin l.

lymphoma *(continued)*
    follicular l.
    giant follicle l.
    Hodgkin l.
    large-cell l.
    malignant l.
    non-Hodgkin l.
    sporadic Burkitt l.

lymphomatosa
    struma l.

lymphomatosum
    cystadenoma l.
    papillary cystadenoma l.

lymphonodular pharyngitis

lymphoplasty

lymphoproliferative
    l. disorder

lymphorrhea

lymphosarcoma

lymphovenous malformation

Lynch suspension laryngoscope

LySonix TTD Design Mercedes

3M
 3M CTRS device
 3M mammary implant
 3M microvascular anasto-
  motic coupling device
 3M syndrome

M4
 M4 Kerr Safety Hedstrom
  instrument
 M4 safety handpiece

MA
 main arteriole
 mental age

mA
 milliampere

MAA
 mandibular advancement
  appliance

Macalister
 ethmoidal spine of M.

MacArthur Communicative De-
 velopment Inventories

McBurney point

McCall
 M. curet
 M. festoon
 M. instrument
 M. scaler

McCollum attachment

McComb procedure

McCraw
 M. gracilis myocutaneous
  flap
 M. technique

McCune-Albright syndrome

maceration
 flap m.
 skin m.

Macewen
 M. sign

Macewen *(continued)*
 M. symptom
 M. triangle

MacFee incision

McGhan
 468 M. Biocell anatomical
  breast implant
 M. fill kit

McGill Pain Questionnaire

McGivney forceps

McGoon technique

McGregor forehead flap

Machida light source connector

machine
 casting m.
 electric casting m.
 MDA ultrasound-assisted lipoplasty m.
 Medicamat ultrasound-as-
  sisted lipoplasty m.
 Mentor ultrasound-assisted
  lipoplasty m.
 Morwel ultrasound-assisted
  lipoplasty m.
 OsteoPower drilling and
  cutting m.
 Sebbin ultrasound-assisted
  lipoplasty m.
 SMEI ultrasound-assisted lipoplasty m.
 Sono-stat Plus EMG m.
 Status-X m.
 Surgitron ultrasound-as-
  sisted lipoplasty m.

machinable apatite-free glass
 ceramic

machining
 computer assisted design/
  computer assisted m.

machinist's gauge

McIndoe
 M. inlay graft

273

McIndoe *(continued)*
 M. method
 M. skin graft
 M. technique
 M. and Reese alar cartilage
   suture fixation

MacKay nasal splint

MacKenty
 M. scissors
 M. septal elevator

MacKenzie syndrome

McKissock
 bilateral M. reduction
   mammaplasty
 M. keyhole areolar template

MacLeod capsular rheumatism

McReynolds pterygium scissors

macrocalcification

macrocephaly

macrocheilia
 port-wine m.

macrochilia *(variant of ma-crocheilia)*

macrodactyly

macrofilled resin

macrofiller

macrogenia

macrogingivae

macroglobulin
 alpha$_2$-m.

macroglobulinemia
 Waldenström m.

macroglossia
 amyloid m.
 unilateral m.

macroglossic

macrognathia
 mandibular m.

macrognathia *(continued)*
 maxillary m.

macrognathic

macroinjection of autologous
 fat

macromastia

macrophage
 blood-borne m.
 chemotactic factor for m.
   (CFM)
 pulpal m.
 tissue m.
 tissue-borne m.

macrophage-activating factor
 (MAF)

macrophage-inhibiting factor
 (MIF)

macrophallus

macrophonia

Macroplastique material

macrorhinia

macroscopic
 m. concavity

macrosmatic

macrosomia

macrostomia

macrotia

macrotooth

macrotrauma

McShirley
 M. electromallet
 M. electromallet condenser

McSpadden
 M. compactor
 M. endodontic technique
 M. method

macula *pl.* maculae
 acoustic m.
 m. adherens

macula *(continued)*
    m. cribrosa media
    m. flava
    medial cribrose m.

macular hair cell

macule
    café au lait m. (CALM)

MAD
    maximum accumulated
        dose

Maestro implant

MAF
    macrophage-activating fac-
        tor
    master apical file

mafenide

Maffucci syndrome

Magan

magenta tongue

Magitot disease

Maglite

Magna-Finder locating device

Magna-Site locating system

magnesium
    m. oxide
    m. salicylate

magnet
    foreign body m.

magnetic
    m. implant
    m. jaw tracking device
    m. resonance angiography
        (MRA)
    m. resonance imaging
        (MRI)
    m. source imaging (MSI)

magnetoencephalography
    (MEG)

Magnevist

magnification
    loupe m.

magnitude
    response m.

magnum
    foramen m.

MAGPI
    meatal advancement and
        glanuloplasty procedure
    meatoplasty and glanulo-
        plasty

Maier sinus

main
    m. arteriole (MA)
    m. venule (MV)

mainstreaming

maintainer
    Mayne space m.

major
    m. anchorage
    aphthae m.
    m. connector
    m. histocompatibility com-
        plex (MHC)
    musculus zygomaticus m.
    pectoralis m. (PM)
    thalassemia m.

make-up
    camouflage m.

mal
    grand m.
    petit m.

malacotic
    m. teeth

maladaptive response

Malaga flap

malaise

malalignment
    vermilion–white line m.

malar
    m. alloplastic augmentation

malar *(continued)*
    m. arch
    m. bag
    m. bag suctioning
    m. bone
    m. deficiency
    m. elevator
    m. eminence
    m. facial augmentation
    m. fat pad
    m. flatness
    m. fold
    m. foramen
    m. fracture
    m. glands
    m. hypoplasia
    m. ligament complex
    m. margin
    m. mound
    m. pad
    m. periosteum-SMAS flap
      fixation suture
    m. prominence
    m. shell augmentation
    m. surface of zygomatic
      bone
    m. tuberosity

malare

malarplasty procedure

malar-zygomatic region

Malassez
    M. debris
    M. epithelial rest

male
    m. abdominoplasty
    m. compression girdle
    m. flank
    m. foreheadplasty
    m. pattern baldness
    m. soprano voice

maleate
    ergonovine m.
    methysergide m.

maleruption

male-to-female transsexual

malformation
    adult Chiari m.
    arrhinia m.
    Arnold-Chiari m.
    arteriovenous m. (AVM)
    Bing-Siebenmann m.
    capillary m.
    capillary vascular m.
    Chiari m. *(types I, II, III, IV)*
    congenital m.
    Dandy-Walker m.
    high-flow arterial m.
    high-flow arteriovenous m.
    holoprosencephalic m.
    lymphatic m.
    lymphovenous m.
    Michel m.
    Mondini m.
    Mondini-Alexander m.
    occult m. of the skull base
    osseous craniofacial arter-
      iovenous m.
    rugose frontonasal m.
    Scheibe m.
    split hand/split foot m.
    vaginal m.
    vascular m.
    venous m.

malfunction

malfunctional occlusion

Malgaigne fossa

Malherbe
    calcifying epithelioma of M.
    epithelioma of M.

malic dehydrogenase

malignancy

malignant
    m. blue nevus
    m. chondroma
    m. dyskeratosis
    m. external otitis
    m. fibroma
    m. fibrous histiocytoma
      (MFH)

malignant *(continued)*
   m. granular cell myoblastoma
   m. hemangiopericytoma
   m. lymphoepithelioma
   m. lymphoma
   m. melanoma (MM)
   m. midline reticulosis
   m. necrotizing otitis externa (MNOE)
   m. neoplasm
   m. odontogenic tumor
   m. pemphigus
   m. pleomorphic adenoma
   m. reticulosis
   m. transformation

malignoma
   thyroid m.

malinger

Maliniac
   M. nasal rasp
   M. retractor

malinterdigitation

MALL
   massive all layer liposuction

malleability

malleable

mallear
   m. fold
   m. ligament

malleolus

malleostapedial assembly

malleotomy

malleovestibulopexy

Mallet
   modified M. scale
   M. scale shoulder external rotation

mallet
   m. finger

mallet *(continued)*
   hard m.

malleus
   caput m.
   fixed m.
   m.-footplate assembly
   handle of m.
   m. head
   head of m.
   m. nipper
   osteoma of m.
   m.-stapes assembly

Mallisol

Mallory-Weiss syndrome

malocclusion
   Ackerman-Proffitt classification of m.
   Angle classification of m.
   class I, II, III, IV m.
   closed-bite m.
   deflective m.
   m. index
   open bite m.
   Simons classification of m.
   teeth m.

malodor

malomaxillary suture

Maloney bougie

malpighian cell

malposition
   bilateral m.
   functional m.
   implant m.
   inferior m.
   superior m.
   teeth m.

malpositioned
   m. tooth

malrelation

malrotation
   philtral m.

malt

Malta fever

maltase

Maltese cross–patterned flap

malturned

Maltz
    M. rasp
    M. saw
    M.-Anderson nasal rasp
    M.-Lipsett nasal rasp

malunion
    fracture with m.
    m. of zygoma

mamelon

mammaplasty (*spelled also*
  mammoplasty)
    Arie reductive m.
    Arie-Pitanguy m.
    augmentation m.
    bilateral McKissock reduc-
      tion m.
    Biesenberger m.
    Biesenberger reduction m.
    devil's incision m.
    endoscopic transaxillary
      submuscular augmenta-
      tion m.
    Goulian m.
    Lejour m.
    periareolar m.
    m. procedure
    reconstructive m.
    reduction m.
    m. reduction technique
    Schatten m.
    Skoog m.
    Strombeck technique for
      reduction m.
    Toronto two-stage m.
    vertical m.
    Wyse pattern for reduc-
      tion m.
    Wyse reduction m.
    Z-m.

mammary
    m. artery

mammary (*continued*)
    m. duct
    m. duct ectasia
    m. fistula
    m. gangrene
    m. implant
    m. prosthesis explantation

mammillaplasty

mammography
    computed tomography la-
      ser m.

Mammopatch
    M. gel self adhesive
    M. gel self-adhesive dress-
      ing
    M. gel self-adhesive scar
      treatment

mammoplasty (*variant of* mammaplasty)

management
    airflow m.
    airway m.
    burn wound m.
    contingency m.
    endovascular m.

mandible
    alveolar limbus of m.
    alveolar margin of m.
    alveolar process of m.
    alveolar surface of m.
    articular fossa of m.
    ascending ramus of m.
    breadth of m.
    cant of occlusal plane of m.
    condyle of m.
    coronoid process of m.
    disappearing m.
    hypoplastic m.
    incisive fossa of m.
    lateral oblique projection
      of m.
    length of m.
    lingula of m.
    mental tubercle of m.
    mylohyoid sulcus of m.
    neck of m.

mandible *(continued)*
m. panogram
peripheral osteoma of m. (POM)
protruding m.
pterygoid tuberosity of m.
m. radiography
ramus of m.
retrognathic m.
retruded m.
m. rim
sagittal splitting of m.
short m.
space of body of m.
symphysial height of m.
temporal process of m.
vertical osteotomy of ramus of m.

mandibula *gen. and pl.* mandibulae
arcus alveolaris mandibulae
capitulum mandibulae

mandibular
m. advancement
m. advancement appliance (MAA)
m. alveolar mucosa
m. alveolus
m. angle
m. angle fracture intraoral open reduction microplate
m. angle fracture intraoral open reduction screw
m. anteroposterior ridge slope
m. arch
m. artery
m. articulation
m. axis
m. base
m. bicuspid
m. bicuspid radiograph
m. block
m. body fracture
m. body length
m. body retractor

mandibular *(continued)*
m. border
m. bridging plate
m. canal
m. cartilage
m. centric relation
m. condylar hypoplasia
m. condyle
m. condyle fracture
m. contour
m. crest
m. cuspid
m. cuspid–first bicuspid radiograph
m. cuspid radiograph
m. cyst
m. defect
m. deficiency
m. dentition
m. depth
m. deviation
m. dislocation
m. distraction
m. distraction osteogenesis
m. distractor
m. equilibration
m. excess
m. fissure
m. foramen
m. forceps
m. fossa
m. functional reconstruction
m. gland
m. glide
m. gliding movement
m. guide-plane prosthesis
m. guide prosthesis
m. head
m. hinge position
m. hypoplasia
m. impression
m. incisor
m. incisor crowding
m. incisor radiograph
m. leiomyosarcoma
m. lingual flange
m. lymph node
m. macrognathia

mandibular *(continued)*
    m. median cyst
    m. micrognathia
    m. miniplate
    m. molar
    m. molar radiograph
    m. nerve
    m. neurovascular canal
    m. notch
    m. occlusal view
    m. osteotomy–genioglossus advancement
    m. overdenture
    m. plane
    m. plane angle
    m. plane to hyoid (MPH)
    m. premolar
    m. process
    m. prognathism
    m. prognathism/protrusion
    m. protraction
    m. protrusion
    m. ramus
    m. ramus fracture
    m. ramus osteotomy
    m. range of motion
    m. reflex
    m. rest position
    m. restriction
    m. retraction
    m. retrognathia
    m. retrognathism
    m. retrognathism/retrusion
    m. retroposition
    m. retrusion
    m. ridge
    m. sagittal deficiency
    m. sagittal split osteotomy
    m. sieving
    m. sling
    m. space
    m. spine
    m. splint
    m. split
    m. staple bone plate (MSBP)
    m. sulcus
    m. surgery
    m. swing approach

mandibular *(continued)*
    m. swing operation
    m. symphysis
    m. symphysis comminution
    m. symphysis fracture
    m. teeth
    m. torus
    m. trusion
    m. vestibule
    m. visceral arch
    m. wiring

mandibulectomy
    anterior m.
    lateral m.
    marginal m.
    right segmental m.
    segmental m.

mandibulofacial
    m. dysostosis

mandibulomasseteric

mandibulomaxillary fixation

mandibulo-oculofacial dyscephaly

mandibulotomy

Mandol

mand operant

mandrel
    disk m.
    endosseous implant needle m.
    Moore m.
    Morgan m.
    snap-on m.

mandril *(variant of* mandrel)

maneuver
    Cairns m.
    Cottle m.
    deglutition m.
    delay m.
    Dix-Hallpike m.
    flexor pollicis longus substitution m.
    Frenzel m.

maneuver *(continued)*
  Hallpike m.
  Heimlich m.
  Hueter m.
  Jahss m.
  Mendelsohn m.
  Moore head-tilt m.
  Schartzmann m.
  Sellick m.
  Valsalva m.

maneuverability

Mangat curvilinear chin prosthesis

Mangoldt
  M. epithelial graft
  M. epithelial grafting

manic reaction

manipulation
  digital m.
  interceptive orthodontic m.
  skin-subcutaneous dissection with SMAS m.
  SMAS m.

manipulator
  Microbeam m.
  Ramirez m.

Mannerfelt syndrome

mannitol

manometer

manometric flame

manometry
  esophageal m.

Mantel-Haenszel analysis

mantle
  blue m.
  m. dentin

manubrium *pl.* manubria

manudynamometer

manufacture

manufacturing
  computer-assisted design/computer-assisted m. (CAD/CAM)

Manz gland

MAP
  Muma Assessment Program

Mapap

mapping
  auditory brain m.
  brain m.
  cognitive m.
  electrophysiologic m.
  nerve m.
  sentinel lymphatic m.

mappy tongue

Maranox

marble bone disease

Marcaine

Marchant zone

Marcillin

Marena by LySonix compression garment

Marezine

Marfan syndrome

Margesic H

margin
  alveolar m.
  alveolar m. of mandible
  bone m.
  carious restoration m.
  cavity m.
  cavosurface m.
  ceramometal m.
  cervical m.
  enamel m.
  eyelid m.
  free m. of eyelid
  free gingival m.

margin *(continued)*
    free gum m.
    gingival m. (GM)
    incisal m.
    infraorbital m.
    malar m.
    metal crown m.
    revised wound m's
    temporal m.
    m. of tongue
    m. trimmer
    vermilion m.
    wound m's
    zygomatic m.

marginal
    m. adaptation
    m. bevel
    m. crest
    m. excess
    m. gingiva
    m. gingivitis
    m. incision
    m. integrity of amalgam
    M. Line Calculus Index
      (MLCI)
    m. mandibular branch
    m. mandibular nerve
    m. mandibular resection
    m. mandibulectomy
    m. nevus
    m. periodontitis
    m. process of malar bone
    m. ridge
    m. ridge fracture
    m. spinning
    m. tubercle
    m. tubercle of zygomatic
      bone
    m. zone

marginalis
    arcus m.
    crista m.

margination

margines *(pl.* of margo)

marginis *(gen. of* margo)

marginoplasty

marginotomy
    inferior m.
    superior m.
    supplementary m.

margo *gen.* mar-
    ginis, *pl.* margines
    m. alveolaris
    m. incisalis
    m. temporalis

Margraf beam aligning film
  holder

marionette line

Marjolin ulcer

mark
    beauty m.
    stretch m's

marked falling curve

markedness theory

marker
    Accu-line Products skin m.
    Allskin m.
    cytokeratin m.
    epithelial m.
    fiducial m.
    Freeman cookie cutter ar-
      eola m.
    I m.
    intentional m.
    K3-7991 Thornton 360 de-
      gree accurate m.
    MIB-1 and PC10 as prog-
      nostic m's for esophageal
      squamous cell carcinoma
    neuroendocrine m.
    neuropeptide m.
    periodontal pocket m.
    phenotypic m.
    Richey condyle m.
    sign m.
    Squeeze-Mark surgical m.
    T4/Leu2a m.
    T4/Leu3a m.
    tumor m.
    Vismark skin m.

marker *(continued)*
 X-act cutaneous x-ray m.

marking
 m. pocket
 skin m's

Mark May sinus disease criteria

Marlex
 M. mesh
 M. mesh closure

Maroteaux-Lamy
 mucopolysaccharidosis
 type VI M.-L. (MPS-VI)

Marquette monitor

Marquis probe

Marritt dilator

marrow
 bone m.
 cancellous cellular m.
 fatty m.
 particulate cancellous bone
 and m. (PCBM)
 m. space

Mars Black artist's acrylic paint

Marshall syndrome

marsh elder

marshmallow

marsupialization
 m. method

Marthritic

Martin
 M. incision
 M. plane
 M. retractor

Marx
 M. classification of microtia
 M. protocol for ORN treat-
 ment

Maryland bridge

Marzola hair restoration surgery

Masera septal organ

mask
 laryngeal m.
 LaserSite facial m.
 m. lift
 Petit facial m.
 Swiss Therapy eye m.

masker
 tinnitus m.
 tunable tinnitus m.

masking
 backward m.
 central m.
 effective m.
 m. efficiency
 forward m.
 initial m.
 m. level difference
 maximum m.
 peripheral m.
 m. technique
 upward m.

masklike
 m. face
 m. facies

masoprocol

masque
 Nouvisage Acne M.
 Nouvisage Anti-Aging M.
 Nouvisage M. for damaged
 or sunburned skin
 Nouvisage M. for normal to
 dry skin
 Nouvisage M. for normal to
 oily skin

Masquelet test

mass
 bisected m.
 exophytic m.
 fungating m.
 hyperintense m.
 incudomalleolar m.
 infra-auricular m.
 lipohypertrophic m.

mass *(continued)*
    multilocular m.
    radiopaque m.
    retroareolar m.
    retromammilar m.
    ropy m.
    salivary gland m.
    sclerotic cemental m.
    soft tissue m.
    Stent m.
    vascular m.

massage
    gingival m.
    glandular m.
    gum m.
    lymphatic m.
    scar m.

Massé breast cream

Masseran trepan bur

masseter
    m. abscess
    m. muscle
    m. muscle flap
    m. muscle hypertrophy
    m. muscle transfer
    m. tendon

masseteric
    m. artery
    m. fascia
    m. hypertrophy
    m. nerve
    m. space

masseter-mandibulopterygoid
    space

massive
    m. all layer liposuction
        (MALL)
    m. hemoptysis
    m. resorption

Masson
    M. trichrome stain

mast cell

mastectomy
    Halsted radical m.

mastectomy *(continued)*
    modified radical m.
    radical m.
    salvage m.
    simple m.
    simultaneous LATRAM
        and m. (SLAM)
    m. skin flap
    skin-sparing m.
    subcutaneous m.
    transareolar m.

master
    m. apical file (MAF)
    m. cast
    m. cone

masticate

masticatory force

mastic varnish

Mastisol

mastitis
    chronic cystic m.
    granulomatous m.
    silicone m.

mastocele
    transareolar m.

mastocytosis
    benign systemic m.

mastoid
    m. abscess
    m. antrum
    artificial m.
    m. bowl
    m. cavity
    m.-conchal suture
    m. cortex
    m. emissary vein
    m. empyema
    m. fascia
    m. foramen
    Kaposi sarcoma of m.
    m. node
    m. notch
    m. obliteration operation
    m. pneumatization
    m. pressure

mastoid *(continued)*
    m. process
    m. tip
    m. tip cell

mastoidectomy
    canal wall-down m.
    canal wall-up m.
    cortical m.
    modified radical m.
    radical m.
    Stacke m.
    tympanoplasty m.

mastoideum
    tegmen m.

mastoiditis
    Bezold m.
    coalescent m.
    Pneumocystis carinii m.
    sclerosing m.
    sclerotic m.

mastopathy

mastopexy
    Benelli m.
    m.–breast augmentation
    dual-pedicle dermoparen-
      chymal m. (DPM)
    Goulain m.
    internal m.
    modified Kiel m.
    Wise pattern m.

mastoplasty
    integrative m.
    Lejour m.

mat
    m. foil
    gingival m.
    m. gold
    Secur-Its silicone cush-
      ion m.

match
    perceptual-motor m.

matching
    impedance m.
    sentence-picture m.

mater
    dura m.

materia *pl.* materiae
    m. alba
    m. dentica

material
    Absorb-its m.
    agar-alginate impression m.
    agar hydrocolloid impres-
      sion m.
    agar impression m.
    alloplastic graft m.
    6AI/4V ELI alloy implant m.
    alginate impression m.
    alloplastic graft m.
    American Society for Test-
      ing and M's
    Aquaplast alloplastic m.
    Aquaplast rapid setting
      splint m.
    autophagocytosed cellu-
      lar m.
    base m.
    baseplate m.
    Biobrane graft m.
    bioceramic implant m.
    biocompatible bone graft
      substitute m.
    biocompatible spacing m.
    Bioglass bone substi-
      tute m.
    Bioglass bone graft substi-
      tute m.
    BioMend periodontal m.
    Bio-Oss corticalis bone
      graft m.
    Bio-Oss spongiosa bone
      graft m.
    Bioplastique augmenta-
      tion m.
    Biovert implant m.
    block-out m.
    Bioglass bone substitute m.
    Bioglass bone graft substi-
      tute m.
    bone implant m.
    brittle m.

material *(continued)*

Canals-N root canal filling m.

carbonaceous m.

cast m.

CeraMed bone grafting m.

chrome-cobalt-molybdenum m.

coating m.

collagen hemostatic m. for wounds

Collastat OBP microfibrillar collagen hemostat m.

colloid impression m.

composite m.

Cranioplastic acrylic cranioplasty m.

Curaderm hydrocolloid dressing m.

Cutinova Cavity wound filling m.

Cyano-Dent m.

dental m.

devascularized m.

ductile m.

Durafill dental restorative m.

Dur-A-Sil ear impression m.

elastic impression m.

elastomeric impression m.

eosinophilic proteinaceous m.

Epoxy Die m.

Fermit-N occlusal hole blockage m.

filling m.

Flexicon m.

Frosted Flex earmold m.

Geristore repair m.

glass ionomer restorative m.

glycolide trimethylene carbonate m.

Gore subcutaneous augmentation m.

Gore-Tex alloplastic m.

Gore-Tex augmentation m. (GTAM)

Gore-Tex periodontal m.

material *(continued)*

Gore-Tex regenerative m.

Hapex bioactive m.

heavy-bodied m.

heavy body impression m.

hemostatic m.

heterologous m.

Hydrocal cast m.

hydrocolloid impression m.

hydroxyapatite implant m.

impression m.

inelastic impression m.

Insta-Mold silicone ear impression m.

intermediate restorative m. (IRM)

irreversible hydrocolloid impression m.

Kerr Permplastic m.

Kerr Traycon m.

light body impression m.

lipoaspirated m.

Macroplastique m.

MediFlex earmold m.

Medpor allograft m.

Medpor alloplastic m.

Medpor block facial structure building m.

Opotow Jelset m.

osteoconductive bone grafting m.

OsteoGen bone grafting m.

OsteoGen HA Resorb implant m.

Osteograf bone grafting m.

Osteograf/D dense bone grafting m.

Osteograf/LD low density bone grafting m.

Osteograf/N natural bone grafting m.

Pacific Coast demineralized bone grafting m.

PerioGlas m.

PermaSoft reline m.

plaster impression m.

plastic restoration m.

plastic wax m.

polyether impression m.

material *(continued)*
    polyether rubber impression m.
    polysulfide impression m.
    polysulfide rubber impression m.
    polyurethane elastomer m.
    Polyviolene polyester suture m.
    Proplast-Teflon m.
    provisionally acceptable m.
    radar absorbent m. (RAM)
    regular body impression m.
    reline m.
    restorative m.
    restorative dental m's
    reversible hydrocolloid impression m.
    rubber impression m.
    semisolid m.
    silicate restorative m.
    silicone impression m.
    silicone rubber impression m.
    Small-Carrion penile implant m.
    spacing m.
    Sta-Tic impression m.
    subcutaneous augmentation m. (S.A.M.)
    Surgamid polyamide suture m.
    Teflon m.
    temporary m.
    temporary endodontic restorative m. (TERM)
    thermoplastic impression m.
    tissue equivalent m.
    tridodecylmethylammonium chloride graft coating m. (TDMAC)
    two-paste polysulfide rubber impression m.
    unacceptable m.
    Uroplastique m.
    Vicryl suture m.
    vinyl polysiloxane impression m.

material *(continued)*
    Vitremer glass-ionomer restorative m.
    wash impression m.
    Xantopren impression m.
    zinc oxide-eugenol impression m.

Materialise computer-aided design software

Mathes and Nahai classification for muscle circulation *(types I–V)*

mathetic
    m. function of language
    m. text

matrix *pl.* matrices
    amalgam m.
    m. band
    bone m.
    celluloid m.
    Class V cervical m.
    Collagraft bone graft m.
    custom m.
    demineralized bone m.
    dentin m.
    dentinal m.
    direct porcelain m.
    enamel m.
    extracellular m. (ECM)
    human tissue collagen m.
    m. metalloproteinase (MMP)
    Mylar m.
    myxochondroid m.
    nuclear m. (NM)
    organic m.
    perilacunar mineral m. (PMM)
    PermaMesh hydroxyapatite woven sheet m.
    plastic m.
    platinum foil m.
    m. pliers
    predentin m. (PDM)
    resin m.
    resin shell m.
    m. retainer

matrix *(continued)*
    m. sentence
    T-band m.

Matsura preparation

matter
    particulate m.

Matthew forceps

mattress
    Akros m.
    D.A.D. m.
    m. stitch
    m. suture
    m. suture otoplasty

mattressed onlay graft

maturation
    enamel m.
    rate of m.
    skeletal m.

maturational lag

maturative stage

mature
    m. bite
    m. dentin
    m. teratoma

maturing temperature

max
    PB m.

Maxaquin

Maxicide

Maxidex

Maxiflor

Maxigold alloy

maxilla *gen. and pl.* maxillae
    alveolar limbus of m.
    alveolar process of m.
    alveolar surface of m.
    anterior surface of m.
    arcus alveolaris maxillae
    conchal crest of m.
    crista conchalis maxillae

maxilla *(continued)*
    crista ethmoidalis maxillae
    facial surface of m.
    greater palatine sulcus
      of m.
    incisive fossa of m.
    infraorbital ridge of m.
    infraorbital sulcus of m.
    infratemporal surface of m.
    juga alveolaria maxillae
    lacrimal groove of m.
    lacrimal sulcus of m.
    limbus alveolaris maxillae
    medial surface of m.
    palatine groove of m.
    palatine lamina of m.
    palatine process of m.
    palatine sulcus of m.
    posterior surface of m.
    m. radiograph
    retrodisplaced maxillae
    septum interalveolaria
      maxillae
    spine of m.
    superior m.
    superolateral surface of m.
    zygomatic process of m.

maxillary
    m. alveolar protrusion
    m. alveolus
    m. angle
    m. anterior tooth
    m. antrum
    m. antrum closure
    m. arch
    m. artery
    m. bicuspid
    m. bicuspid radiograph
    m. bite plate
    m. bone
    m. buttress
    m. canal
    m. canine
    m. cuspid
    m. cuspid radiograph
    m. cyst
    m. deficiency
    m. dentition
    m. depth

maxillary *(continued)*
  m. division
  m. downgrafting
  m. excess
  m. expansion
  m. first molar alveolus
  m. fissure
  m. foramen
  m. forceps
  m. fossa
  m. fracture
  m. hypoplasia
  m. impression
  m. incisor
  m. incisor radiograph
  m. incisor retraction
  m. intrusion
  m. ligament
  m. lymph node
  m. macrognathia
  m. malignant mesenchy-
    moma
  m. median anterior cyst
  m. micrognathia
  m. molar
  m. molar radiograph
  m. neoplasm
  m. nerve
  m. occlusal view
  m. osteotomy
  m. ostium
  m. posterior tooth
  m. process
  m. process of zygomatic
    bone
  m. prognathism/protrusion
  m. prominence
  m. prosthesis
  m. protraction
  m. protrusion
  m. rampart
  m. removal implant-re-
    tained denture
  m. removal and reinsertion
  m. restoration
  m. retardation
  m. retrognathia
  m. retroposition
  m. retrusion

maxillary *(continued)*
  m. sinus
  m. sinus carcinoma
  m. sinusoscopy
  m. sinus cyst
  m. sinus Foley catheter bal-
    loon placement technique
  m. sinusitis
  m. sinus mucocele
  m. sinus radiograph
  m. sinus roentgenogram
  m. stent
  m. surface
  m. surface of great wing
  m. surface of perpendicular
    plate of palatine bone
  m. surgery
  m. teeth
  m. trusion
  m. tuberosity
  m. vein
  m.-zygomatic hypoplasia

maxillectomy
  composite bilateral infra-
    structure m.
  endoscopic medial m.

maxillitis

maxilloalveolar
  m. breadth
  m. index
  m. length

maxillodental

maxillofacial
  m. abnormality
  m. anomaly
  m. and facioproximal sur-
    face toothbrushing
  m. fracture
  m. injury
  m. prosthesis
  m. prosthodontics
  m. reconstruction
  m. skeletal advancement
  m. surgery

maxillofrontale

maxillojugal

maxillomandibular
  m. anchorage
  m. disharmony
  m. dysplasia
  m. elastic
  m. fixation (MMF)
  m. record
  m. registration
  m. relation
  m. traction

maxillonasal dysostosis

maxillopalatal and palatoproximal surface toothbrushing

maxillopalatine

maxillotomy

maxillozygomatic complex

maximal
  m. contrast
  M. Static Response Assay (MSRA)
  m. static response assay of facial motion
  m. stress

maximum
  m. accumulated dose (MAD)
  m. acoustic output
  m. amplitude
  m. bite force
  m. duration of phonation
  m. duration of sustained blowing
  m. frequency range
  m. intercuspation
  m. interincisal distance (MID)
  m. masking
  m. movement
  m. permissible dose (MPD)
  m. power output (MPO)
  m. stimulation test (MST)

Maximum Strength Anbesol

Maximum Strength Desenex antifungal cream

maximus
  gluteus m.

Maxipime

Maxitrol

Maxivate

Maxon suture

Mayer
  M. nasal splint
  M. reflex
  M. view
  M.-Rokitansky syndrome
  M.-Rokitansky-Küster-Hauser syndrome (MRKHS)

mayfly

Mayne
  M. muscle control appliance
  M. space maintainer

Mayo
  M. scissors
  M. stand

mazopexy

MBD
  minimal brain dysfunction
  MBD syndrome

MC
  mesenchymal chondrosarcoma

MCL-N
  midclavicular line to nipple

MCP
  metacarpophalangeal
  MCP joint

MCT
  motor coordination test
  mucociliary transport

McXIM file

MDA ultrasound-assisted lipoplasty machine

M.D. Forte

Mead
    M. forceps
    M. rongeur

mean
    m. rejection grading (MRG)
    m. residual gap (MRG)

measles
    German m.
    three-day m.
    m. virus

measurement
    anthropometric m.
    Breslow m's
    carpal height m.
    m. control handle
    facial excursion m.
    m. film
    nasion-pogonion m.

measuring
    precise lesion m. (PLM)
    m. wire

meatal
    m. advancement and glanu-
        loplasty procedure
        (MAGPI)
    m. atresia
    m. stenosis

meatoplasty
    m. and glanuloplasty
        (MAGPI)

meatorrhaphy

meatoscope

meatoscopy

meatotome

meatotomy

meatus *pl.* meatus
    anterior middle m.
    inferior m.
    middle m.
    superior m.
    urinary m.

mebendazole

MEC
    mucoepidermoid carci-
        noma

mechanical
    m. avulsion
    m. condenser
    m. creep of skin
    m. labyrinthectomy
    m. perforation
    m. retention
    m. separator
    m. strain
    m. tooth separation
    m. triturator

mechanically balanced occlu-
    sion

mechanics
    wrist m.

mechanism
    palatopharyngeal m.

mechanoactivation

mechanoreceptor

mechanotherapy
    multibanded m.

Meckel
    M. cartilage
    M. cave
    M. cavity
    M. ganglion
    lesser ganglion of M.
    internal zygomatic foramen
        of M.
    M. rod

meclizine

meclofenamate

Mectra irrigation/aspiration
    system

Med

MedDev gold eyelid implant

media
    acute otitis m. (AOM)

media *(continued)*
    adhesive otitis m.
    aerotitis m.
    barotitis m.
    catarrhal otitis m.
    chronic cholesteatomatous
        otitis m.
    chronic granulation oti-
        tis m.
    chronic otitis m. (COM)
    chronic suppurative oti-
        tis m. (CSOM)
    macula cribrosa m.
    mucoid otitis m.
    necrotizing otitis m.
    noncholesteatomatous
        chronic suppurative oti-
        tis m.
    nonsuppurative otitis m.
    otitis m.
    purulent otitis m.
    reflux otitis m.
    scala m.
    secretory otitis m.
    serous otitis m. (SOM)
    suppurative otitis m.
    tuberculous otitis m.
    tunica m.

medial
    m. antebrachial cutaneous
        nerve
    m. brachial cutaneous
        nerve
    m. canthal fissure
    m. canthoplasty
    m. canthus
    m. collateral ligament
    m. cribrose macula
    m. crus
    m. cutaneous thigh flap
    m. distally based fasciocu-
        taneous flap
    m. elevation
    m. forearm flap
    m. geniculate
    m. incudal fold
    m. nasal concha
    m. oblique and low lateral
        osteotomy

medial *(continued)*
    m. plantar sensory flap
    m. pterygoid muscle
    m. pterygoid plate
    m. rectus muscle
    m. slip
    m. surface
    m. surface of maxilla
    m. turbinate bone
    m. upper arm flap
    m. vestibular nucleus
    m. wall of agger nasi cell

medialis
    lamina m.
    vastus m.

medialization
    fracture m.
    greenstick m.
    incomplete m.
    vocal cord m.

medialized

medial-to-lateral tumor removal

median
    m. alveolar cyst
    m. anterior maxillary cyst
    m. cleft face syndrome
    m. cleft lip
    m. facial cleft
    m. forehead flap
    m. glossoepiglottic fold
    m. jaw relation
    m. labiomandibular glosso-
        tomy
    m. laryngotomy
    m. line
    m. lingual sulcus
    m. longitudinal raphe
    m. mandibular cyst
    m. mandibular point
    m. maxillary anterior alveo-
        lar cleft
    m. nerve (MN)
    m. nerve compression test
    m. occlusal position
    m. palatal cyst
    m. palatine suture
    m. raphe plane

median *(continued)*
    m. retruded relation
    m. rhinoscopy
    m. rhomboid glossitis
    m. sagittal plane
    m. thyrohyoid fold
    m. thyrohyoid ligament

mediastinal dissection

mediastinitis
    descending necrotizing m.
        (DNM)
    fulminant m.

mediastinoscope
    Carlens m.
    Tucker m.

mediastinoscopy

mediastinum

mediator
    pain-related m.

Medicamat
    M. ultrasound-assisted lipo-
        plasty machine
    M. ultrasound device

medicamentosa
    dermatitis m.
    rhinitis m.
    stomatitis m.

medication-induced hyperplasia

medicinal
    m. leech
    m. preparation

medicine
    evidence-based m. (E-BM)

medicodental

Medicon
    M. ultrasonic liposuction
        device
    M. US liposuction device

MediFlex earmold material

mediodens

medionasal process

mediotrusion

Medipain 5

Medipatch Gel Z adhesive
    dressing

Mediplast Plaster

Medipore H surgical tape

Medi-Quick topical ointment

Mediskin hemostatic sponge

Mediterranean fever

MedLite
    M. Q-Switched neodymium-
        doped yttrium-aluminum-
        garnet laser
    M. Q-Switched YAG laser

MedMorph
    M. III patient video imaging
    M. III software

Medpor
    M. allograft material
    M. alloplastic material
    M. Biomaterial wedge
    M. block facial structure
        building material
    M. facial implant
    M. malar implant
    M. reconstructive implant
    M. surgical implant

medrysone

Medtronics Sequestra 1000 au-
    totransfusion system

medulla
    m. oblongata

medullary
    m. artery
    m. fixation

medullated nerve fiber

medullogram
    sternal puncture m.

Med-Wick nasal pack

Meek island sandwich graft

MEG
    magnetoencephalography

megadont

megadontia

megadontism

megadontismus

MegaDyne
    M. arthroscopic hook elec-
        trode
    M. electrocautery pencil

megaesophagus

megaglossia

megagnathia

megalodont

megalodontia

megaloglossia

megalourethra

meibomian gland

Meige
    M. disease
    M. syndrome

meiopragic bone

Meissner
    M. corpuscles
    M. ganglion
    M. tactile corpuscle

Meisterschnitt incision

mel

Melaleuca

Melanex

melanin

melanization

melanoameloblastoma

melanocyte
    cultured autologous m.

melanocyte-stimulating hor-
    mone
    m.-s. h.–inhibiting factor

melanocytic
    m. atypia
    m. lesion

melanocytoma
    compound m.

melanoderma
    Riehl m.
    senile m.

melanogenesis

melanoglossia

melanoma
    acral lentiginous m.
    benign juvenile m.
    cutaneous m.
    desmoplastic m.
    halo m.
    lentigo maligna m.
    malignant m. (MM)
    neurotropic m.
    nodular m.
    sinonasal m.
    m. in situ (MIS)
    subungual m.
    superficial malignant m.
    superficial spreading m.

melanonychia
    longitudinal m.
    m. striata (MS)

melanoplakia

melanosarcoma

melanosis
    circumscribed precancer-
        ous m. of Dubreuilh
    dermal m.
    m. diffusa congenita
    laryngeal m. (LM)
    mucocutaneous m.
    Riehl m.

melanosome

melanotic
  m. neuroectodermal tumor
  m. neuroectodermal tumor of infancy
  m. whitlow

melanotrichosis
  m. linguae

melasma

melatonin

Meleney ulcer

melitis

Melkersson
  M. syndrome
  M.-Rosenthal syndrome

mellitus
  diabetes m.

melocervicoplasty

melolabial flap

melonoplasty (*variant of* melo-plasty)

meloplasty
  intraoral m.
  laser m.
  m. procedure

melphalan

membrana eboris

membrane
  adamantine m.
  adventitious m.
  alveolodental m.
  barrier m.
  basement m.
  basilar m.
  BioBarrier m.
  Bio-Gide resorbable barrier m.
  Bio-Gide resorbable bilayer barrier m.
  BioMend m.
  bioresorbable guided tissue m.

membrane *(continued)*
  Brunn m.
  cloacal m.
  cricothyroid m.
  cricovocal m.
  dentinoenamel m.
  drum m.
  enamel m.
  ePTFE m.
  ePTFE augmentation m.
  fibroelastic m.
  Golgi m's
  Gore Resolut regenerative tissue m.
  Gore-Tex m.
  Gore-Tex augmentation m. (GTAM)
  Huxley m.
  hyaline basement m.
  hyoglossal m.
  Imtec BioBarrier m.
  internal elastic m.
  ivory m.
  labyrinthine m.
  mucous m.
  mucous m. of lip
  mucous m. of tongue
  Nasmyth m.
  oropharyngeal m.
  otolithic m.
  peridental m.
  periodontal m. (PM)
  plasma m.
  pseudoserous m.
  pulpodentinal m.
  quadrangular m.
  Reissner m.
  resorbable bilayer collagen m.
  Rivinus m.
  salpingopalatine m.
  salpingopharyngeal m.
  schneiderian m.
  schneiderian respiratory m.
  Schultze m.
  Shrapnell m.
  stylomandibular m.
  subepithelial m.
  subimplant m.

membrane *(continued)*
    submucous m.
    synovial m.
    tectorial m.
    TefGen-FD guided tissue re-
        generation m.
    TefGen-FD plastic m.
    thyrohyoid m.
    tympanic m.
    unilaminar m.
    unit m.
    vestibular m.
    von Brunn m.

membranous
    m. gingivostomatitis
    m. labyrinth
    m. laryngitis
    m. pharyngitis
    m. stomatitis

Meme implant

memocouple

memory
    immunologic m.

Menadol

mendelian theory

Mendelsohn maneuver

Ménétrier disease

Meniere
    M. disease
    M. quadrad
    M. syndrome

meningeal artery

meningioma
    cutaneous m.
    m. en plaque
    extracranial m.
    posterior cranial fossa m.

meningismus

meningitis
    AIDS-related cryptococ-
        cal m.
    bacterial m. (BM)

meningitis *(continued)*
    cryptococcal m.
    otitic m.

meningocele

meningoencephalocele
    frontoethmoidal m.

meningoencephalomyelitis
    mumps m.

meningothelial cell

meningovascular syphilis

meniscus *pl.* menisci
    triangular fibrocartilage m.

menogingivitis
    periodic transitory m.

menstruation gingivitis

mental
    m. age (MA)
    m. artery
    m. block injection
    m. extraoral radiography
    m. foramen
    m. height
    m. muscle
    m. nerve
    m. point
    m. process
    m. projection
    m. protuberance
    m. region
    m. retardation
    m. ridge
    m. spine
    m. tubercle
    m. tubercle of mandible
    m. V-Y island advancement
        island flap

mentalis
    m. band
    m. muscle

mentolabial
    m. sulcus

menton

mentoplasty

Mentor
  M. breast implant
  M. Contour Genesis ultrasonic assisted lipoplasty system
  M. H/S Siltex implant
  M. 1600 implant
  M. ultrasound-assisted lipoplasty machine
  M. ultrasound device

mentum

mepenzolate

Mepergan

Mepitel
  M. dressing
  M. nonadherent silicone dressing

meprobamate

merbromin

Mercedes
  M. cannula
  M. incision
  LySonix TTD Design M.
  M. tip

mercurial
  m. line
  m. stomatitis

mercuric oxide

mercurochrome

mercuroscopic expansion

Merendino technique

Merit-B periodontal probe

Merkel
  M. cell
  M. cell carcinoma
  M. corpuscles
  M. filtrum ventriculi
  M. fossa

Merocel
  M. epistaxis packing
  M. nasal packing

meropenem

Merrem I.V.

Merrifield knife

Mershon arch

Mersilene
  M. mesh
  M. suture

Mersol

Merthiolate

Merz-Vienna nasal speculum

Mesalt sodium chloride impregnated dressing

mesencephalon

mesenchyma

mesenchymal
  m. cell
  m. chondrosarcoma (MC)
  m. cleft
  m. neoplasm
  m. sarcoma
  m. tumor

mesenchyme
  perifollicular m.

mesenchymoma
  maxillary malignant m.

mesenteric arcade

mesh
  Dexon surgically knitted m.
  Dumbach mini m.
  Dumbach regular m.
  Dumbach titanium m.
  Gore-Tex m.
  m. graft
  m. graft urethroplasty
  Marlex m.
  Mersilene m.

298   meshed split-thickness skin graft

mesh *(continued)*
    micro m.
    mixed m.
    polyamide m.
    polypropylene m.
    polytetrafluoroethylene m.
    Prolene m.
    skin m.
    skin graft m.
    skin graft expander m.
    Supramid polyamide m.
    synthetic m.
    TiMesh cranial m.
    TiMesh orbital m.
    TiMesh titanium m.
    Vicryl m.
    zippered m.

meshed split-thickness skin graft

mesher
    Tanner m.

meshwork
    coagulation m.

mesioangular
    m. impaction
    m. position

mesioaxial

mesioaxiogingival

mesioaxioincisal

mesiobuccal (MB)
    m. alveolus
    m. developmental groove
    (MBDG)
    m. line angle

mesiobucco-occlusal (MBO)
    m. point angle

mesiobuccopulpal (MBP)

mesiocervical

mesioclination

mesioclusion
    bilateral m.
    unilateral m.

mesiodens *pl.* mesiodentes

mesiodistal
    m. clasp
    m. fracture
    m. plane
    m. width

mesiodistocclusal (MOD)

mesiogingival (MG)

mesioincisal

mesioincisodistal (MID)

mesiolabial (MLA)
    m. bilobed transposition
    flap
    m. line angle

mesiolabioincisal (MLAI)
    m. point angle

mesiolingual (ML)
    m. developmental groove
    (MLDG)
    m. fossa (MLF)
    m. groove (MLG)
    m. line angle

mesiolinguoincisal (MLI)
    m. point angle

mesiolinguo-occlusal (MLO)
    m. point angle

mesiolinguopulpal (MLP)

mesio-occlusal (MO)
    m. line angle

mesio-occlusion

mesio-occlusodistal (MOD)

mesiopalatal

mesioplacement

mesiopulpal (MP)

mesiopulpolabial (MPLA)

mesiopulpolingual (MPL)

mesioversion

mesoderm

mesodermal
   m. core
   m. somite
   m. tumor

mesodont

mesodontia

mesodontic

mesodontism

mesognathic

mesognathous

meson
   pi m's

mesostomia

mesostructure
   m. bar
   m. conjunction bar
   implant m.
   m. implant
   integral intraoral bilateral
     posterior m.

mesotaurodontism

mesotympanum

Messerklinger technique

META
   methacryloxyethyl trimel-
     litic anhydride

metabolic sialadenosis

metacarpal
   rudimentary m.

metacarpophalangeal (MCP,
  MP)
   m. joint

metachronous
   m. metastasis
   m. tumor

metacone

metaconid

metaconule

metaidoioplasty (*spelled also*
  metoidioplasty)

metal
   alloy-forming m.
   Babbitt m.
   m. base
   m. bracket
   m. bucket-handle prosthe-
     sis
   d'Arcet m.
   implant m.
   m. interface
   m. opaquer
   m. reconstruction plate
   m. and rubber block
   m. scleral shield
   wrought m.

metallic
   m. frontal needle
   m. implant
   m. oxide paste
   m. restoration
   m. stain

metallic-dense shadow

metalloproteinase
   matrix m. (MMP)

metal-plated die

metamerism

metamorphosis
   calcific m.

Metamucil

metaphor

metaphysis

metaplasia
   cystic oncocytic m.
   m. of pulp
   sebaceous m.

metapragmatic

metaproterenol

metarteriole

metastasis *pl.* metastases
    cervical m.
    cutaneous m.
    hematogenous m.
    intraparotideal m.
    lymphatic m.
    metachronous m.
    precocious m.
    septic m.
    skip m.
    synchronous m.
    tumor-to-tumor m.

metastasize

metastatic
    m. basal cell carcinoma
    m. carcinoma
    m. neoplasm

metatarsal
    m. bone
    m. free vascularized graft
    m. joint

metatarsophalangeal (MTP, MP)
    m. joint

metathesis

metaxalone

methacrylate
    bisphenol A-glycidyl m.
      (bis-GMA)
    butyl m.
    dimethyl m.
    ethyl m.
    hydroxyethyl m.
    2-hydroxyethyl m. (HEMA)
    methyl m.
    poly-2-hydroxyethyl m.
      (poly-HEMA)
    polymethyl m. (PMMA)
    vinyl ethyl m.

methacryloxyethyl trimellitic
    anhydride (META)

methadone

methantheline bromide

methanthelinium

methazolamide

methemoglobinemia

methicillin

methimazole

methocarbamol and aspirin

method
    acoupedic m.
    acoustin m.
    analytic m.
    apneic m.
    artificial m.
    auditory m.
    Bass m.
    bimodal m.
    biotechnologic m.
    bisensory m.
    Blue Peel chemical m.
    Bobath m.
    breathing m.
    Brown-Brenn staining m.
    Bruhn m.
    Callahan m.
    carbon dioxide snow m.
    Carpue m.
    Charters m.
    Chayes m.
    chloropercha m.
    combined m.
    consonant-injection m.
    conventional m.
    Converse m.
    Cronin m.
    cross-consonant injec-
      tion m.
    Dieffenbach m.
    Eicken m.
    ethnographic m.
    expanded two-flap m. for
      microtia reconstruction
    finite element m. (FEM)

method *(continued)*
    foam and dome m.
    Fones m.
    formal m.
    French m.
    French-line m.
    fusion temperature wire m.
    German m.
    grammatic m.
    Gruver m.
    Hagedorn-Le Mesurier m.
      of cleft lip repair
    hanging chain m.
    Hirschfield m.
    Howe silver precipita-
      tion m.
    Indian m.
    indirect restorative m.
    informal m.
    inhalation m.
    injection m.
    injection-molded m.
    Italian m.
    Jena m.
    Johnston m.
    Karapandzic m.
    key word m.
    kinesthetic m.
    Kinzie m.
    Kitano and Okada m.
    Krause m.
    logical m.
    manual m.
    marsupialization m.
    McIndoe m.
    McSpadden m.
    modified Frost m.
    modified Wardill m.
    mother m.
    Mueller-Walle m.
    natural m.
    Needles split cast m.
    Ninhydrin-Schiff m.
    Nitchie m.
    numerical cipher m.
    odd-even m.
    Ollier m.
    online assessment m.

method *(continued)*
    oral-aural m.
    Partsch I m.
    plateau m.
    plosive-injection m.
    Politzer m.
    prolabial unwinding flap m.
    retrofilling m.
    Reverdin m.
    Rochester m.
    rotation-advancement m.
    Roux m.
    Sargenti m.
    shadowing m.
    silver cone m.
    simultaneous m.
    Skoog m.
    sniff m.
    Song and Song m.
    split cast m.
    Stillman m.
    swallow m.
    synthetic m.
    systematic m.
    Thiersch m.
    threshold shift m.
    Tweed m.
    unilateral V-Y m.
    verbotonal m.
    vertical-cut m.
    visual m.
    von Koss m.
    Warthin-Starry staining m.
    Waterson m.
    water sorption/desorp-
      tion m.
    Weber-Fergusson m.
    Wolfe m.
    zigzag m.
    Zisser-Madden m. of upper
      lip reconstruction

methodology
    Cutler-Ederer life-table m.

methyl
    m. cellulose paste
    m. ethyl ketone
    m. methacrylate

methyl *(continued)*
 m. methacrylate ear stent
 m. methacrylate polymer

methylcellulose
 gelatin, pectin, and m.
 hydroxypropyl m.

methyldopa

methylene
 m. blue
 m. blue line

methylprednisolone

methylsulfate
 diphemanil m.

methysergide maleate

Meticorten

Metimyd Ophthalmic

metipranolol

metoclopramide

metodontiasis

metoidioplasty *(variant of* me-taidoioplasty)*

Metol

metonymy

metopic
 m. synostosis
 m. synostosis reoperation

metopoplasty

metrizamide

metroplasty

Mettelman prejowl chin implant

Metz
 M. recruitment test

Metzenbaum scissors

Meurmann external ear anomaly grade

Meyenburg
 M. disease

Meyenburg *(continued)*
 M.-Altherr-Uehlinger syndrome

Meyer
 M. cartilage
 M. organ

Meyerding
 M. finger retractor
 M. skin hook
 M. skin hook and retractor

Mezlin

mezlocillin

MF
 mitogenic factor

MFH
 malignant fibrous histiocytoma

MF-Y gold

MG
 mesiogingival

MGJ
 mucogingival junction

MHC
 major histocompatibility complex

MHN
 Mohs hardness number

MIB-1 and PC10 as prognostic markers for esophageal squamous cell carcinoma

Mibelli angiokeratomas

Michel malformation

Michigan probe

miconazole

Micro
 M. Link endoscope fiber
 M. oral surgery handpiece
 M. Plus plating system

micro
 m. mesh

microabrasion

microabscess

micro-adaption plate

microanastomosis

microbar

Microbeam manipulator

microbial
    m. pathogen
    m. plaque

micro-bicinchoninic acid protein assay kit

microbiology
    quantitative m.

microblade
    Sharptome m.

Microbond NP

microbrachycephaly

microcephaly

microcheilia

microchilia (variant of microcheilia)

microcirculation
    peripheral m.

microclamp
    disposable m.

micrococcus pl. micrococci

microcoil
    platinum m.

microcrack

microcrystalline wax

microcystic
    m. adnexal carcinoma

microdebrider
    Hummer m.
    Wizard m.

microdensitometric

MicroDigitrapper

microdirect laryngoscopy

microdissection

microdont

microdontia
    relative generalized m.
    single-tooth m.
    true generalized m.

microdontism

microdrill

microdrilling guide

microdroplet
    silicone m.

microembolization

microetcher

microetching technique

microfibrillar
    m. collagen
    m. collagen hemostat

Microfil
    M. injection
    M. silicone-rubber injection
      compound
    M. solution

Microfine
    Prisma M.

microfixation

Micro-Flow compactor (MFC)

microfoam

microfracture

microgenia

microglossia

microglossic

micrognathia
    adult acquired m.
    mandibular m.
    maxillary m.

micrognathia *(continued)*
    m. with peromelia

micrognathic
    m. appearance

micrograft
    m. dilator
    m. punctiform technique

Micro-Halogen otoscope

microhandpiece

microischemia

microknife

microlaryngeal surgery

microlaryngoscopy
    suspension m.

microleakage

Micro-Lok implant

MicroLux video camera system

micromandible

micromanipulator
    microscope-mounted m.
    microspot m.
    UniMax 2000 laser m.

micromat

micromaxilla

MicroMax speed drill

micromechanical retention

micrometastasis *pl.* micrometastases

micrometastatic disease

MicroMirror gold sensor

micro-mosquito
    m. curved scissors
    m. straight scissors

microneurolysis

microneurorrhaphy

microneurosurgery

Micronor

microorganism
    gram-negative m.
    gram-positive m.
    pathogenic m.

microparticle

MicroPeel

Micro-Pen handpiece

micropenis

microphallus

microphonic
    cochlear m.

microphonoscope

microphthalmos

micropigmentation handpiece

micropipette

microplate
    AO-Titanium m.
    m. fixation
    mandibular angle fracture
      intraoral open reduction m.

Micropore
    M. dressing
    M. tape

microporosity

microprocessor

microradiograph

microradiography

microreconstruction

microscope
    confocal m.
    EIE 150F operating m.
    electron m.
    JedMed TRI-GEM m.
    m.-mounted micromanipulator
    operating m.

microscope *(continued)*
    Protégé Plus m.
    scanning electron m.
    Seiler MC-M900 surgical m.
    stereoscopic m.
    tonsillectomy with opera-
      ting m.
    transmission electron m.
      (TEM)
    Welch Allyn LumiView por-
      table binocular m.
    Wild operating m.
    Zeiss m.
    Zeiss/Jena surgical m.
    Zeiss operating m.

microscopy
    binocular m.
    light m. (LM)
    scanning electron m. (SEM)
    transmission electron m.
      (TEM)

microscrew
    forehead elevation and fixa-
      tion with percutaneous
      m's
    percutaneous m.

microserrefine
    Storz m.

microsomatic

microsomia
    craniofacial m.
    hemifacial m. (HFM, HM)

microsomy

microspectroscopy

Microsponge delivery system

microspot micromanipulator

Microstat handpiece

microstomia

Microstone

microsurgery

microsurgical
    m. procedure

microsyringe

Microtek Heine otoscope

microtia

microtome
    Leitz 1600 Saw m.

microtrauma

microtubule

microvascular
    m. anastomosis
    m. bone transfer
    m. clip
    m. decompression (MVD)
    m. free flap transfer
    m. free gracilis transfer
    m. free posterior interos-
      seous flap
    m. free tissue transfer
    m. graft
    m. surgery
    m. thrombosis

microvascularize

Micro-Vent
    M. implant
    M. implant system

Micro-Vent2 implant

microvesicle
    Novasome m.

microvessel density (MVD)

microvillar cell

microvillus *pl.* microvilli

micturition

MID
    maximum interincisal dis-
      tance

Midas
    M. alloy
    M. Rex instrumentation

midazolam

midbrain

Midchlor

midclavicular line to nipple
  (MCL-N)

midconcha cymba

middle
    m. constrictor pharyngeal
      muscle
    m. cranial fossa
    m. cranial fossa line
    m. ear
    m. ear cleft
    m. ear effusion (MEE)
    m. ear infection
    m. ear muscle reflex
    m. ear neoplasm
    m. fossa approach
    m. fossa plate
    m. fossa retractor
    m. fossa syndrome
    m. fossa vestibular neurec-
      tomy
    m. latency response (MLR)
    m. meatal antrostomy
    m. meatus
    m. meningeal artery
    m. nasal concha
    m. pharyngeal constrictor
    m. thyroid vein
    m. turbinate
    m. vault deformity
    m. zone

midface
    m. alloplastic augmentation
    m. avulsion flap
    m. fracture
    m. hypoplasia
    m. lift
    m. trauma

mid-face lift
    subperiosteal m. l.

midfacial
    m. breadth
    m. degloving
    m. fracture
    m. hypoplasia
    m. retrusion

midfoot

midge
    nimitti m.

Midigold alloy

midlamellar cicatricial retraction

midline
    m. of the columella
    m. cranio-orbital clefting
    m. disharmony
    m. forehead flap
    m. lethal granuloma
    m. malignant reticulosis
      granuloma

midpalatal
    m. opening
    m. suture opening

midpalatine raphe

mid-penile hypospadias

Midrin

midroot

midsagittal

mid-to-deep dermal peel

Miescher cheilitis granulomatosa

MIF
    macrophage-inhibiting fac-
      tor
    migration-inhibiting factor

migraine
    basilar artery m.
    m. equivalent
    m. headache

migrans
    erythema m.
    glossitis m.

migrated tooth

migration
    epithelial m.

migration *(continued)*
    physiologic mesial m.
    postoperative m.
    tooth m.
    m. of tooth

migration-inhibiting factor (MIF)

Mikamo double-eyelid operation

Mikulicz
    M. aphthae
    M. cells
    M. disease
    M. pad
    M. syndrome
    M.-Vladimiroff amputation

Miles Magic Mixture

milium *pl.* milia
    colloid m.

Millard
    M. bilateral cleft lip repair
    M. clamp
    M. creed
    M. flap
    M. forked flap technique
    M. graft augmentation
    M. Lite-Pipe
    M. modification of Kernahan and Elsahy striped Y classification for cleft lip and palate
    M. mouth gag
    M. rotation-advancement unilateral cleft lip repair
    M. thimble retractor
    unilateral M. repair

Miller-Fisher variant of Guillain-Barré syndrome

milliampere (mA)

milling-in

Miltex
    M. blepharoplasty scissors
    M. saber-back rhytidectomy scissors

Miltex *(continued)*
    M. stitch scissors
    M. tenaculum hook
    M. undermining scissors

Miltown

mimetic
    m. hyperkinesis
    m. modulation
    m. muscle

mimic
    facial m.
    m. speech

mimicry
    molecular m.

mimmation

mineral
    m. salt
    m. trioxide aggregate (MTA)
    m. wax

mineralization
    calcospherite m.
    capsular m.
    dystrophic m.

mineralized tissue

miniabdominoplasty
    open m.

miniature
    m. carrier
    m. plugger

Mini-Blade
    Beaver M.

Minidyne

mini–face-lift

Mini-Fibralux pocket otoscope

Minigold alloy

minigraft
    m. dilator

Minilux pocket otoscope

minimal brain dysfunction
  (MBD)

minimastopexy

Mini-Matic implant

minimus
    gluteus m.

miniplate
    Champy m.
    m. fixation
    8-hole m.
    L-shaped m.
    mandibular m.
    Storz m.
    titanium m.
    two-holed m.

miniscrew

mini trephine

Mini-Würzburg
    M. Flexplates craniomaxil-
      lofacial plating system
    M. standard craniomaxillo-
      facial plating system
    Leibinger M. plate

Minnesota retractor

minor
    aphthae m.
    m. connector
    m. gland obstruction
    m. salivary glands
    teres m.

Mirault-Blair-Brown method of
  cleft lip repair

mirror
    m.-based reflective optics
    curved laryngeal m.
    curved magnifying m.
    DenLite illuminated hand-
      held m.
    fiberoptic lighted m.
    frontal m.
    head m.
    mouth m.
    Neovision micro m.

mirror *(continued)*
    straight laryngeal m.
    straight magnifying m.

MIS
    melanoma in situ

misarticulation

misdirection
    facial nerve m.

mismatch
    m. negativity (MMN)
    pigmentation m.
    vessel caliber m.

misphonia

missile-caused wound

missing tooth

mist
    GraftCyte hydrating m.

Mitek
    M. anchor
    M. GII suture anchor
    M. Mini GII anchor

Mithracin

mitigated echolalia

mitochondrial oxidative enzyme

mitochondrion *pl.* mitochondria

mitogenic factor (MF)

mitomycin-C

mitosis

mitotic figure

mitoxantrone

Mittelman implant

Mitutoyo Digimatic calipers

Mitz procedure

mixed
    m. dentition
    m. failure
    m. hemangioma

mixed *(continued)*
 m. hypertrophy
 m. laterality
 m. mesh
 m. nasality
 m. odontoma
 m. tumor
 m. tumor of salivary gland
 m. type parapharyngeal
  schwannoma

mixture
 eutectic m. of local anesthetics (EMLA)
 Miles Magic M.

ML
 mesiolingual

MLA
 mesiolabial

Mladick
 M. abdominoplasty
 M. ear reconstruction

MLAI
 mesiolabioincisal

MLCI
 Marginal Line Calculus Index

MM
 malignant melanoma

MMC
 myelomeningocele

MMF
 maxillomandibular fixation

MMN
 mismatch negativity

MMS
 Mohs micrographic surgery

MND
 modified neck dissection

MNOE
 malignant necrotizing otitis
  externa

MO
 myositis ossificans

Moberg
 M. arthrodesis
 M. pickup test
 M. volar advancement flap

Mobidin

mobility
 breast m.

mobilization
 bony m.

Möbius syndrome

mode
 Hexascan m.

model
 casting m.
 immunocompetent squa-
  mous cell cancer m.
 implant m.
 m. plaster
 m. plaster Grade A
 m. trimmer
 Westmore m.

modeling
 bilateral fronto-orbital m.
 m. composition
 m. compound
 m. plastic
 m. plastic impression

moderately
 m. differentiated neuroendocrine carcinoma

modification
 activator m.
 appliance m.
 Bardach m.
 behavior m.
 bracket m.
 cingulum m.
 Goldner m.
 interference m.
 O'Leary m.
 Salyer m. of Obwegeser
  mandibular osteotomy
 Webster m. of Bernard-Burow cheiloplasty

modified
- m. abdominoplasty
- m. anterior scoring technique
- m. Bernard-Burow technique
- m. cast
- m. Chopart amputation
- m. desmosome
- m. flap operation
- m. Frost method
- m. Frost suture
- m. junctional complex
- m. Kiel mastopexy
- m. Krukenberg procedure
- m. lateral pharyngotomy
- m. Mallet scale
- m. neck dissection (MND)
- m. pen grasp
- m. polymer
- m. Pulvertaft classification for mutilating injuries (*categories 1–5*)
- m. radical mastectomy
- m. radical mastoidectomy
- m. Singapore flap
- m. Skoog technique
- m. somatic perception questionnaire (MSPQ)
- m. submental retractor, flared tip
- m. Wardill method
- m. Weber-Fergusson incision
- m. Weber-Fergusson procedure
- m. zinc oxide-eugenol cement

modifier
- biologic response m.

modiolus labii

modulation
- immune m.
- mimetic m.

Moe alar hook

Moeller glossitis

mogiarthria

mogilalia

Mohr-Tranebjaerg syndrome

Mohs
- M. chemosurgery
- M. defect
- M. excision
- M. fresh tissue chemosurgery technique
- M. hardness
- M. hardness number (MHN)
- M. hardness scale
- M. hardness test
- M. index
- M. micrographic surgery (MMS)
- M. micrographic surgery by fixed-tissue technique
- M. resection
- M. surgery
- M. wound

moiré topography index

molar
- mandibular m.
- maxillary m.

mold
- AquaNot swim m.
- casting m.
- m. guide
- inlay m.
- mother matrix m.
- Swyris swim m.
- Teflon m.

molding
- border m.
- compression m.
- injection m.
- m. temperature
- tissue m.

mole
- atypical m.
- hairy m.
- m. melanoma syndrome

mole *(continued)*
   pigmented m.
   spider m.

molecular mimicry

molecule
   cell adhesion m. (CAM)
   collagen m.
   neurotransmitter m.
   polymerized mucopolysac-
     charide m.
   tropocollagen m.

molilalia

Molina
   M. mandibular distractor
   M. mandibular distractor
     set

Möller disease

Moll glands

Mollison rongeur

molluscum contagiosum

Mölnlycke

Molt
   M. mouth gag
   M. No. 4 elevator

Monahan-Lewis knife

Mona Lisa smile

monangle hoe

Mondini
   M. deafness
   M. deformity
   M. dysplasia
   M. malformation
   oral M.
   M.-Alexander malformation

Mondor disease

mongolism

monitor
   Accutorr m.
   Accutorr bedside m.
   blood perfusion m.

monitor *(continued)*
   Colin STBP-780 stress test
     blood pressure m.
   Criticare m.
   Criticare 507N noninvasive
     blood pressure m.
   Criticare 507O pulse oxime-
     ter/NIBP m.
   Criticare comprehensive vi-
     tal sign m.
   Criticare POET TE end-tidal
     CO_2 respiration m.
   Haemogram blood loss m.
   laser Doppler perfusion m.
   Laserflo BPM laser Dop-
     pler m.
   Marquette m.
   m. muscle flap
   MRL blood pressure m.
   Multinex ID gas m.
   Neurosign 100 nerve m.
   Passport bedside m.
   perfusion m.
   Porta-Resp m.
   Stat-Temp II liquid crystal
     temperature m.
   Transonic laser Doppler
     perfusion m.
   VISA multi-patient m.

Monks-Esser island flap

monoangle chisel

monoangled

monobloc
   m. advancement
   m. appliance

monochromatic radiation

Monocid

monoclonal antibody

monocortical
   m. bone
   m. screw

Monocryl suture

monocyte

monocytoid cell

monofascicular nerve

monofilament
  m. nylon suture
  Semmes-Weinstein nylon m. (SWMF)
  m. suture
  m. test

Mono-Gesic

monomaxillary

monomorphic
  m. adenoma
  m. pattern

Mononine

mononucleosis
  infectious m.

monoplegia
  m. masticatoria

monopodal
  m. ankylotic stapes

monostotic
  m. fibrous dysplasia
  m. lesion

monostructure implant

Monro abscess

Monson curve

mons pubis

Montague plane

montan wax

Montgomery
  M. glands
  M. laryngeal keel
  M. speaking valve
  M. thyroplasty implant system
  M. T tube
  M. tubercles

Moore
  M. head-tilt maneuver
  M. mandrel

moorean ulcer

Moorehead
  M. cheek retractor
  M. retractor

Morand foot

morbidity
  perinatal m.

morbid obesity

morcel

morcellation

morcellizer
  Rubin septal m.

Morel ear

Morgagni
  M. cartilage
  M. concha
  M. foramen
  sinus of M.
  M. ventricle

Morgan
  M. fold
  M. mandrel

Moro reflex

morphea

morpheaform
  m. basal cell carcinoma

morphogen

morphogenic stage

morphographemic rule

morphology
  Antoni classification of schwannoma m.
  craniofacial m.

morphotype

Morquio
  mucopolysaccharidosis type IV M.
  M. syndrome

Morrison toe flap

morselized cartilage

morsicatio

mortality
    perinatal m.

Morwel
    M. ultrasound-assisted lipo-
       plasty machine
    M. ultrasound device

Mosher nasal speculum

mosquito
    m. forceps
    m. clamp
    m. hemostat

Moss balloon triple-lumen gas-
    trostomy tube

mother
    m. matrix mold
    m. method

motility

motion
    active range of m. (AROM)
    brownian m.
    cartwheel m.
    ciliary m.
    lunotriquetral m.
    mandibular range of m.
    maximal static response as-
       say of facial m.
    range of m. (ROM)
    range of m. of the wrist
    scapholunate m.
    short arc m. (SAM) proto-
       col

motivating operation

motivation

motokinesthetics

motor
    m. aphasia
    m. area
    m. control test

motor *(continued)*
    m. coordination test (MCT)
    m. disorder
    m. endplate
    fine m.
    gross m.
    m. impairment
    m. nerve
    m. nerve of tongue
    m. neuron
    m. roots of submandibular
       ganglion
    m. root of trigeminal nerve

moulage
    facial m.

mould *(variant of* mold)

Moult curet

mound
    malar m.

mount
    Adamount pocket m's
    split cast m.

moustache *spelled also* mus-
    tache
    m. dressing
    m.-like flap

mouth
    m. breathing
    carp m.
    denture sore m.
    depressor muscle of angle
       of m.
    dry m.
    floor of m. (FOM)
    m. flora
    m. gag
    m. guard
    m. hygiene
    m. lamp
    levator muscle of angle
       of m.
    lymphatic vessels of m.
    m. mirror
    numerary m.
    orbicular muscle of m.
    orifice of the m.

mouth *(continued)*
    phlegmon of floor of m.
    m. preparation
    m. prop
    putrid sore m.
    m. rehabilitation
    roof of m.
    m. stick
    trench m.
    vestibule of m.
    white m.

movability

movable-arm clasp

movement
    ballistic m.
    Bennett m.
    bodily m.
    border tissue m.
    brownian m.
    compensatory m.
    cutting m.
    dentogenic m.
    distal m.
    empty m.
    eruptive tooth m.
    extraneous m.
    Facial Grading System voluntary m. (FGSM)
    free mandibular m.
    functional mandibular m.
    gliding m.
    grinding m.
    hinge m.
    intermediary m.
    jaw m.
    labial m.
    lateral m.
    laterotrusive m.
    lingual m.
    mandibular gliding m.
    masticatory mandibular m.
    maximum m.
    nonfunction mandibular m.
    opening mandibular m.
    oral commissure m.
    pendulum m.
    posterior border m.
    protrusive m.
    random m.

movement *(continued)*
    retrusive m.
    rotational m.
    sagittal mandibular m.
    smooth-pursuit eye m.
    tipping m.
    translatory m.
    volition oral m.

moving two-point discrimination

Mozart ear

MP
    metacarpophalangeal
        MP joint arthroplasty
    metatarsophalangeal
        MP joint arthroplasty

MPAPC
    mucus-producing adenopapillary carcinoma

MPD
    maximum permissible dose
    myofascial pain-dysfunction
        MPD syndrome

MPH
    mandibular plane to hyoid

M-plasty

MPO
    maximum power output

MPS
    mucopolysaccharidosis
        MPS-IH
        MPS-IHS
        MPS-II
        MPS-IIIA
        MPS-IIIB
        MPS-IIIC
        MPS-IS
        MPS-IV
        MPS-VI
        MPS-VII
    myofascial pain syndrome

MRA
    magnetic resonance angiography

MRG
mean rejection grading
mean residual gap

MRI
magnetic resonance imaging
coronal MRI of wrist
FISP-3D (fast-imaging steady precession sequence three-dimensional) MRI
MRI scan
surface-coil MRI

MRKHS
Mayer-Rokitansky-Küster-Hauser syndrome

MRL blood pressure monitor

MS
melanonychia striata

MSBP
mandibular staple bone plate

MSI
magnetic source imaging

MSPQ
modified somatic perception questionnaire

MST
maximum stimulation test

MTA
mineral trioxide aggregate

MTP
metatarsophalangeal

mucicarmine

mucigen granule

mucinase

mucinosis
cutaneous focal m.
oral focal m.

mucinous
m. cell adenocarcinoma

mucinous (continued)
m. plaque

mucobuccal
m. fold
m. reflection

mucocele
frontal sinus m.
maxillary sinus m.
retention m.
sinus m.

mucochondrocutaneous flap

mucociliary
m. drainage pathway
m. flow
m. transport (MCT)

mucocutaneous
m. junction
m. leishmaniasis
m. lymph node syndrome
m. melanosis

mucoepidermoid
m. carcinoma (MEC)
m. carcinoma of parotid
m. carcinoma of the tongue
m. lesion
m. tumor

mucogingival
m. junction (MGJ)
m. line
m. surgery

mucoid
m. otitis media

mucolabial fold

Mucolube

mucolytic

mucoperichondrial
m. elevation
m. flap

mucoperichondrium
septal m.

mucoperiosteal
m. flap technique
m. lining

mucoperiosteal *(continued)*
   m. periodontal flap
   m. periodontal graft
   m. sliding flap

mucoperiosteum

mucopolysaccharide
   acid m.
   m. keratin dystrophy

mucopolysaccharidosis (MPS)
   pl. mucopolysaccharidoses
   m. type I Hurler (MPS-IH)
   m. type I Hurler-Scheie
     (MPS-IHS)
   m. type II Hunter (MPS-II)
   m. type III Sanfilippo A
     (MPS-IIIA)
   m. type III Sanfilippo B
     (MPS-IIIB)
   m. type III Sanfilippo C
     (MPS-IIIC)
   m. type I Scheie (MPS-IS)
   m. type VII Sly (MPS-VII)
   m. type VI Maroteaux-Lamy
     (MPS-VI)
   m. type IV Morquio (MPS-
     IV)

mucopurulent
   m. hemorrhagic effusion

mucopus

mucopyelocele

mucopyocele

mucormycosis
   rhinocerebral m.
   rhinoorbital m.
   rhinoorbitocerebral m.

mucosa
   alveolar m.
   alveolar ridge m.
   bladder m.
   buccal m.
   conchal m.
   dorsal lingual m.
   ethmoidal m.
   free graft from urinary
     bladder m.
   friable m.

mucosa *(continued)*
   gastric m.
   gingival m.
   hypermobile m.
   hyperplastic m.
   lingual m.
   lining m.
   mandibular alveolar m.
   masticatory m.
   nasal m.
   oral m.
   palatal m.
   palatine m.
   reflecting m.
   respiratory m.
   retromolar m.
   retrotuberosity m.
   septal m.
   specialized m.
   sublingual m.
   vestibular m.
   vomer m.

mucosae
   lipoidosis cutis et m.

mucosal
   m. blood vessel
   m. coat
   m. collar
   m. cyst
   m. excision
   m. grafting
   m. horn
   m. implant
   m. insert
   m. patch replacement
   m. periodontal flap
   m. periodontal graft
   m. prelaminated flap
   m. relaxing incision tech-
     nique
   m. transudate

mucosalize

mucositis
   radiation m.
   xerostomic m.

mucosobuccal fold

mucostatic

mucous
m. alveolus
m. blanket
m. cell
m. cyst
m. gland
m. membrane
m. membrane of lip
m. membrane of tongue
m. otitis
m. patch
m. plaque
m. plug
m. retention cyst
m. retention phenomenon
m. tubule

mucoviscidosis

mucus
glairy m.
nasal m.
olfactory m.
salivary m.

mucus-producing adenopapillary carcinoma (MPAPC)

mucus-secreting cell

Muehrcke band

Mueller
M. test
M.-Walle method

muffled voice

muffle furnace

Muhlmann
M. appliance

Mulder
angle of M.

Muldoon retractor

Müller
ganglion of M.

müllerian
m. dimple
m. duct

müllerian (continued)
m. duct aplasia

mulling

Multicenter Selective Lymphadenectomy trial

multicentric glomus tumor

multichannel cochlear implant

Multicide

multicultural family

Multidimensional Body-Self Relations Questionnaire

multidirectional distractor

Multi-fil

multifocal lymphocytic infiltrate

Multi-Form dual purpose impression paste

multiforme
erythema m.

MULTIGUIDE mandibular distractor

multilaminar

MultiLase D copper vapor laser

multilocular
m. cyst
m. mass

multiloculated

Multinex ID gas monitor

multinodular goiter

multinucleated
m. dentinoblastic cell
m. giant cell

multipara

multiphase
m. appliance
m. attachment
m. bracket

multiplanar
  m. endoscopic facial reju-
    venation technique
  m. upper facial rejuvena-
    tion technique

multiple
  m. abutment
  m. abutment support
  m. anchorage
  m. clasp
  m. diastemata
  m. endocrine neoplasia
  m. exostoses of jaw
  m. foramina
  m. hamartoma syndrome
  m. loop archwire
  m. loop wiring
  m. myeloma
  m. papillomatosis
  m. primary
  m. retainer
  m. sclerosis

multiplex
  dysostosis m.
  steatocystoma m.

multiply handicapped

multipoint contact plate

multipolar neuron

multiprong rake retractor

multirooted
  m. abutment

multiscope
  roaming optical access m.
    (ROAM)

multisensory

multivacuolated

multivesicular body

Muma Assessment Program
  (MAP)

mumps
  m. encephalitis
  m. meningoencephalomye-
    litis

mumps *(continued)*
  m. virus

Munro classification of orbital
  hypertelorism *(types A–D)*

mural ameloblastoma

muromonab-CD3

muscle
  abductor hallucis m.
  abductor pollicis longus m.
  m.-access abdominoplasty
  adductor longus m.
  adductor magnus m.
  Aeby m.
  alar m.
  anconeus m.
  ansa hypoglossus m.
  antagonistic m.
  anterior auricular m.
  anterior superficialis m.
  antitragicus m.
  aryepiglottic m.
  arytenoid m.
  auricular m.
  m. belly
  bipennate m.
  Bochdalek m.
  Bovero m.
  Bowman ciliary m.
  brachialis m.
  brachioradialis m.
  Brücke m.
  buccal m.
  buccinator m.
  m. bundle
  canine m.
  cheek m.
  chin m.
  chondroglossus m.
  chondropharyngeal m.
  cleft m. of Veau
  compressor m. of naris
  constrictor pharyngeal m.
  constrictor m. of pharynx
  m. contraction
  m. contraction headache
  corrugator m.
  corrugator supercilii m.
  cremaster m.

muscle *(continued)*
   cricoarytenoid m.
   cricopharyngeus m.
   cricothyroid m.
   dartos m.
   denervated m.
   depressor m. of angle of
     mouth
   depressor anguli oris m.
   depressor labii inferioris m.
   depressor labii oris m.
   depressor septi m.
   digastric m.
   dilator naris m.
   epicranius m.
   extensor carpi radialis
     brevis m.
   extensor carpi radialis lon-
     gus (ECRL) m.
   extensor carpi ulnaris
     (ECU) m.
   extensor digiti minimi m.
   extensor digitorum m.
   extensor digitorum lon-
     gus m.
   extensor hallucis longus m.
   extensor indicis m.
   extensor pollicis brevis m.
   extensor pollicis longus
     (EPL) m.
   extralaryngeal m.
   extraocular m.
   extrinsic m. of tongue
   facial m.
   facial mimetic m.
   fast-twitch fatigable skele-
     tal m.
   flexor carpi ulnaris m.
   flexor digitorum brevis m.
   flexor digitorum longus m.
   flexor digitorum profundus
     (FDP) m.
   flexor digitorum superfici-
     alis (FDS) m.
   flexor hallucis longus m.
   flexor pollicis longus
     (FPL) m.
   frontalis m.
   Gantzer m.
   gastrocnemius m.

muscle *(continued)*
   genioglossus m.
   geniohyoglossus m.
   geniohyoid m.
   glossopalatine m.
   gracilis m.
   greater zygomatic m.
   m. hernia
   Horner m.
   hyoglossal m.
   hyoglossus m.
   hyperactive m.
   hyperactive glabellar m.
   hypertonic m.
   hypotonic m.
   iliocostalis dorsi m.
   iliocostalis lumborum m.
   m. implantation
   incisive m.
   inferior constrictor pharyn-
     geal m.
   inferior longitudinal m. of
     tongue
   inferior oblique m.
   inferior rectus m.
   infrahyoid m.
   infrahyoid strap m.
   infraspinatus m.
   interarytenoid m.
   intercostalis externus m.
   intercostalis internus m.
   internal pterygoid m.
   intrinsic m. of tongue
   lateral cricoarytenoid m.
   lateral pterygoid m.
   lateral rectus m.
   latissimus dorsi m.
   levator m.
   levator m. of angle of
     mouth
   levator anguli oris m.
   levator costae m.
   levator glandulae thyro-
     idea m.
   levator labii superioris m.
   levator labii superioris
     alaeque nasi m.
   levator palatini m.
   levator veli palatini m.
   longitudinalis inferior m.

muscle *(continued)*
   longitudinalis superior m.
   longitudinal m. of tongue
   longus capitis m.
   longus colli m.
   masseter m.
   mastication m.
   masticatory m.
   medial pterygoid m.
   medial rectus m.
   mental m.
   mentalis m.
   middle constrictor pharyn-
     geal m.
   mimetic m.
   m. moment arm length
   musculus transversus
     menti m.
   mylohyoid m.
   nasal m.
   nasalis m.
   nasolabial m.
   oblique m.
   oblique arytenoid m.
   obliquus abdominis exter-
     nus m.
   obliquus abdominis inter-
     nus m.
   obliquus inferior m.
   obliquus superior m.
   occipitofrontalis m.
   omohyoid m.
   orbicularis m.
   orbicularis oculi m.
   orbicularis oris m.
   orbicular m. of mouth
   palatal m.
   palatoglossal m.
   palatoglossus m.
   palatopharyngeal m.
   palatopharyngeus m.
   palmar interosseous m.
   palmaris longus m.
   paravertebral m.
   pectoralis major m.
   pectoralis minor m.
   perioral m.
   periorbital orbicularis ocu-
     li m.
   m.-periosteal flap

muscle *(continued)*
   peroneus tertius m.
   pharyngeal constrictor m.
   pharyngopalatinus m.
   platysma m.
   posterior cricoarytenoid m.
   procerus m.
   pronator quadratus m.
   pronator teres m.
   pterygoid m.
   quadrate m. of lower lip
   quadrate m. of upper lip
   quadratus labii inferioris
     muscle
   quadratus labii superi-
     oris m.
   quadratus lumborum m.
   rectus abdominis m.
   rectus capitis m.
   rectus femoris m.
   rectus labii m.
   rectus medialis m.
   rectus superioris m.
   m. relaxant
   m. repositioning
   risorius m.
   salpingopharyngeal m.
   salpingopharyngeus m.
   Santorini m.
   sartorius m.
   scalenus anterior m.
   scalenus medius m.
   scalenus posterior m.
   scalp m.
   semimembranosus m.
   semimembranous m.
   serratus anterior m.
   serratus posterior infer-
     ior m.
   serratus posterior super-
     ior m.
   short extensor m.
   short flexor m.
   short radial extensor m.
   m. sling
   slow-twitch fatigue-resis-
     tant skeletal m.
   smooth m.
   Soemmering m.
   soleus m.

muscle *(continued)*
    spastic m.
    m. spindle
    splenius capitis m.
    square m. of lower lip
    stapedius m.
    sternoclavicularis m.
    sternocleidomastoid m.
    sternocleidomastoideus m.
    sternohyoid m.
    sternohyoideus m.
    sternothyroid m.
    sternothyroideus m.
    strap m.
    styloglossus m.
    stylohyoid m.
    stylopharyngeal m.
    stylopharyngeus m.
    subclavius m.
    subcostal m.
    subcostalis m.
    superior auricular m.
    superior constrictor m.
    superior constrictor phar-
        yngeal m.
    superior longitudinal m. of
        tongue
    superior rectus m.
    superior tarsal m.
    supinator m.
    suprahyoid m.
    temporal m.
    temporalis m.
    m. tension headache
    tensor fasciae latae m.
    tensor tympani m.
    tensor veli palatini m.
    teres major m.
    teres minor m.
    thyroarytenoid m.
    thyroepiglottic m.
    thyrohyoid m.
    thyropharyngeal m.
    tibialis anterior m.
    tibialis posterior m.
    m. tonus
    trachealis m.
    transpalpebral corruga-
        tor m.
    m. transposition

muscle *(continued)*
    transverse arytenoid m.
    transverse m. of tongue
    transversus abdominis m.
    transversus linguae m.
    transversus perinei profun-
        dus m.
    transversus thoracis m.
    trapezius m.
    triangular m.
    m. trimming
    tympanic m.
    uvula m.
    uvular m.
    Valsalva m.
    vastus lateralis m.
    vastus medialis m.
    vastus medialis obli-
        quus m.
    verticalis linguae m.
    vertical m. of tongue
    vocal m.
    vocalis m.
    zygomatic m.
    zygomaticomandibular m.
    zygomaticus m.
    zygomaticus major m.
    zygomaticus minor m.

muscle-plasty
    V-Y m.

muscle transfer
    free m. t.
    gracilis free m. t.
    island frontalis m. t.
    masseter m. t.
    pectoralis minor m. t.
    rectus abdominis m. t.
    regional m. t.
    staged m. t.

muscular
    m. bolster
    m. dystrophy
    m. graft
    m. sclerosis
    m. torticollis

musculature
    aponeurotic m.

musculature *(continued)*
    contralateral m.
    facial mimetic m.

musculoaponeurotic
    m. control
    m. layer
    m. plication
    m. system

musculocutaneous
    m. flap
    m. flap skin paddle
    m. perforator
    rectus abdominis m. (RAM) flap
    transverse rectus abdominis m. (TRAM) flap

musculofascial flap

musculomucosal
    facial artery m. (FAMM) flap

musculoperitoneal
    transversus and rectus abdominis m. (TRAMP) composite flap

musculotendinous aponeurosis

musculovascular pedicle

musculus
    m. helicis major
    m. helicis minor
    m. levator anguli oris
    m. levator labii superioris
    m. risorius
    m. tensor fasciae latae
    m. transversus menti muscle
    m. vastus lateralis
    m. zygomaticus major

Musgrave and Dupertuis graft augmentation

mustache *(variant of* moustache)

Mustardé
    M. lateral cheek rotation flap

Mustardé *(continued)*
    M. otoplasty
    M. rotation-advancement flap
    M. suture
    M. technique

mutacism

mutagen

mutagenic

mute

mutilation
    dorsal m.
    jugomasseteric m.
    labiogeniomandibular m.
    orbitopalpebral m.

mutism
    elected m.
    elective m.
    voluntary m.

Muti technique

"mutton chop" flap

MV
    main venule

MVD
    microvascular decompression
    microvessel density

myasthenia
    m. gravis
    m. laryngis

My-Bond Carbo cement

Mycelex
    M.-7
    M.-G
    M. Troche

mycelium *pl.* mycelia

mycetoma
    Vincent white m.

mycobacteria *(pl.* of mycobacterium)

mycobacterial
  m. infection
  m. lymphadenitis
  m. nodal infection

mycobacterium *pl.* mycobacteria
  atypical m.
  nontuberculous m. (NTM)

mycomyringitis

mycophenolate

mycosis
  antral m.
  m. fungoides
  m. leptothrica
  systemic m.

Mycostatin

mycotic
  m. disease
  m. stomatitis

Myco-Triacet II

Mydriacyl

mydriasis

mydriatic

myectomy

myelinated
  m. axon
  m. nerve fiber
  m. sensory nerve fiber

myelination

myelinization

myelin sheath

myeloblastoma
  granular cell m.

myeloma
  multiple m.

myelomeningocele (MMC)

myiasis
  aural m.
  nasal m.
  oral m.

Mylar
  M. matrix
  M. strip

mylohyoid
  m. line
  m. muscle
  m. nerve
  m. region
  m. ridge
  m. sulcus
  m. sulcus of mandible

myoblastoma
  granular cell m.
  malignant granular cell m.

Myobock artificial hand

myocardial infarction

myocutaneous
  m. flap
  transverse rectus abdominis m. (TRAM) flap

myodermal flap

myoelastic acrodynamic theory of phonation

myoelastic theory

myoepithelial
  m. cell
  m. cell island
  m. cell process
  m. sialadenitis

myoepithelioma

myofascial
  m. flap
  m. pain-dysfunction (MPD)
  m. pain-dysfunction disorder
  m. pain-dysfunction syndrome
  m. pain syndrome (MPS)

myofasciitis
  necrotizing m.

myofiber atrophy

myofibrositis

myofunctional
m. therapy

myogaleal

myogenic

myognathus

myograph
palate m.

myography

myoma

Myo-monitor centric

myomucosal flap

myonecrosis

myoneural blocking agent

myoneurotization

myopathic
m. paralysis

myopathy
thyrotoxic m.

myoplastic

myoplasty

myosarcoma
angiomatoid m.

myositis
m. ossificans (MO)
m. ossificans progressiva

myospherulosis

myotactic

myotatic
m. irritability
m. reflex

myotomy
cricopharyngeal m.
hyoid m.
procerus muscle m.

myotonia
acquired m.

myotonia *(continued)*
congenital m.
dystrophic m.

myringeal web

myringectomy

myringitis
m. bullosa
bullous m.

myringodermatitis

myringomycosis

myringoplasty

myringostapediopexy

myringotome

myringotomy
m. and grommet insertion
m. knife

myrinx

mytacism

myxedema
m. voice

myxochondroid
m. matrix
m. stroma

myxofibroma
odontogenic m.

myxoid
m. crystal
m. liposarcoma
m. lobule
m. neurofibroma
m. stroma

myxolipoma

myxoma
fibro-osteogenic m.
nerve sheath m. (NSM)
odontogenic m.
osteogenic m.

myxomatous degeneration

myxosarcoma

Nabers probe

NAC
nipple-areola complex

Naga sore

Nager
N. acrofacial dysostosis
N. syndrome

Nahai
N. tensor fasciae latae flap
N.-Mathes classification of
fasciocutaneous flaps
(*types A–C*)
N.-Mathes fasciocutaneous
flap (*types A–C*)

nail
n. fold
Grosse-Kempf interlock-
ing n.
n. plate

Nance
N. analysis of arch length
N. leeway space

nape of neck flap

naris *pl.* nares
anterior n.
nares constriction
constrictor n.
nares internae
posterior n.

narrow-field laryngectomy

nasal
n. accessory artery
n. airway
n. airway obstruction
n. antrostomy
n. artery
n. bone
n. cavity
n. cross-sectional area
n. dome
n. dorsum
n. dysplasia

nasal *(continued)*
n. floor
n. fossa
n. fracture
n. height
n. lisp
n. muscle
n. nerve
n. process
n. recess
n. septal perforation
n. septa reconstruction
n. septum
n. stenosis
n. tip
n. tip deformity
n. tip-plasty
n. wing

nasality
excessive n.
mixed n.

nasal-labial furrow

nasal-septal fracture

nasion
basion-n. (Ba-N) plane
orbitale n.
n. perpendicular
n. point
sella-n. (S-N) plane
n. soft tissue

nasion-alveolar point line

nasion-pogonion measurement

Nasmyth membrane

nasoalveolar cyst

nasobregmatic arc

nasociliary nerve

nasoethmoidal fracture

naso-ethmoid-orbital fracture

nasofacial
n. analysis
n. groove

nasofrontal
n. angle
n. duct
n. orifice
n. suture

nasojugal fold

nasolabial
n. angle
n. cyst
n. flap
n. fold (NLF)
n. ligament
n. line
n. muscle
n. rotation flap
n. stigma
n. sulcus

nasolacrimal duct

nasomalarmaxillary

nasomandibular
n. fixation
n. ligament

nasomaxillary
n. balloon
n. buttress
n. dysplasia

nasomental reflex

naso-ocular
n. cleft

naso-oral

nasoorbitoethmoid (NOE)
n. fracture

nasopalatine
n. cyst
n. duct
n. duct cyst
n. foramen
n. injection
n. nerve

nasopharyngeal
n. abscess
n. angiofibroma

nasopharyngeal *(continued)*
n. carcinoma (NPC)
n. cyst
n. fibroma

nasopharyngectomy

nasopharyngolaryngoscope

nasopharynx
carcinoma of n. (types a–c)

nasoplasty

Naso-Tamp nasal packing
sponge

Nassif parascapular flap

Nataf
N. lateral flap
superiorly based N. lateral
flap

natal
n. cleft

NaturaLase
N. Erbium laser
N. Er:YAG laser

natural-feel breast prosthesis

Natural Profile abutment system

Nd:YAG
neodymium:yttrium-alumi-
num-garnet
Nd:YAG laser

near-total laryngectomy

neck
bur n.
condylar n.
n. of condyle
congenital cartilaginous
rest of the n. (CCRN)
fiddler n.
n. flap
functional assessment of
cancer therapy—head
and n. (FACT-HN)
implant n.
n. implant substructure

neck *(continued)*
    implant superstructure n.
    n. jowl
    n. of mandible
    n. of middle turbinate
    osteotomy of condylar n.
    ridge of mandibular n.
    sulcus of mandibular n.

neck dissection
    bilateral n. d.
    discontinuous n. d.
    elective n. d. (END)
    functional n. d.
    modified n. d. (MND)
    radical n. d.
    selective n. d. (SND)
    suprahyoid n. d.
    supraomohyoid n. d.
    tongue-jaw-n. d.
    Wookey radical n. d.

necrobiosis lipoidica

necropsy

necrosis
    acute tubular n.
    aseptic n.
    avascular n. (AVN)
    caseous n.
    coagulation n.
    colliquative n.
    coronal n.
    cortical n.
    epidermal n.
    fat n.
    fibrinoid n.
    flap n.
    gummatous n.
    ischemic n.
    liquefactive n.
    radiation n.
    rim n.
    septal n.
    skin edge n.
    spot n.
    subcutaneous fat n.
    tendon n.
    tumorlike n.
    wound n.

necrotizing
    n. external otitis
    n. fasciitis (NF)
    n. myofascial fungal infection
    n. myofasciitis
    n. soft tissue infection (NSTI)

needle
    Agnew tattooing n.
    aspirating n.
    aspiration biopsy n.
    atraumatic n.
    biopsy n.
    Brown cleft palate n.
    catgut n.
    Colorado microdissection n.
    fine n.
    Hagedorn suture n.
    Halle septal n.
    harelip n.
    Keith n.
    Klein infiltration n.
    Lukens n.
    metallic frontal n.
    Permark micropigmentation n.
    Reverdin n.
    swaged n.
    Wright n.

needle holder
    Axhausen n. h.
    Baumgartner n. h.
    Converse n. h.
    Converse-Gillies n. h.
    Gillies n. h.
    Gillies-Sheehan n. h.
    Hagedorn n. h.
    Webster n. h.

Needles split cast method

negativity
    mismatch n. (MMN)

Neiman nasal splint

Neivert knife guide and retractor

neoclitoris *pl.* neoclitorides
    vascularized sensate n.

neoclitoroplasty
    sensate pedicled n.

neoglottic reconstruction

neoglottis

neomeatus urethrae

neophallus

neoplasia
    endocrine n.
    multiple endocrine n.

neoplasm
    benign epithelial n.
    benign mesenchymal n.
    connective tissue n.
    cranial base n.
    epithelial n.
    expansible osseous n.
    glandular n.
    infratentorial n.
    laryngeal n.
    malignant n.
    maxillary n.
    mesenchymal n.
    metastatic n.
    middle ear n.
    neural sheath n.
    neuroendocrine n.
    salivary n.
    salivary gland n.
    vascular n.

neoplastic

neosphincter
    electrically stimulated n.

neosulcus
    submammary n.

neoumbilicoplasty

neovagina

neovaginal
    n. cavity
    n. introitus

neovaginoplasty

neovascularization

neovasculature

nerve
    abducent n.
    acousticofacial n.
    n. action potential
    afferent n.
    alveolar n.
    ampullary n.
    n. anastomosis
    anterior auricular n.
    anterior ethmoidal n.
    n. approximator
    Arnold n.
    auditory n.
    auricular n.
    auriculotemporal n.
    avulsion of n.
    n. block
    n. branch
    branchial n.
    buccal n.
    buccinator n.
    n. bundle
    carotid n.
    n. cell
    cervical sympathetic n.
    n. compression
    n. compression syndrome
    n. of Cotunnius
    cranial n's (I–XII)
    n. crush injury
    dead n.
    deep peroneal n.
    deep petrosal n.
    dorsal antebrachial cuta-
      neous n.
    EBSL n.
    efferent n.
    n. ending
    ethmoidal n.
    n. evulsion
    n. excitability test
    external branch of the su-
      perior laryngeal n.
    external nasal n.
    facial n. (FN)
    n. factor

nerve *(continued)*
   n. fascicle
   femoral cutaneous n.
   n. fiber
   n. fiber bundle
   fibroma of n.
   n. force
   frontal n.
   frontalis n.
   furcal n.
   Galen n.
   n. gap
   genitofemoral n.
   gingival n.
   glossopharyngeal n.
   n. graft
   great auricular n.
   greater palatine n.
   greater petrosal n.
   greater superficial petro-
     sal n.
   n. growth factor (NGF)
   hypoglossal n.
   iliohypogastric n.
   ilioinguinal n.
   n. impulse
   incisive n.
   inferior alveolar n. (IAN)
   inferior laryngeal n.
   inferior nasal n.
   infraorbital n.
   infratrochlear n.
   intercostal n.
   intermediary n.
   intermediate n.
   internal branch of the su-
     perior laryngeal (IBSL) n.
   intertubular n.
   intratubular n.
   Jacobson n.
   laryngeal n.
   lateral antebrachial cuta-
     neous n.
   lateral femoral cuta-
     neous n.
   lesser petrosal n.
   lesser superficial petrosal n.
   lingual n.
   n. loss
   mandibular n.

nerve *(continued)*
   marginal mandibular n.
   masseteric n.
   masticator n.
   maxillary n.
   medial antebrachial cuta-
     neous n.
   medial brachial cuta-
     neous n.
   median n. (MN)
   mental n.
   monofascicular n.
   motor n.
   motor n. of tongue
   mylohyoid n.
   nasal n.
   nasociliary n.
   nasopalatine n.
   nonmyelinated n.
   nonrecurrent laryngeal n.
   obturator n.
   ocular n.
   oculomotor n.
   olfactory n.
   ophthalmic n.
   optic n.
   palatine n.
   palmar cutaneous n.
   palmar digital n's
   peroneal n.
   petrosal n.
   phrenic n.
   polyfascicular n.
   posterior ampullary n.
     (PAN)
   posterior ethmoidal n.
   posterior inferior nasal n.
   posterior superior nasal n.
   posterosuperior alveolar n.
   postganglionic n.
   predentinal n.
   pterygoid n.
   radial n.
   recurrent laryngeal n.
     (RLN)
   saccular n.
   saphenous n.
   secretory n.
   sensory n.

nerve *(continued)*
    n. sharing
    n. sheath
    n. sheath myxoma (NSM)
    n. sheath tumor
    somatic motor n.
    special somatic sensory n.
    sphenopalatine n.
    spinal accessory n.
    spinal tract of trigeminal n.
    splayed facial n.
    n. stump
    stylohyoid n.
    stylopharyngeal n.
    sublingual n.
    submandibular n.
    submaxillary n.
    superficial petrosal n.
    superficial radial n.
    superior alveolar n.
    superior laryngeal n. (SLN)
    superior maxillary n.
    superior nasal n.
    supraorbital n.
    supratrochlear n.
    sural n.
    sympathetic n.
    temporal n.
    temporal facial n.
    temporofacial n.
    temporomalar n.
    tensor tympani n.
    terminal n.
    thoracic n.
    thoracodorsal n.
    n. transfer
    trigeminal n.
    trochlear n.
    n. trunk
    n. twig
    tympanic n.
    upper cervical n.
    vagus n.
    Valentin n.
    variant n.
    vestibular n.
    vestibulocochlear n.
    vidian n.

nerve *(continued)*
    zygomatic frontal n.
    zygomaticofacial n.
    zygomaticotemporal n.

nerve block
    external nasal n. b.
    inferior alveolar n. b.
    infraorbital n. b.
    intercostal n. b.
    local n. b.
    mandibular n. b.
    median n. b.
    mental n. b.
    nasopalatine n. b.
    phrenic n. b.
    radial n. b.
    Spaeth facial n. b.
    supraorbital n. b.
    supratrochlear n. b.
    thoracic n. b.
    ulnar n. b.

nervus intermedius

netting
    Dacron n.

network
    dermal n.
    terminal capillary n. (TCN)

Neubauer artery

Neumann
    N. cell
    N. sheath

neural
    n. crest cell
    n. element
    n. filament
    n. plate
    n. sheath neoplasm
    n. sheath tumor
    n. tube

neuralgia
    atypical facial n.
    auriculotemporal n.
    buccal n.
    causalgia n.

neuralgia *(continued)*
 facial n.
 n. facialis vera
 geniculate n.
 geniculate ganglion n.
 genitofemoral n.
 glossopharyngeal n.
 Hunt n.
 iliohypogastric n.
 ilioinguinal n.
 occipital n.
 paratrigeminal n.
 paroxysmal n.
 postherpetic n.
 postsurgical n.
 posttraumatic n.
 Sluder n.
 sphenopalatine n.
 temporomandibular n.
 trifacial n.
 trigeminal n.
 vidian n.

neuralgia-inducing cavitational osteonecrosis (NICO)

neurapraxic lesion

neurectomy
 middle fossa vestibular n.
 pharyngeal plexus n.
 retrosigmoid vesicular n.
 vestibular n.

neurilemma

neurilemmatosis
 familial n.

neurinoma
 facial n.

neuritis
 fallopian n.
 peripheral n.
 retrobulbar n.
 vestibular n.

neuroadventitia
 perivascular n.

neuroanastomosis
 hypoglossal-facial n.

neurocutaneous flap

neuroendocrine
 n. carcinoma
 n. marker
 n. neoplasm
 n. tumor
 n. tumor of larynx

neurofibroma
 n. of larynx
 myxoid n.
 paranasopharyngeal n.
 plexiform n.
 solitary n.

neurofibromatosis (NF) *(types 1 and 2)*
 cranio-orbital n.
 Recklinghausen n.
 segmental n.
 variant n.

neurofibrosarcoma

neurogenic
 n. dysarthria
 n. dysphagia
 n. factor
 n. sarcoma
 n. tumor

neurological
 n. dysfunction
 n. pinwheel

neurolysis

neuroma
 amputation n.
 cutis n.
 n. excision
 palisaded encapsulated n.
 subcutaneous n.
 traumatic n.
 Verneuil n.

Neuromeet nerve ending approximator

neuromotor

neuromuscular
 n. choristoma
 n. hamartoma

neuromuscular *(continued)*
  n. junction
  n. pacification (NMP)
  n. pedicle graft
  n. retraining

neuromyography

neuron
  motor n.
  multipolar n.

neuronal
  n. circuit
  n. survival

neuronitis
  vestibular n.

neuropathic incontinence

neuropathy
  diabetic n.
  ischemic n.
  optic n.
  postherniorrhaphy n.

neuroplasty

neuropolyendocrine syndrome

neurosensorial free medial
  plantar flap

neurosensory flap

Neurosign 100 nerve monitor

neurotomy
  bilateral temporal n.
  vestibular n.

neurotropic
  n. environment
  n. melanoma

neurovascular
  n. bundle
  n. cross compression
    (NVCC)
  n. free flap
  n. infrahyoid island flap for
    tongue reconstruction
  n. island flap
  n. pulpal plexus

nevocellular

nevus *pl.* nevi
  agminated blue n.
  atypical n.
  balloon cell n.
  basal cell n.
  Becker n.
  benign n.
  benign cellular blue n.
  blue n.
  blue rubber bleb n.
  capillary n.
  cellular blue n.
  Clark nevi
  comedones epidermal n.
  common n.
  common blue n.
  compound n.
  congenital n.
  connective tissue n.
  cutaneous blue n.
  developmental n.
  dysplastic n.
  epidermal n.
  eruptive blue n.
  extensive blue n.
  n. flammeus
  faun tail n.
  n. fibrosus
  flammeus n.
  n. flammeus
  n. flammeus neonatorum
  giant n.
  giant congenital n.
  giant pigmented n.
  hairy n.
  halo n.
  halo blue n.
  inflammatory linear verru-
    cous epidermal n. (ILVEN)
  intradermal n.
  Ito n.
  junctional n.
  juvenile n.
  locally invasive congenital
    cellular blue n. of scalp
  malignant blue n.

nevus *(continued)*
    marginal n.
    nevocellular n.
    oral epithelial n.
    organoid n.
    Ota n.
    pigmented cellular n.
    n. pigmentosus
    plaque-type blue n.
    n. sanguineus
    scarf n.
    sebaceous n.
    n. sebaceus
    speckled lentiginous n.
    spider n.
    Spitz n.
    n. spongiosus albus muco-
      sae
    strawberry n.
    Sutton n.
    n. tardus
    n. unius lateris
    vascular n.
    verrucous n.
    Werther n.
    white sponge n.
    woolly-hair n.

new
    n. dermis
    n. skin

New Beginnings GelShapes silicone gel sheeting

NF
    necrotizing fasciitis
    neurofibromatosis
        NF1
        NF2

NGF
    nerve growth factor

NICO
    neuralgia-inducing cavita-
      tional osteonecrosis

nicotina
    stomatitis n.

nicotine stomatitis

nidus
    vascular n.

nigra
    dermatosis papulosa n.
    lingua n.

nigrities
    n. linguae

Ninhydrin-Schiff method

nipper
    malleus n.

nipple
    n.-areola complex (NAC)
    boxing of n.
    donor n.
    n. inversion
    shared n.
    n. sharing
    sternal notch to n. (SN-N)
    supernumerary n.

nipple-areolar
    n.-a. amputation
    n.-a. reconstruction

Nissenbaum surgical exposure

Nitchie method

NLF
    nasolabial fold

NMP
    neuromuscular pacification

Nobelpharma implant

nocardiosis
    primary soft-tissue n.
    soft tissue n.

node
    accessory n.
    axillary n.
    buccal lymph n.
    calcified n.
    calcified lymph n.
    deep facial lymph n.

node *(continued)*
  deep lateral n.
  deep parotid n.
  Delphian n.
  draining lymph n.
  facial n.
  hard subcutaneous n.
  hot n.
  inferior deep cervical n.
  jugular chain lymph n.
  jugular lymph n.
  jugulodigastric n.
  jugulo-omohyoid n.
  lingual lymph n.
  lymph n.
  mandibular lymph n.
  mastoid n.
  maxillary lymph n.
  nuchal n.
  occipital lymph n.
  parotid lymph n.
  periparotid lymph n.
  postauricular n.
  posterior auricular n.
  postglandular n.
  preauricular lymph n.
  preglandular n.
  prelaryngeal n.
  pretracheal n.
  Ranvier n's
  n's of Ranvier
  regional lymph n.
  retroauricular lymph n.
  retroparotid lymph n.
  retropharyngeal n.
  retropharyngeal lymph n.
  sentinel lymph n.
  singer's n's
  spinal accessory chain
    lymph n.
  subdigastric lymph n.
  submandibular n.
  submandibular lymph n.
  submaxillary lymph n.
  submental lymph n.
  subparotid lymph n.
  superficial parotid n.
  superior deep cervical n.
  supraclavicular lymph n.

node *(continued)*
  suprahyoid n.
  supramandibular n.
  teachers' n's
  transverse cervical n.
  Virchow sentinel n.

nodular
  n. fasciitis
  n. melanoma

nodule
  Bohn n's
  calcified n.
  cutaneous n.
  cutaneous-subcutaneous n.
  fibrocystic n's
  fibrous n.
  lymph n.
  lymphatic n.
  red n.
  satellite n.
  sharply circumscribed n.
  singer's n's
  solitary n.
  subcutaneous n.
  subcutaneous granuloma-
    tous n.
  thyroid n.

nodulosis
  rheumatoid n.

nodulo-vegetating keratoacanthoma

NOE
  nasoorbitoethmoid
    NOE fracture

nonabsorbable
  n. mattress suture

nonautologous implant

noncornified epithelium

nondistinctive feature

nondyskeratotic leukoplakia

nonepithelial bone cyst

nonfebrile-associated vesicular
  eruption

nonfunction mandibular movement

nonhealing wound

nonhornified epithelium

noninflamed

nonkeratinization

nonkeratinize

nonkeratinized epithelium

nonkeratinizing
    n. carcinoma

nonneoplastic
    n. tumorlike lesion

nonoccluding earmold

nonocclusive dressing

nonoculoplastic surgeon

nonopportunistic infection

nonpurulent

nonresorbable fixation

nonseptate cavity

nonsynostotic plagiocephaly

nontraumatized full-thickness specimen

nontuberculous mycobacterium (NTM)

nonunion
    fibrous n.
    fracture with n.

nonvascularized
    n. bone graft (NVBG)
    n. fibular strut graft

nonvolitional facial expression

Nord
    N. appliance
    N. expansion plate

normodivergent facial pattern

Northbent suture scissors

nose
    bifid n.
    bilateral cleft lip–associated n.
    bottom-shaped n.
    brandy n.
    n. cleft
    cleft lip n.
    columellar jut of n.
    copper n.
    Cyrano n.
    dog n.
    external n.
    hammer n.
    Pinocchio n.
    platyrrhine n.
    potato n.
    rum n.
    saddle n.
    toper's n.
    unilateral cleft lip n.

nosegay
    Riolan n.

notch
    antegonial n.
    Carhart n.
    n. correction
    craniofacial n.
    ethmoidal n.
    hamular n.
    Hutchinson crescentic n.
    interarytenoid n.
    intertragic n.
    labial n.
    mandibular n.
    mastoid n.
    palatine n.
    parotid n.
    pterygomaxillary n.
    rivinian n.
    Rivinus n.
    sigmoid n.
    sphenopalatine n. of palatine bone
    sternal n. to nipple (SN-N)
    sternoclavicular n.
    superior thyroid n.

notch *(continued)*
  supraorbital n.
  suprasternal n.
  supratragal n.
  thyroid n.
  tragal n.
  trigeminal n.

notching
  antegonial n.
  vermilion n.

notch-shaped erosion

Nouvisage
  N. Acne Masque
  N. Anti-Aging Masque
  N. Deep-Hydration body
    patch
  N. Deep-Hydration glove
  N. Deep-Hydration neck
    patch
  N. Masque for damaged or
    sunburned skin
  N. Masque for normal to
    dry skin
  N. Masque for normal to
    oily skin
  N. transdermal beauty
    product

NOVA DPM 9003 skin testing instrument

Novagold mammary implant

Nova jaw hook

NovaPulse
  N. CO_2 laser
  N. laser
  N. laser system

Novasome microvesicle

NPC
  nasopharyngeal carcinoma

N2-Sargenti technique

NSM
  nerve sheath myxoma

NSTI
  necrotizing soft tissue in-
    fection

NTM
  nontuberculous mycobac-
    terium

Nucleus
  N. 22 cochlear implant
  N. multichannel cochlear
    implant

nucleus
  angular vestibular n.
  Deiters n.
  inferior vestibular n.
  medial vestibular n.

Nuhn glands

Nu-Hope skin barrier strip

number
  Mohs hardness n. (MHN)

numbness

Nurolon suture

Nu-Vois artificial larynx

NVCC
  neurovascular cross com-
    pression

NVBG
  nonvascularized bone graft

nystagmus
  caloric n.
  labyrinthine n.

Obagi
- O. Blue Peel
- O. Blue Peel skin peel treatment
- O. controlled variable-depth peel
- O. Nu-Derm skin care program
- O. Nu-Derm system
- O. sign

obesity
- morbid o.

oblique
- o. arytenoid muscle
- o. facial cleft
- o. fiber
- o. flap in mucogingival surgery
- o. line
- o. muscle
- o. septum
- o. subcondylar osteotomy

obliquus
- o. abdominis externus muscle
- o. abdominis internus muscle
- o. inferior muscle
- o. superior muscle

obliterans
- keratosis o.
- thromboangiitis o.

obliteration
- posterior sulcus o.
- total ear o.

oblongata
- medulla o.

O'Brien
- O'B. akinesia
- O'B. fixation forceps
- O'B. stitch scissors
- O'B. tissue forceps

obstruction
- airway o.

obstruction *(continued)*
- ductal o.
- laryngeal o.
- minor gland o.
- nasal o.
- nasal airway o.
- ostial o.
- papillary o.
- parotid o.
- salivary duct o.
- sublingual o.
- submandibular o.

obturans
- keratosis o.

obturator
- o. appliance
- o. nerve
- palatal o.
- Thermafil Plus o.

obturatoria stapedis fold

Obwegeser
- O. orthognathic surgery instrument
- O. sagittal split osteotomy

OC
- occlusocervical

occipital
- o. anchorage
- o. artery
- o. bone
- o. condyle
- o. condyle syndrome
- o. lobe
- o. lymph node
- o. neuralgia

occipitofrontalis
- o. muscle
- venter frontalis musculi o.

occipitomeatal view

occipitosphenoidal synchondrosis

occipitotemporal

occlude

337

occluded lisp

occlusal
- o. adjustment
- o. analysis
- o. balance
- o. cephalometric analysis
- o. clearance
- o. contouring
- o. correction
- o. curvature
- deflective o.
- o. disharmony
- o. disturbance
- o. embrasure
- o. form
- o. function
- o. harmony
- o. imbalance
- interceptive o.
- o. interference
- o. perception
- o. pivot
- o. plane
- o. plane angle
- o. plane plate
- o. position
- o. pressure
- o. recontouring
- o. rehabilitation
- o. relation
- o. relationship
- o. rest angle
- o. splint
- o. stability
- o. stent
- o. sulcus
- o. surface
- o. therapy
- o. trauma
- o. vertical dimension

occlusion
- abnormal o.
- acentric o.
- adjusted o.
- adjustment o.
- afunctional o.
- o. analysis

occlusion *(continued)*
- anatomic o.
- Andrews six keys to normal o.
- anterior o.
- o. balance
- balanced o.
- bilateral balanced o.
- bimaxillary protrusive o.
- buccal o.
- central o.
- centrally balanced o.
- centrically balanced o.
- centric o.
- class I, II, III o.
- convenience o.
- crossbite o.
- curve of o.
- dental o.
- distal o.
- eccentric o.
- faulty eccentric o.
- ideal o.
- labial o.
- lateral o.
- line of o.
- lingual o.
- malfunctional o.
- mechanically balanced o.
- neutral o.
- normal o.
- postnormal o.
- prenormal o.
- protrusive o.
- retrusive o.
- skeletal o.
- spherical form of o.
- transfemoral balloon o.
- trauma from o.
- traumatic o.
- traumatogenic o.
- two-plane o.
- working o.

occlusive dressing

occlusocervical (OC)

occlusogingival

occlusorehabilitation

occult
  o. cholelithiasis
  o. cleft palate
  o. malformation of the skull
    base
  o. primary
  o. spina bifida
  o. trauma

Ochsenbein
  O. gingivectomy
  O.-Luebke flap

Ocoee scalp cleansing unit

O'Connor
  O'C. lid clamp
  O'C. tenotomy hook

Octa-Hex implant

OCTR
  open carpal tunnel release

ocular
  o. adnexa
  o. dysmetria
  o. dysmetria test
  o. dystopia
  o. headache
  o. hypotelorism
  o.-mucous membrane syn-
    drome
  o. nerve
  o. prosthesis
  o. torticollis

oculi
  orbicularis o.

oculodento-osseous dysplasia

oculomandibulodyscephaly

oculopharyngeal syndrome

odontalgia
  o. dentalis

odontectomy

odontoma
  mixed o.

Ogsten-Luc operation

Ohngren line

oil
  croton o.

ointment
  Cavilon barrier o.
  Medi-Quick topical o.

old man's beard

O'Leary modification

olfactory
  o. foramen
  foramina for o. nerves

Olivecrona conchotome

Oliver retractor

Ollier
  O. disease
  O. graft
  O. method
  O.-Thiersch graft

Olympian forehead

O'Malley jaw fracture splint

OMENS
  orbit, mandible, ear, cranial
    nerves, and soft tissue
    OMENS score

omental
  o. filler
  o. flap
  o. skin graft
  o. transposition
  o. transposition flap

omentoplasty

omentum
  transposed o.

Omni laser tip

omocervical flap

omohyoid
  o. muscle

omphalocele

OMS
    oral and maxillofacial sur-
        gery
OMU
    ostiomeatal unit
oncocyte
oncocytic
    o. adenoma
    o. epithelial cell
    o. schneiderian papilloma
        (OSP)
oncocytoid
    o. carcinoid
    o. change
oncocytosis
oncologic
    o. mandibular resection
oncologist
    surgical o.
oncology
    radiation o.
oncotaxis
    inflammatory o.
one-piece lip retractor
one-stage esthetic correction
onion peel appearance
onlay (ON)
    o. bone graft
    o. bone grafting
    composite o.
    single cortical bone o.
    o. splint
    o. technique
    o. tip graft
onychomycosis nigricans
onychoplasty
opacification
    corneal o.

opaquer
    metal o.
open
    o. capsulotomy
    o. carpal tunnel release
        (OCTR)
    o. coronal brow lift
    o. dressing
    o. earmold
    o. flap
    o. flap technique
    o. foreheadplasty
    o. fracture
    o. miniabdominoplasty
    o. osteotomy
    o. reduction
    o. reduction and internal
        fixation (ORIF)
    o. rhinoplasty
    o. sky procedure
    o. sky rhinoplasty
opening
    access o.
    bony caval o.
    choanal o.
    o. flap
    interincisal o.
    lateral deviation on o.
    midpalatal o.
    midpalatal suture o.
    vertical mandibular o.
operant
    mand o.
operated cleft
operation
    Abbe o.
    Abbe-Estlander o.
    accessory feminizing o.
    Adams ectropion o.
    Agee fiberoptic carpal tun-
        nel o.
    Alexander o.
    Allport o.
    Alsus-Knapp o.
    Alvis o.
    Angelucci o.

operation *(continued)*
Arie-Pitanguy o.
Arie-Pitanguy mammary
ptosis o.
Arlt o.
Arlt-Jaesche o.
Asch o.
Auclair o.
Bauer-Tondra-Trusler o. for
syndactylism
Beard-Cutler o.
Becker o.
Bell o.
Berke o.
Bernard o.
Bernard-Burow o.
Biesenberger o.
Binne o.
Blair o.
Blair-Brown o.
Blair ptosis correction o.
Blasius lid o.
Blaskovics o.
Blasius o.
bloodless o.
Bossalino o.
Brophy o.
Brown-Blair o.
Burow o.
Burow flap o.
Caldwell-Luc o.
Caldwell-Luc window o.
Carmody-Batson o.
Carpue o.
Chopart o.
combined o.
Converse o.
double eyelid o.
Dupuy-Dutemps o.
Edlan-Mejchar o.
Esser o.
Estlander o.
eyelid o.
Fasanella-Servat blepharop-
tosis o.
Fasanella-Servat o. for lid
ptosis
fenestration o.
flap o.

operation *(continued)*
Foley o.
Fomon o.
Friedenwald-Guyton o.
Frost o.
Gabarro o.
Gaillard o.
Gillies o.
Gillies-Fry o.
Gillies-Kilner o.
Hagerty o.
Heath o.
Hess eyelid o.
Hess ptosis o.
Hinsberg o.
Hotchkiss o.
Hughes eyelid o.
Hummelsheim o.
Indian o.
Italian o.
Jansen o.
Kazanjian o.
Killian o.
King o.
Langenbeck o.
Luc o.
mandibular swing o.
mastoid obliteration o.
Mikamo double-eyelid o.
modified flap o.
motivating o.
Ogsten-Luc o.
orthognathic o.
palatal pushback o.
Partsch o.
pedicle flap o.
plastic o.
pull-through o.
Randall o.
Randall-Tennison o.
Reese ptosis o.
Reverdin o.
Ridell o.
Rosenburg o.
Savin o.
Sayoc o.
Schimek o.
Schönbein o.
Schuchardt-Pfeifer o.

operation *(continued)*
  Sédillot o.
  Serre o.
  Simon o.
  Sistrunk o.
  Smith eyelid o.
  Snellen ptosis o.
  Sorrin o.
  Sourdille ptosis o.
  Spaeth ptosis o.
  Stallard flap o.
  tagliacotian o.
  Tansley o.
  Tennison o.
  Tessier craniofacial o.
  Tessier facial dysostosis o.
  Thiersch o.
  Thiersch graft o.
  Toti o.
  Trainor-Nida o.
  Tripier o.
  Truc o.
  Ulloa o.
  Van Milligen o.
  Veau o.
  Veau-Axhausen o.
  Veau-Wardill-Kilner push-
    back o.
  Verwey eyelid o.
  Vogel o.
  von Blaskovics-Doyen o.
  Wagner o.
  Wardill-Kilner-Veau o.
  Webster o.
  Wheeler o.
  Wicherkiewicz o.
  Wies o.
  Wolfe o.
  Wolfe ptosis o.
  Wolff o.
  Worth o.
  Wright o.
  W-Y o.
  Wynn cleft lip o.

opercular fold

opisthocheilia

opisthogenia

opisthognathism

Opmilas laser system

Opotow Jelset material

opponensplasty

opportunistic infection

oral
  o. anomaly
  o. antimicrobial prophy-
    laxis
  o. arch
  o. atresia
  o. cancer
  o. candidiasis
  o. cavity cancer
  o. commissuroplasty
  o. hairy leukoplakia
  o. leukoplakia
  o. and maxillofacial surgery
    (OMS)
  o. Mondini
  o. plate
  o. rongeur forceps
  o. squamous carcinoma
  o. squamous cell carci-
    noma (oral SCC)
  o. surface
  o. surgeon
  o. surgery
  o. trauma

Orban knife

orbicular
  o. muscle of mouth
  o. retractor

orbicularis
  o. laxity
  o. muscle
  o. oculi
  o. oculi muscle
  o. oris
  o. oris muscle

orbit
  bony o. of eye
  exenterated o.
  harlequin o.

orbit *(continued)*
  hollow sunken o.

orbital
  o. abscess
  o. apex
  o. blow-in fracture
  o. blow-out fracture
  o. cellulitis
  o. compartment syndrome
  o. decompression
  o. fat
  o. fissure
  o. hematoma
  o. hypotelorism
  o. line
  o. lipectomy
  o.-palpebral furrow
  o. plane
  o. process
  o. rim
  o. rim reconstruction
  o. roof
  o. support

orbitale nasion

orbitomaxillary defect

orbitomaxillectomy

orbitopalpebral mutilation

orbito-temple distance

orbitotomy
  Krönlein o.
  lateral o.

orchiectomy

orchioplasty

organ
  Jacobson o.
  Masera septal o.
  Meyer o.
  vomeronasal o. (VNO)

Oriental sore

ORIF
  open reduction and internal fixation

orifice
  o. of the mouth
  nasofrontal o.

oris
  orbicularis o.

orocutaneous fistula

orodigitofacial dysostosis

orofacial
  o. dysfunction syndrome
  o. fistula
  o. muscle imbalance
  o. reconstruction

oromandibular
  o. defect
  o. dystonia
  o. lesion
  o. rehabilitation

oromaxillary

oronasal fistula

oropharyngeal
  o. defect
  o. membrane
  o. pack
  o. ulcer

oropharynx

orthodontics
  corrective o.
  cosmetic o.
  interceptive o.
  preventive o.
  prophylactic o.
  surgical o.

orthognathia

orthognathic
  o. operation
  o. surgery

orthognathism

orthognathous

orthognathus

orthopaedic (*variant of* orthopedic)

orthopaedics (*variant of* orthopedics)

orthopedic (*spelled also* orthopaedic)

orthopedics (*spelled also* orthopaedics)
    dentofacial o.
    functional jaw o.
    gnathologic o.

orthosis
    SOMI (sternal-occipital-
    mandibular immobi-
    lizer) o.

orthostatic hypotension

orthosurgical

orthotopic
    o. bone graft
    o. graft

Orticochea
    O. flap
    O. pharyngoplasty
    O. procedure
    O. scalping technique

Osada two-stage palatoplasty

oscheoplasty

oscillation
    laryngeal o.

Osler
    O. hemangiomatosis
    O.-Weber-Rendu syndrome

OSP
    oncocytic schneiderian
    papilloma

osseocartilaginous craniofacial
    skeleton

osseoprosthesis

Osseotite
    O. dental implant
    TG O. single-stage proce-
    dure implant

Osseotite (*continued*)
    O. two-stage procedure im-
    plant

osseous
    o. craniofacial arteriove-
    nous malformation
    o. dysplasia
    o. fixation
    o. grafting
    o. labyrinth
    o. surgery

ossification
    heterotopic o.
    labyrinthine o.
    reactive o.

osteitis
    alveolar o.
    sclerosing o.

osteoarthritis (OA)
    generalized o. (GOA)
    rheumatoid o.
    temporomandibular joint o.
    (TMJ-OA)

osteoarthropathy
    hypertrophic o.

osteocartilaginous
    o. excision
    o. exostosis
    o. framework

osteochondrodystrophy
    familial o.

osteoclasia
    interseptal o.

osteoclast
    o.-activating factor

osteocutaneous
    o. fillet flap
    o. scapular flap

osteodystrophy
    Albright hereditary o.
    (AHO)

osteofibroma

osteofibrosis
    periapical o.

OsteoGen
    O. bone graft
    O. bone grafting material
    O. HA Resorb implant material

osteogenesis
    distraction o. (DO)
    o. imperfecta
    mandibular distraction o.

osteogenic
    o. fibroma
    o. myxoma
    o. sarcoma

Osteograf
    O. binder
    O. bone grafting material
    O./D dense bone grafting material
    O./LD low density bone grafting material
    O./N natural bone grafting material

Osteo implant

osteoma
    cutis o.
    o. of malleus
    peripheral o. of the mandible (POM)

osteomicrotome
    Tessier o.

Osteomin freeze-dried bone

osteomyelitis
    Garré o.
    suppurative o.
    zygomatic o.

osteomyocutaneous flap

osteonecrosis
    neuralgia-inducing cavitational o. (NICO)

osteoperiostitis

osteopetrosis

osteopetrotic scar

osteoplastic
    o. craniotomy
    o. frontal sinus procedure
    o. reconstruction

osteoplasty

osteoporosis
    o. circumscripta
    periarticular o.

Osteoplate implant

OsteoPower drilling and cutting machine

osteosynthesis
    distraction o.
    wire o.

osteotome
    alar o.
    Converse o.
    Cottle-Medicon o.
    Rubin nasofrontal o.
    sinus lift o.
    Tessier o.

osteotomized

osteotomy
    bijaw o.
    bijaw segmental dentoalveolar setback o.
    bilateral mandibular sagittal split o.
    bilateral sagittal split o. (BSSO)
    bilateral sagittal split advancement o.
    blind o.
    block o.
    buccal o.
    C-form o.
    closed o.
    o. of condylar neck
    Converse guarded o.
    C sliding o.

osteotomy *(continued)*
  cuneiform o.
  cup-and-ball o.
  hinge o.
  horizontal o.
  horseshoe Le Fort I o.
  inverted-L o.
  Le Fort I o.
  Le Fort I–type o.
  Le Fort II o.
  Le Fort II–type midface o.
  Le Fort III advancement o.
  Le Fort maxillary o.
  L-form o.
  linear o.
  mandibular o.–genioglossus advancement
  mandibular ramus o.
  mandibular sagittal split o.
  maxillary o.
  medial oblique and low lateral o.
  oblique subcondylar o.
  oblique subcondylar ramus o.
  Obwegeser sagittal split o.
  open o.
  perforation o.
  periodontal o.
  posterior maxillary segmental o.
  proximal o.
  radial wedge o.
  Reverdin o.
  reverse facial o.
  rotation o.
  rotational advancement o.
  Rubin o.
  sagittal ramus o.
  sagittal split o. (SSO)
  sagittal split mandibular o.
  sagittal split ramus o. (SSRO)
  Salyer modification of Obwegeser mandibular o.
  segmental alveolar o.
  sliding o. in mandibular reconstruction

osteotomy *(continued)*
  sliding oblique o.
  subapical o.
  Tessier o.
  total midface o.
  vertical o.
  vertical o. of ramus of mandible
  vertical ramus mandibular o.
  visor o.
  zygomaticomaxillary o.

osteum internum

ostiomeatal
  o. complex
  o. stent
  o. unit (OMU)

ostium
  accessory o.
  anterior o.
  ethmoidal o.
  frontal o.
  maxillary o.
  sphenoidal o.

Ota nevus

otitis
  acute o. media (AOM)
  adhesive o. media
  benign necrotizing o. externa (BNOE)
  catarrhal o. media
  chronic cholesteatomatous o. media
  chronic granulation o. media
  chronic o. media (COM)
  chronic suppurative o. media (CSOM)
  malignant external o.
  malignant necrotizing o. externa (MNOE)
  o. media
  mucoid o. media
  mucous o.
  necrotizing external o.
  necrotizing o. media

otitis *(continued)*
  noncholesteatomatous
    chronic suppurative o.
    media
  nonsuppurative o. media
  purulent o. media
  reflux o. media
  secretory o. media
  serous o. media (SOM)
  suppurative o. media
  tuberculous o. media

otomandibular dysostosis

otoplasty
  Adams o.
  Alexander o.
  anterior-posterior o.
  Furniss o.
  incisionless o.
  mattress suture o.
  Mustardé o.
  Peled knifeless o.
  Stenstrom o.
  Stenstrom technique in o.
  Straith o.
  Tan o.
  Vogel o.

otoscope
  Micro-Halogen o.
  Microtek Heine o.
  Mini-Fibralux pocket o.
  Minilux pocket o.

output
  maximum acoustic o.
  maximum power o. (MPO)

over-and-out cheek flap

overbite
  deep o.
  excessive o.
  vertical o.

overcorrection

overdenture
  mandibular o.

overexposure

overextend

overextension

overgrafting
  dermal o.

overgrowth
  skeletal o.

overhang
  excess o.

overlap
  deep vertical o.
  septal o.

overprojecting nasal tip

overrotation

overzealous flaring

Owen's line

oximeter
  Accusate pulse o.
  Datascope pulse o.
  pulse o.

oxygen
  hyperbaric o. (HBO)

pachyblepharon

pachyblepharosis

pachycephaly

pachycheilia

pachydactyly

pachyderma
p. circumscripta
p. laryngis
p. lymphangiectatica

pachydermatous

pachydermoperiostosis

pachyglossia

pachygnathous

pachymucosa

pachynsis

pachyonychia
p. congenita

pachyotia

pachyperiosteoderma

pachysomia

Pacific Coast
P. C. demineralized bone
grafting material
P. C. demineralized cortical
bone powder
P. C. flexible laminar bone
strip

pacification
neuromuscular p. (NMP)

Pacini corpuscles

pacinian corpuscles

pack
Adaptic gauze p.
Flents breast comfort p.
Med-Wick nasal p.
nasopharyngeal p.

pack *(continued)*
oropharyngeal p.
pressure p.
wax p.

packer
Balshi p.

packing
Adaptic gauze p.
Algiderm wound p.
Gelfoam p.
ice p.
intranasal p.
Merocel epistaxis p.
Merocel nasal p.
nasal p.
Rhino Rocket nasal p.
p. strip
Vaseline petrolatum p.
Weimert epistaxis p.
wet p.

Pac-Man flap for closure of
pressure sores

pad
ABD p.
abdominal p.
Bichat fat p.
buccal fat p.
Chaston eye p.
cheek p.
eye p.
fat p.
Gelfoam p.
herniated fat p.
knuckle p's
labial p.
laparotomy p.
malar p.
masticatory fat p.
Mikulicz p.
nasal drip p.
Passavant p.
pharyngoesophageal p's
Pro-Ophtha eye p.
ptotic malar fat p.
retromolar p.
scaphoid fat p.
submental fat p.

pad *(continued)*
- sucking p.
- suctorial p.
- Telfa p.
- Telfa sterile adhesive p.
- thumb p.
- TopiFoam gel-backed self-adhering foam p.
- volar p.

paddle
- boomerang-shaped skin p.
- crescentic-shaped skin p.
- cutaneous p.
- elliptical transverse skin p.
- fleur-de-lis–shaped skin p.
- horizontal-shaped skin p.
- musculocutaneous flap skin p.
- sentinel skin p.
- skin p.
- thin-skin p.
- Y-shaped skin p.

Padgett
- P. blade
- P. dermatome
- P. endoscope
- P. mesh skin graft
- P. prosthesis
- P.-Hood dermatome

Pad Medipatch Gel Z self-adhesive scar treatment

PAF
- platelet-activating factor
- platelet-aggregating factor

Paget
- P. cells
- P. disease
- P. disease of bone
- P. disease of nipple
- extramammary P. disease
- P. I syndrome
- P. II syndrome

pagetoid

pain
- ghost p.
- incisional p.

pain *(continued)*
- myofascial p.-dysfunction (MPD)
- phantom p.
- preauricular p.
- referred p.
- sialogenic p.
- ulnar wrist p.

Paine
- P. carpal tunnel retinaculotome
- P. syndrome

paint
- Mars Black artist's acrylic p.

Pairolero classification of sternotomy wound infection *(types I–III)*

Palant-Feingold-Berkman syndrome

palatal
- p. aponeurosis
- p. arch
- p. bar
- p. bone
- p. cleft
- p. closure
- p. connector
- p. dimple
- p. distraction
- p. edema
- p. expansion
- p. expansion appliance
- p. fistula
- p. fronting
- p. gland
- p. height index
- p. insufficiency
- p. island flap
- p. length
- p. lengthening procedure
- p. lift
- p. linguoplate
- p. mucoperiosteal flap
- p. mucosa
- p. muscle
- p. obturator

palatal *(continued)*
> p. papillomatosis
> p. paralysis
> p. plate
> p. prosthesis
> p. pushback operation
> p. ramping
> p. root
> p. seal
> p. shelf
> p. split
> p. strap
> transverse p. suture

palate
> artificial p.
> bilateral cleft p.
> bilateral cleft lip and p. (BCLP)
> p. bone
> bony p.
> bony hard p.
> breadth of p.
> Byzantine arch p.
> cleft p. (CP)
> cleft lip and p. (CLP)
> complete cleft p.
> falling p.
> gothic p.
> hard p.
> hard cleft p.
> height of p.
> incomplete cleft p.
> length of p.
> longitudinal ridge of hard p.
> longitudinal suture of p.
> occult cleft p.
> partial cleft p.
> pendulous p.
> pillar of soft p.
> p. plate
> posterior nasal spine to soft p. (PNSP)
> premaxillary p.
> p. reconstruction
> p. retractor
> secondary p.
> smoker's p.
> soft p.
> soft cleft p.

palate *(continued)*
> submucosal cleft p.
> submucous cleft p.
> subtotal cleft p.
> total cleft p.
> unilateral cleft lip and p.

palate-splitting appliance

palatine
> p. aponeurosis
> p. arch
> p. artery
> p. block anesthesia
> p. bone
> p. canal
> p. durum
> p. fold
> p. foramen
> p. glands
> p. groove
> p. groove of maxilla
> p. mucosa
> p. nerve
> p. notch
> p. papilla
> p. papilla cyst
> p. process of maxilla
> p. protuberance
> p. raphe
> p. recess
> p. reflex
> p. ridge
> p. root
> p. ruga
> p. shelf
> p. spines
> p. sulcus
> p. sulci of maxilla
> p. surface
> p. suture
> p. tonsil
> p. torus
> p. uvula
> vertical plate of p.
> p. velum
> p. vessel

palatoalveolar fistula

palatoethmoid suture

palatoethmoidal suture

palatoglossal
p. arch
p. band
p. muscle

palatognathous

palatomaxillary
p. arch
p. canal
p. cleft
p. groove
p. groove of palatine bone
p. suture

palatonasal

palatopharyngeal
p. closure
p. fold
p. mechanism
p. muscle
p. ring

palatopharyngcus
p. muscle

palatopharyngoplasty

palatopharyngorrhaphy

palatoplasty
alveolar extension p.
Brown push-back p.
Delaire p.
diathermy p.
four-flap p.
Frolova primary p.
Furlow double-opposing
Z-plasty p.
laser p.
mucoperiosteal push-
back p.
Osada two-stage p.
pharyngeal flap p.
p. pushback operation
posterior p.
Samonara p.
two-flap p. repair
Veau p.
Veau-Wardill-Kilner p.
V-Y p.
W-Y p.

palatoplegia

palatoproximal

palatorrhaphy
functional p.
Langenbeck p.
Langenbeck with pharyn-
geal flap p.
primary p.
V-Y pushback p.

palatoschisis

palatovaginal canal

palatum pl. palata
p. durum
p. durum osseum
p. fissum
p. molle
p. ogivale
p osseum

Palfyn
P. sinus
P. suture

palisaded
p. encapsulated neuroma

palmar
p. advancement flap
p. aponeurosis
p. arch
p. beak ligament
p. contraction
p. crease
p. cutaneous nerve
deep p. arch
p. digital arteries
p. digital nerves
p. digital veins
p. dysesthesia
p. fascia
p. fasciitis
p. flap
p. flexion
p. incision
p. interosseous muscle
p. ligaments
p. metacarpal arteries
p. pulley

palmar *(continued)*
    p. pulp
    p. skin bridge
    p. space
    superficial p. arch

palmaris
    p. brevis
    p. longus
    p. longus composite flap
    p. longus muscle
    p. longus tendon

Palmaz stent

palpebra *pl.* palpebrae
    p. inferior
    p. superior

palpebral
    p. commissure
    p. fascia
    p. fissure
    p. furrow
    p. raphe

palpebronasal fold

palsy
    Bell p.
    cerebral p.
    Erb p.
    Erb-Duchenne p.
    facial p.
    high median nerve p.
    high ulnar nerve p.
    House grade facial p.
    Klumpke p.
    low median nerve p.
    low median/ulnar nerve p.
    low ulnar nerve p.
    posterior interosseous
      nerve p.
    radial nerve p.
    tardy p.
    tardy median p.
    ulnar nerve p.

PAN
    posterior ampullary nerve

Panas ptosis correction technique

Pancoast suture

pancraniomaxillofacial fracture

Panelipse panoramic radiograph

Panex panoramic radiograph

panfacial fracture

panniculectomy

panniculitis
    septal p.

panniculus
    p. adiposus
    hanging p.
    histiocytic cytophagic panniculitis

pannus
    abdominal p.

panogram
    mandible p.

panoramic
    p. radiograph
    p. roentgenogram
    p. series
    p. view

Panorex
    P. radiograph
    P. view

papilla *pl.* papillae
    arcuate papillae of tongue
    atrophied p.
    calciform p.
    capitate papillae
    circumvallate p.
    clavate p.
    conic papillae
    conoid papillae of tongue
    papillae of corium
    corolliform papillae of
      tongue
    dermal papillae
    filiform p.
    foliate papillae
    fungiform papillae
    hair p.
    hypertrophied p.

papilla *(continued)*
  incisive p.
  lacrimal p.
  lingual p.
  papillae linguales
  p. mammae
  palatine p.
  parotid p.
  p. pili
  retrocuspid p.
  p. of Santorini
  sublingual p.
  tactile p.
  vallate p.
  p. of Vater
  vestibular p.

papillary
  p. adenocarcinoma
  p. cyst
  p. dermal peel
  p. ectasia
  p. hyperplasia
  p. keratosis
  p. pedicle graft
  p. thyroid carcinoma

papilloma *pl.* papillomas
  basal cell p.
  cutaneous p.
  fibroepithelial p.
  intracanalicular p.
  intracystic p.
  inverted ductal p.
  inverted schneiderian p.
  inverting p.
  keratotic p.
  oncocytic schneiderian p.
    (OSP)
  sinonasal p.
  soft p.
  squamous p.
  squamous cell p.
  villous p.

papillomatosis
  confluent and reticulated p.
  florid cutaneous p.
  inflammatory p.
  laryngeal p.
  malignant p.

papillomatosis *(continued)*
  multiple p.
  palatal p.

Papillon-Léage and Psaume syndrome

Papillon-Lefèvre syndrome

Papineau
  P. bone graft staging
    (stages I–III)
  P. cancellous graft
  P. graft
  P. technique

papular
  p. acne
  p. acrodermatitis
  p. fibroplasia

papule
  indurated p.
  keratotic p.
  red p.
  split p.

papulosa
  acne p.
  p. nigra dermatosis

papulosis
  atrophic p.
  bowenoid p.
  lymphomatoid p.
  malignant p.
  malignant atrophic p.

papulosquamous
  p. dermatitis
  p. lesion

papulovesicular
  p. lesion
  p. rash

papyraceous scar

paraffin
  p. gauze
  p.-impregnated gauze

paraganglioma
  laryngeal p.

paraglossia

paragnathus

Paragon
    P. implant
    P. laser

parakeratinized epithelium

parakeratosis

paralysis
    adductor p.
    bilateral abductor p.
    bilateral adductor p.
    bilateral facial p.
    central facial p.
    cricothyroid p.
    facial p.
    facial nerve p.
    faucial p.
    frontalis muscle p.
    hypoglossal p.
    idiopathic facial p.
    incomplete p.
    incomplete facial p.
    labioglossolaryngeal p.
    laryngeal motor p.
    laryngeal sensory p.
    lingual p.
    myopathic p.
    palatal p.
    Ramsay Hunt facial p.
    sensory p.
    soft palate p.
    trigeminal nerve p.
    unilateral abductor p.
    unilateral adductor p.
    unilateral vocal cord p.
      (UVCP)
    Volkmann ischemic p.
    X p.

paramedian forehead flap

parameter
    baseline p's

paraneoplastic acrokeratosis

paraneural
    p. anesthesia
    p. block

parapharyngeal
    p. fat

parapharyngeal *(continued)*
    p. space abscess
    p. tumor

PARAS
    postauricular and retroau-
      ricular scalping

parascapular flap

Par Decon

parenchyma
    breast p.

paresthesia
    laryngeal p.
    lip p.

Paré suture

parieto-occipital flap

Parkes
    P. rasp
    P.-Weber hemangiomatosis
    P.-Weber syndrome

Parkland fluid requirement formula for burn patients

Parona space

paronychia
    herpetic p.

parotid
    p. capsule
    p. carcinoma
    p. cyst
    p. duct
    p. duct ligation
    p. duct transposition
    p. fascia
    p. gland abscess
    mucoepidermoid carci-
      noma of p.
    p. notch
    p. obstruction
    p. sialodochoplasty
    p. tumor

parotidectomy
    facial nerve–preserving p.
    lateral p.
    p. procedure

parotidectomy *(continued)*
    radical p.
    superficial p.
    total p.

parrot
    p. beak
    p. beak deformity
    p. beak flap

Parrot sign

Parsonage Turner syndrome

partial laryngopharyngectomy (PLP)

partial-thickness flap

particulate cancellous bone and marrow (PCBM)

Partsch
    P. I method
    P. operation

Pasini
    atrophoderma of P. and Pierini

Passavant
    P. bar
    circular with P. ridge pattern of closure
    P. cushion
    P. pad
    P. ridge

passer
    Carter-Thomason suture p.
    Gore suture p.
    tendon p.

Passport bedside monitor

paste
    Abbot p.
    metallic oxide p.
    methyl cellulose p.
    Multi-Form dual purpose impression p.

patagium
    cervical p.

patch
    cotton-wool p.

patch *(continued)*
    Gore-Tex soft-tissue p.
    mucous p.
    Nouvisage Deep-Hydration body p.
    Nouvisage Deep-Hydration neck p.
    p. graft
    salmon p.
    smoker's p.
    vascularized fascial p.

path
    condylar p.
    p. of insertion

pathogen
    blood-borne p.
    microbial p.

pathology
    craniofacial p.

pathway
    afferent-efferent p.
    mucociliary drainage p.
    sensory p.

patient
    hyperdivergent p.

pattern
    acanthomatous p.
    arborization p.
    circular with Passavant ridge p. of closure
    class III ring avulsion injury p.
    cribriform p.
    ground-glass p.
    fleur-de-lis breast reconstruction p.
    gull-wing p.
    hyperdivergent facial p.
    hyperdivergent skeletal p.
    incremental appositional p.
    monomorphic p.
    normodivergent facial p.
    reticular p.
    SLAC (scapholunate advanced collapse) p. of degenerative change

pattern *(continued)*
    stellate p.
    submucosal vascular p.
    Wise p.
    Wise p. in breast reduction
    Wolfe mammographic parenchymal p's
    Wyse p. for reduction mammaplasty

Paulus midfacial plate

Pautrier abscess

Payr sign

PBI
    PBI Medical copper vapor laser
    PBI MultiLase D copper vapor laser

PCBM
    particulate cancellous bone and marrow

PCR
    progressive condylar resorption

PD
    probing depth

PDGF
    platelet-derived growth factor

PDL
    periodontal ligament

PDS
    polydioxanone
        PDS suture

PE
    pharyngoesophageal

peak
    Cupid's bow p.
    lingual p.

pearl
    epithelial p.

peau d'orange

pectoralis
    p. major (PM)
    p. major flap
    p. major muscle
    p. major myocutaneous flap
    p. minor
    p. minor flap
    p. minor muscle
    p. myocutaneous flap
    p. myofascial flap

pectus
    p. carinatum
    p. excavatum

pedicle
    circumflex scapular p.
    dermal vascularized p.
    dominant p.
    fasciovascular p.
    Filatov-Gillies tubed p.
    p. flap
    p. flap donor site
    p. graft
    inferior p.
    latissimus dorsi segmental musculovascular p.
    musculovascular p.
    Pontén-type tubed p.
    superior dermal p.
    thoracoacromial p.
    vascular p.

pedicled
    p. cartilage graft
    p. galeal frontalis flap
    p. latissimus flap
    p. mucosa flap
    p. myocutaneous flap
    p. pericranial flap
    p. tibial bone flap

pedunculated

peel
    Blue P. chemical p.
    chemical p.
    chemosurgical superficial dermatologic p.

peel *(continued)*
  feather the p.
  full-face p.
  glycolic skin p.
  Jessner solution p.
  mid-to-deep dermal p.
  Obagi Blue P.
  Obagi controlled variable-
    depth p.
  papillary dermal p.
  skin p.
  trichloroacetic acid
    (TCA) p.
  upper reticular dermal p.

peeling
  chemical p.
  chemical face p.
  glycolic acid p.
  phenol p.

Peet nasal rasp

peg
  epithelial p.
  epithelial rete p.

Peled knifeless otoplasty

pemphigoid
  benign mucous mem-
    brane p.
  bullous p.

pemphigus
  benign p.
  benign familial chronic p.
  malignant p.

pen
  Skin Skribe p.

pencil
  Blaisdell skin p.
  MegaDyne electrocau-
    tery p.

pendulous
  p. abdomen
  p. palate

penetration
  upper reticular dermal p.

penile
  p. agenesis
  p. flap
  p. girth enhancement
  p. hypospadias
  p. lengthening
  p. skin inversion vagino-
    plasty

penis
  buried p.

penoscrotal
  p. edema
  p. hypospadias

perception

perforation
  Bezold p.
  iatrogenic p.
  lateral p.
  mechanical p.
  nasal septal p.
  septal p.

perforator
  fascial p.
  fasciocutaneous p.
  musculocutaneous p.
  periumbilical p.
  segmental p's
  septocutaneous p.
  septomuscular p.
  p. vessel

perforator-based flap

perfusion
  p. monitor
  regional p.

periarticular
  p. osteoporosis
  p. soft tissue swelling

periareolar
  p. incision
  p. mammaplasty
  p. scar

periauricular

perichondrial flap

perichondritis
    arytenoid p.
    laryngeal p.

perichondrocutaneous graft

pericyte
    vascular p. of Zimmerman

perilunar instability (PLI)

perilunate dislocation

perilymphatic duct

perineal
    p. artery axial flap
    p. hypospadias
    p. reconstruction
    p. tear

perineoplasty
    Hierst p.
    single-stage castration,
        vaginal construction, p.
    Tait p.

perineural
    p. fibroblastoma
    p. anesthesia
    p. channels

perineurial suture

perineurium

periocular
    p. festooning
    p. pigmentation
    p. rhytids

periodontal ligament (PDL)

periodontitis
    marginal p.

PerioGlas
    P. material
    P. synthetic bone graft

Perio Med

perioral flaw

periorbital
    p. fat

periorbital *(continued)*
    p. orbicularis oculi muscle

periosteal
    p. cyst
    p. elevation
    p. elevator
    p. flap
    p. graft
    p. release

periosteum *pl.* periostea
    alveolar p.
    lingual p.
    lingual mandibular p.

periostitis
    ethmoidal p.

Periotest implant

periotic duct

peripheral
    p. osteoma of the mandible
        (POM)
    p. temporomandibular joint
        remodeling

peritoneoplasty

periumbilical perforator

PermaMesh hydroxyapatite woven sheet matrix

Permark
    P. micropigmentation handpiece
    P. micropigmentation needle
    P. micropigmentation system

PermaRidge alveolar ridge augmentation

PermaSoft reline material

peromelia

peroneus
    p. brevis flap
    p. longus flap

peroral
    p. endoscopy

perpendicular
    nasion p.

Perroncito
    apparatus of P.

perseveration
    infantile p.

Personna Plus MicroCoat sur-
    geon's blade

pes
    p. anserinus

Petit
    P. canal
    P. facial mask

petrolatum
    p. gauze

petrosal
    p. artery
    p. nerve
    p. ridge
    p. sulcus

petrosquamous fissure

petrotympanic
    p. fissure
    p. suture

Peyer glands

Pfeiffer syndrome

phalanx
    buckling fracture of the p.
    distal p.
    floating distal p.
    shaft of p.

Phalen sign

phalloplasty procedure

phallourethroplasty

pharyngeal
    p. bursa
    p. hypophysis
    p. wall

pharyngitis
    atrophic p.

pharyngitis (continued)
    lymphonodular p.
    membranous p.

pharyngocutaneous fistula

pharyngoepiglottic fold

pharyngoesophageal (PE)
    p. defect
    p. diverticulum
    p. reconstruction

pharyngoesophagoplasty

pharyngoinfraglottic duct

pharyngomaxillary fissure

pharyngoplasty
    Barsky p.
    Hynes p.
    Orticochea p.
    sphincter p.
    Wardill p.

pharyngotomy
    lateral p.
    modified lateral p.

pharynx
    vault of p.

phase
    acute p. of burn injury
    horizontal growth p.
    remodeling p. of wound
      healing

Phemister graft

phenol

phenomenon
    autoimmune p.
    Bell p.
    jaw-winking p.
    Kasabach-Merritt p.
    mucous retention p.

philtral
    p. column
    p. column elevation
    p. dimple
    p. height
    p. malrotation

philtral *(continued)*
    p. symmetry
    p. tubercle
    p. unit
    p. vermilion

philtrum *pl.* philtra
    rotation of p.

pHisoHex facial wash

phlegmon
    p. of floor of mouth

photoaging

photocoagulation
    intralesional laser p. (ILP)

photocoagulator
    argon laser p.
    Coherent argon laser p.

PhotoDerm
    P. PL laser
    P. T laser
    P. T10 laser
    P. T laser system
    P. V laser
    P. VL laser
    P. VLS pulsed dye laser

PhotoGenica
    P. LPIR with TKS laser
    P. T10 laser
    P. V laser
    P. VLS pulsed dye laser

photothermolysis
    selective p.

Pickerill imbrication line

Pierce cheek retractor

Pierre Robin sequence

Piffard dermal curet

pigmentary
    p. changes
    p. dyschromia

pigmentation
    bear track p.
    bismuth p.

pigmentation *(continued)*
    brown/black p.
    p. mismatch
    periocular p.

pigmented
    p. basal cell carcinoma
    p. cellular nevus
    p. lesion
    p. linear streak

pigmentosus
    nevus p.

pillar
    anterior p. of fauces
    p. of fauces
    p. of soft palate

pillow
    Carter p.

pin
    apex p.
    biphasic p.
    distraction p.
    Hoffman transfixion p.
    Roger Anderson p.
    Steinmann p. with ball
      bearing
    Steinmann calibration p.
    Steinmann p. with Crowe
      pilot point
    Steinmann fixation p.

pinch
    functional p.
    p. graft
    lateral p.
    three-point p.

pinching
    supra-alar p.

pinna
    bifid p.

Pinocchio
    P. nose
    P. tip
    P. tip deformity

Pinto superficial dissection cannula

pinwheel
  neurological p.

PIP
    proximal interphalangeal
      PIP joint

pipestem artery

Pirie bone

piriform
  p. angle
  p. aperture stenosis
  p. fossa
  p. rim
  p. sinus

pit
    commissural p.
    labial p.
    lip p.

pityriasis
  atypical p. rosea

Pitanguy abdominoplasty

pivot
  occlusal p.

placement
    eyelid sulcus p.
    lingual p.

plagiocephaly
    compensational frontal p.
    deformational frontal p.
    frontal p.
    lambdoid synostotic p.
    nonsynostotic p.
    occipital p.
    p. without synostosis
    synostotic frontal p. (SFP)
    unilateral p.

plane
    Aeby p.
    auriculoinfraorbital p.
    axial p.
    basion-nasion (Ba-N) p.
    Bolton p.
    Bolton-Broadbent p.

plane (continued)
    Bolton nasion p.
    Camper p.
    cephalometric p.
    coronal p.
    cranial base p.
    p. of dissection
    extended supraplatysmal p.
      (ESP)
    facial p.
    fascial p.
    Frankfort horizontal p.
      (Po-Or)
    Frankfort mandibular p.
    frontal p.
    labiolingual p.
    mandibular p.
    mandibular p. to hyoid
    Martin p.
    maxillary p.
    median raphe p.
    median sagittal p.
    mesiodistal p.
    Montague p.
    nasion-pogonion facial
      axis p.
    nasion–point A p.
    nasion–point B p.
    occlusal p.
    orbital p.
    palatal p.
    pocket p.
    sagittal p.
    sella-nasion (S-N) p.
    subfascial p.
    subgaleal p.
    subperiosteal vomerine-
      ethmoidal p.
    subplatysmal p.
    tangential p.
    temporal p.
    tissue p.
    von Ihring p.

planer
    Rubin bone p.
    Rubin cartilage p.

plantar
    p. arch

plantar *(continued)*
>   deep p. arch
>   p. flexion
>   p. foot defect
>   p. forefoot ulcer
>   p. metatarsal arteries
>   superficial p. arch

plaque
>   microbial p.
>   mucinous p.
>   mucous p.

plaster
>   Mediplast P.
>   model p.
>   model p. Grade A

plastic
>   modeling p.

plate
>   alloplastic p.
>   atresia p.
>   bony atretic p.
>   Brophy p.
>   buccal alveolar p.
>   Coffin split p.
>   compression p.
>   condylar lag screw p.
>   cortical bone p.
>   cribriform p.
>   cribriform p. of alveolar
>   process
>   dynamic compression p.
>   (DCP)
>   ethmoid p.
>   ethmoidomaxillary p.
>   genial advancement p.
>   fibrocartilage p.
>   horizontal p. of palatine
>   bone
>   infraorbital p.
>   Jaeger bone p.
>   Jaeger lid p.
>   lateral pterygoid p.
>   Leibinger 3-D bone p.
>   Leibinger Micro Plus p.
>   Leibinger Mini-Würzburg p.
>   lingual p.
>   lingual cortical p.

plate *(continued)*
>   Luhr fixation p.
>   Luhr Vitallium micro-
>   mesh p.
>   mandibular bridging p.
>   mandibular staple bone p.
>   (MSBP)
>   maxillary bite p.
>   medial pterygoid p.
>   metal reconstruction p.
>   micro-adaption p.
>   middle fossa p.
>   multipoint contact p.
>   nail p.
>   neural p.
>   Nord expansion p.
>   occlusal plane p.
>   oral p.
>   palatal p.
>   palate p.
>   Paulus midfacial p.
>   perpendicular p. of eth-
>   moid
>   pterygoid p.
>   resorbable p. and screw
>   Senn bone p.
>   Sherman p.
>   Sherman bone p.
>   Sherman p. and screws
>   staple bone p.
>   supraorbital p.
>   tarsal p.
>   TiMesh orthognathic
>   strap p.
>   titanium hollow-screw os-
>   seointegrating reconstruc-
>   tion plate (THORP)-type
>   mandibular reconstruc-
>   tion p.
>   urethral p.
>   vertical p. of palatine
>   vestibular oral p.
>   Vitallium p.
>   volar p.
>   wing p.
>   Y bone p.

platelet
>   p.-activating factor (PAF)
>   p.-aggregating factor (PAF)

platelet *(continued)*
    p.-derived growth factor
      (PDGF)
    p. tissue factor

plating
    Leibinger p.

Platinum 5000 micropigmentation handpiece

platysma
    cervical p.
    p. flap
    p. myocutaneous flap
    p. resection
    p. rhytidectomy

platysmal
    p. band
    p. imbrication
    p. transection

platysmaplasty
    corset p.

pledget
    cotton p.
    Gelfoam p.

pleomorphic adenoma

pleomorphism
    cellular p.

plexus
    areolar venous p.
    arterial p.
    basilar p.
    brachial p.
    capillary p.
    carotid p.
    cervical p.
    common carotid p.
    dermal vascular p.
    Haller p.
    hypoglossal p.
    intermediate p.
    Jacobson p.
    Kiesselbach p.
    lingual p.
    neurovascular pulpal p.
    pterygoid p.
    ranine vein p.

plexus *(continued)*
    Sappey p.
    Stensen p.
    subepithelial nerve p.
    submucosal venous p.
    suboccipital p.
    thyroid p.
    venous p.

PLI
    perilunar instability

plica *pl.* plicae
    p. nasi
    p. semilunaris
    p. sublingualis

plication
    endoscopic muscle p.
    fascial p.
    fusiform p.
    galea aponeurosis p.
    midline p. of the anterior
      rectus sheath
    musculoaponeurotic p.
    musculofascial p.
    Rehne-Delorme p.
    SMAS p.
    p. suture
    tongue p.
    vertical rectus p.

pliers
    debonding p. (DP)
    lingual arch-forming p.
    matrix p.

PLM
    precise lesion measuring

PLP
    partial laryngopharyngec-
      tomy

plug
    Freeman punctum p.
    mucous p.
    umbrella punctum p.

plugger
    miniature p.

Plummer-Wilson syndrome

plumper
  lip p.

PM
  pectoralis major
  periodontal membrane

PMMA
  polymethyl methacrylate

pneumatization
  mastoid p.

PNSP
  posterior nasal spine to
    soft palate

POC
  presurgical orthopedic cor-
    rection

pocket
  absolute p.
  deepening p.
  p. depth
  p. epithelium
  expander p.
  infrabony p.
  infracrestal p.
  intra-alveolar p.
  intrabony p.
  marking p.
  submuscular p.

pogonion
  bony p.

point
  auricular p.
  chin p.
  cleft high p's
  Crowe pilot p.
  ethmoid registration p.
  high p. of Cupid's bow
  jugomaxillary p.
  McBurney p.
  median mandibular p.
  mental p.
  nasion p.
  p. of proximal contact

Poirier glands

Poland syndrome

pole
  p. of the breast
  p. of the hamate
  lateral condylar p. of the
    TMJ

Politzer method

pollicization
  index finger p.
  p. procedure

polly beak
  cutaneous p. b.
  p. b. deformity
  fibrous p. b.
  p. b. nasal deformity

polydactylism

polydactyly
  index finger p.
  thumb p.

Polydek suture

polydioxanone suture (PDS)

polyethylene
  ultra-high-molecular-
    weight p. (UHMWP)

poly-HEMA
  poly-2-hydroxyethyl meth-
    acrylate

polymer
  Bioplastique p.
  modified p.

polymethyl methacrylate
  (PMMA)

polyp
  choanal p.
  laryngeal p.

polysyndactyly
  complex p.

polytetrafluoroethylene (PTFE)
  expanded p. (ePTFE)

Polytec LaseAway Q-switched ruby laser

Polyviolene polyester suture material

POM
peripheral osteoma of the mandible

Pontén-type tubed pedicle

ponticulus
p. auriculae

Po-Or
Frankfort horizontal plane

Porex implant

Porges Neoflex dilator

porion *pl.* poria

port
endoscopic access p. (EAP)

Porta-Resp monitor

Porta-Stat cephalostat

Porzett splint

position
anatomic p.
angular p. of the ramus
calibrated p.
centric p.
condylar hinge p.
forehead-nose p.
Jahss p.
jaw-to-jaw p.
mandibular hinge p.
mandibular rest p.
median occlusal p.
mesioangular p.
occlusal p.
retruded p.
Rose p.
semi-Fowler p.
semirecumbent p.

positioner
forehead p.

postalveolar cleft palate fistulation (CPF)

postauricular and retroauricular scalping (PARAS)

posterior
p. ampullary nerve (PAN)
p. auricular flap
p. nasal spine to soft palate (PNSP)
p. skin flap

post implant

postinflammatory hypopigmentation

postpeel
p. hyperpigmentation
p. hypopigmentation

posturing
anterior mandibular p.

potential
nerve action p.

Potter facies

pouch
branchial p.
cheek p.
dermal p.

Poupart ligament

powder
Cranioplastic p.
demineralized cortical bone p.
hyCURE hydrolyzed protein p. and exudate absorber
Pacific Coast demineralized cortical bone p.
Ultimatics demineralized cortical bone p.

power
suspension p.

PowerStar bipolar scissors

preauricular
    p. crease
    p. fistula
    p. incision

prechamber
    ethmoidal p.

precise lesion measuring (PLM)

Preiser disease

premaxilla
    floating p.
    loose p.

premolar
    mandibular p.

preparation
    access p.
    Matsura p.
    medicinal p.
    mouth p.

press
    Cali-Press graft p.

Press Lift chin strap

pressure
    arterial p.
    back p.
    capillary p.
    compartment p.
    p. dressing
    mastoid p.
    occlusal p.
    P. Ulcer Scale for Healing
       (PUSH) Tool

prestyloid recess

presurgical orthopedic correc-
    tion (POC)
    p.o.c. device

pretarsal fold

primary
    multiple p.
    occult p.

primer
    Kadon p.

principle
    Gibson p.

Prisma Microfine

probe
    blunt lacrimal p.
    calibrated p.
    lacrimal p.
    Marquis p.
    Merit-B periodontal p.
    Michigan p.
    Nabers p.

probing depth (PD)

procedure
    ablative p.
    adipofascial sural flap p.
    adjunctive p.
    Allport ptosis correction p.
    autogenous fascia lata
       sling p.
    Alvis ptosis correction p.
    anchorage p.
    autogenous fascia lata
       sling p.
    Bilhaut-Cloquet p.
    Brockman clubfoot p.
    cervicofacial rhytidecto-
       my p.
    chin-contouring p.
    Cutler-Beard bridge flap p.
    Cyclops p.
    dacryocystorhinostomy p.
    Darrach p.
    Davis-Kitlowski p.
    dermoplasty p.
    Ely's p.
    endoscopic p.
    fenestration p.
    fillet flap p.
    four-flap p.
    free flap p.
    frontalis sling p.
    Furlow p.
    genioplasty p.
    Giannestras step-down p.
    Gillies cocked hat p.
    Gillies elevation p.

procedure *(continued)*
  Goulian p. to harvest skin graft
  Hoffman and Mohr p.
  Hueston flap p.
  Ilizarov p.
  Killian frontoethmoidectomy p.
  Kole p.
  Krukenberg p.
  Kuhnt-Szymanowski ectropion repair p.
  laryngopharyngoesophagectomy p.
  lateral tarsal strip p.
  Le Fort I p.
  Le Fort II p.
  Le Fort III p.
  Le Fort osteotomy p.
  McComb p.
  malarplasty p.
  meatal advancement and glanuloplasty p. (MAGPI)
  meloplasty p.
  microsurgical p.
  Mitz p.
  modified Krukenberg p.
  modified Weber-Fergusson p.
  open sky p.
  Orticochea p.
  osteoplastic frontal sinus p.
  palatal lengthening p.
  parotidectomy p.
  phalloplasty p.
  pollicization p.
  pushback p.
  reduction-augmentation p.
  reversed extensor digitorum muscle island flap p.
  rotation-transposition cleft lip p.
  Sauve-Kapandji p.
  second-look p.
  Sistrunk p.
  SMAS (superficial musculoaponeurotic system) plication p.
  staged p.

procedure *(continued)*
  sternum turnover p.
  toe fillet flap p.
  transblepharoplasty p.
  uvulopalatoplasty p.
  vaginoplasty p.
  Van Nes p.
  V-Y p.
  V-Y pushback p.
  Wardill-Kilner p.
  Wassmund p.
  Weber-Fergusson p.

process
  alveolar p.
  alveolar p. of mandible
  alveolar p. of maxilla
  anterior clinoid p.
  burn p.
  clinoid p.
  condyloid p.
  coronoid p. of mandible
  fibro-osseous p.
  frontal p.
  frontal p. of maxilla
  frontonasal p.
  hamular p.
  inflammatory p.
  intercellular matrix p.
  lacrimal p.
  mandibular p.
  marginal p. of malar bone
  mastoid p.
  maxillary p.
  maxillary p. of zygomatic bone
  medial nasofrontal p.
  medionasal p.
  mental p.
  myoepithelial cell p.
  nasal p.
  orbital p.
  palatine p.
  palatine p. of maxilla
  radial styloid p.
  septic p.
  sphenoid p.
  sphenoidal p.
  styloid p.
  temporal p. of mandible

process *(continued)*
    temporal p. of zygomatic
      bone
    uncinate p.
    vaginal p. of sphenoid bone
    xiphoid p.
    zygomatic p.
    zygomatic p. of frontal
      bone
    zygomatic p. of maxilla
    zygomatic p. of temporal
      bone

Proctor retractor

product
    blood p.
    Nouvisage transdermal
      beauty p.
    skin care p.

profile
    facial p.
    retrognathic p.

profilometer
    Straith p.

progeria
    Hutchinson-Gilford p.

prognathism
    basilar p.
    bimaxillary p.
    mandibular p.
    mandibular p./protrusion
    maxillary p./protrusion
    retromaxillary p.

prognathous

program
    ENZA laser skin care p.
    Muma Assessment P.
      (MAP)
    Obagi Nu-Derm skin care p.

progressive perilunar instability
  (stages I–IV)

projection
    axial p.
    basilar p.
    Caldwell p.
    cross-sectional p.

projection *(continued)*
    frontal p.
    horizontal p.
    lateral jaw p.
    lateral oblique p. of mandi-
      ble
    mental p.
    sagittal p.
    submentovertical axial p.
    tangential p.
    Templeton-Zim carpal tun-
      nel p.
    tip p.

Prolene
    P. mesh
    P. mesh sheet
    P. mesh silo
    P. stitch
    P. suture

proliferation
    epithelial p.
    lymphoepithelial p.
    synovial p.
    vascular p.

prominence
    bony p.
    canine p.
    laryngeal p.
    malar p.
    maxillary p.

Pro-Ophtha eye pad

ProOsteon
    P. 500 bone implant graft
    P. Implant 500 granule

prop
    mouth p.

property
    viscoelastic p. of skin

prophylaxis
    antibiotic p.
    oral antimicrobial p.

Proplast
    P. allograft
    P. implant
    P.-Teflon disk implant
    P.-Teflon material

prosopoanoschisis

prosopodiplegia

prosopodysmorphia

prosoponeuralgia

prosopoplegia

prosopoplegic

prosoposchisis

prosopospasm

prosthesis
    alloplastic p.
    Anderson columella p.
    articulated chin p.
    Ashley breast p.
    auricular p.
    Becker breast p.
    Becker mammary p.
    breast p.
    cable-operated hand p.
    cleft palate p.
    combination gel and inflat-
        able mammary p.
    cranial p.
    Cronin Silastic mammary p.
    definitive p.
    dual-chambered p.
    facial p.
    Fredricks mammary p.
    Georgiade breast p.
    glottic p.
    heterograft p.
    Heyer-Schulte breast p.
    Heyer-Schulte chin p.
    Heyer-Schulte mammary p.
    Heyer-Schulte testicular p.
    Hinderer malar p.
    hinged great toe replace-
        ment p.
    Hydroflex penile p.
    implant-borne p.
    Lezinski Flex-HA PORP os-
        sicular chain p.
    Mangat curvilinear chin p.
    mandibular guide p.
    mandibular guide-plane p.

prosthesis (continued)
    maxillary p.
    maxillofacial p.
    metal bucket-handle p.
    myeloelectric hand p.
    natural-feel breast p.
    ocular p.
    Padgett p.
    palatal p.
    PTFE (polytetrafluoroethyl-
        ene) p.
    removable expansion p.
    screw-retained p.
    Silastic penile p.
    Silastic chin p.
    Silastic mammary p.
    Silastic otoplasty p.
    silicone gel p.
    Silima breast p.
    wire-Gelfoam p.

prosthetic
    p. dislocation
    p. fracture

prosthodontics
    maxillofacial p.

Protégé Plus microscope

protection
    barrier p.

protector
    Cottle alar p.

protein
    bone-inductive p.
    bone morphogenic p.
        (BMP)
    bone morphogenic p.-2
        (BMP-2)
    recombinant human bone
        morphogenetic p.
        (rhBMP-2)

protocol
    Marx p. for ORN treatment
    short arc motion (SAM) p.

protraction
    mandibular p.
    maxillary p.

protrusion
  beaklike p. of nose
  bimaxillary p.
  bimaxillary dentoalveo-
    lar p.
  double p.
  jaw p.
  mandibular p.
  mandibular prognathism/p.
  maxillary alveolar p.
  maxillary p.
  maxillary prognathism/p.

protuberance
  Bichat p.
  bony p.
  chin p.
  mental p.
  palatine p.

proximal
  p. interphalangeal (PIP)
  p. interphalangeal (PIP)
    joint

Proximate disposable skin stapler

prune belly syndrome

pseudoepithelioma
  squamous cell p.

pseudoepitheliomatous hyperplasia

pseudohermaphroditism
  female p.
  male p.

pseudo-Kaposi sarcoma

pseudolymphoma
  Spiegler-Fendt p.

pseudomallet deformity

pseudomelanoma

pseudoscar
  spontaneous p.
  stellate p.

pseudotumor cerebri

pseudovaginal hypospadias

pterygium
  cervical midline p.
  p. colli

pterygoid
  p. hamulus
  p. plate
  p. plexus
  p. tuberosity of mandible

pterygomandibular
  p. fold
  p. raphe
  p. space abscess

pterygomaxillary
  p. buttress
  p. fissure
  p. fossa

pterygopalatine canal

PTFE
  polytetrafluoroethylene
    PTFE-containing im-
      plant
    PTFE prosthesis

ptosis
  breast p. (grades I–IV)
  brow p.
  p. of the chin
  eyebrow p.
  eyelid p.
  p. of lacrimal glands
  p. of submandibular glands

ptotic
  p. brow
  p. earlobe
  p. eyebrow
  p. malar fat pad

pucker
  lip p.

Pulec and Freedman classification of congenital aural atresia

pulley
  annular p.
  cruciate p.
  p's in fibro-osseous tunnel
  palmar p.
  palmar aponeurosis p.
  p. reconstruction

pulp
  dental p.
  finger p.
  palmar p.

pulpa dentis

pulsed dye laser
  Candela p. d. l.
  flashlamp-excited p. d. l.
  flashlamp p. d. l. (FLPD la-
    ser)
  flashlamp-pumped p. d. l.
    (FPPDL) 510 nm
  flashlamp-pumped p. d. l.
    (FPPDL) 585 nm
  PhotoDerm VLS p. d. l.
  PhotoGenica VLS p. d. l.
  tunable flashlamp-excited
    p. d. l.
  Vbeam p. d. l.

Pulvertaft
  modified P. classification
    for mutilating injuries
    (categories 1–5)

pump
  Klein p.

punch
  backward-biting ostrum p.
  biopsy p.
  biting p.
  Goldman cartilage p.
  hair transplant p.
  Hajek-Koffler sphenoidal p.
  Hajek-Skillern sphenoidal p.

punch (continued)
  Hardy sellar p.
  Schmithhuisen sphenoid p.
  Takahashi nasal p.

punctum lacrimale

puncture
  lumbar p.

pupil
  blown p.

PUSH
  Pressure Ulcer Scale for
    Healing
      PUSH Tool

pushback
  Dorrance palatal p.
  palatal p.
  p. procedure
  Veau-Wardill palatal p.
  V-Y p.

pustule
  sterile p.

pyeloplasty
  capsular flap p.

pyoderma
  blastomycosis-like p.
  bullous hemorrhagic p.
    gangrenosum
  hemorrhagic p. gangreno-
    sum
  superficial granuloma-
    tous p.

pyramidal
  p. eminence
  p. fracture
  p. tuberosity of palatine
    bone

pyramid cannula

Q

QS
Q-switched
QS alexandrite laser
QS neodymium:yt-
trium-aluminum-gar-
net (Nd:YAG) laser
QS ruby laser
QS ruby/YAG laser

Q-switched (QS)
Q-s. alexandrite laser
Q-s. neodymium:yttrium-
aluminum-garnet (Nd:
YAG) laser
Q-s. ruby laser
Q-s. ruby/YAG laser

Quadcat wire

quadrad
Meniere q.

quadrangular
q. cartilage
q. fontanelle
q. membrane
q. space

quadrant
anterosuperior q.

quadrantectomy
q., axillary dissection, and
radiotherapy (QUART)

quadrapod flap

quadrate
q. muscle of lower lip
q. muscle of upper lip

quadratus
q. labii inferioris
q. labii inferioris muscle
q. labii superioris
q. labii superioris muscle
q. lumborum muscle
q. menti

quadriceps
q. atrophy

quadricuspid

quadriga syndrome

quadrilateral
q. cartilage
q. space

quadrilobed flap

quadriplegia

quadrisected
q. graft dilator
q. minigraft dilator

QUART
quadrantectomy, axillary
dissection, and radiotherapy

qualitative
q. analysis
q. melanin test

Quant sign

quantitative
q. analysis
q. microbiologic bacterial
count
q. microbiology

quantity
absolute q.

Quatrefage angle

quartile

quenching
thermal q.

question
q. mark ear
q. tag

questionnaire
McGill Pain Q.
modified somatic percep-
tion q. (MSPQ)
Multidimensional Body-Self
Relations Q.

Queyrat
erythroplasia of Q.

quick-mount face-bow articulator

quiescent

quilting stitch

Quimby scissors

Quisling intranasal hammer

quinsy
    lingual q.

R

RA
    rheumatoid arthritis

rabbit sniffing exercise

raccoon eyes

racemose

rad

radial
    r. abduction
    r. artery
    r. column
    r. deviation
    r. forearm flap
    r. forearm osteocutaneous
      flap
    r. mutilation injury
    r. nerve
    r. nerve block
    r. nerve palsy
    palmar r. arch
    resisted r. wrist extension
    r. sensory compression
    r. shortening
    r. styloid process
    r. tunnel syndrome
    r. wedge osteotomy
    r. wrinkle

Radial Jaw biopsy forceps

radial-ulnar deviation axis

radiation
    r. absorbed dose
    r. burn
    r. dermatitis
    r. dermatosis
    r.-induced ulceration
    r. injury
    monochromatic r.
    r. mucositis
    r. necrosis
    r. oncology
    r. therapy
    r. wound

radical
    r. excision
    r. hemimaxillectomy

radical *(continued)*
    r. mastectomy
    r. mastoidectomy
    r. neck dissection
    r. parotidectomy
    r. subtotal resection

radiocarpal
    r. arch
    r. articulation
    r. fusion
    r. joint
    r. joint capsule
    r. ligament
    volar r. ligament

radiocarpus

radiodensity

radiodermatitis

radioepidermatitis

radiograph
    bisected angle r.
    bregma-menton r.
    Brewerton view r.
    cephalometric r.
    composite r.
    density r.
    inferior-superior zygomatic
      arch r.
    jaw r.
    lateral oblique r.
    lateral sinus r.
    lateral skull r.
    long-cone r.
    mandibular bicuspid r.
    mandibular cuspid r.
    mandibular cuspid–first bi-
      cuspid r.
    mandibular incisor r.
    mandibular molar r.
    maxilla r.
    maxillary bicuspid r.
    maxillary cuspid r.
    maxillary incisor r.
    maxillary molar r.
    maxillary sinus r.
    occlusal cross section r.
    Panelipse panoramic r.

radiograph *(continued)*
    Panex panoramic r.
    panoramic r.
    Panorex r.
    posteroanterior mandible r.
    posteroanterior sinus r.
    posteroanterior skull r.
    reverse Robert view r.
    Robert view r.
    straight-on r.
    temporomandibular joint r.
    transcranial temporoman-
      dibular joint r.
    Waters view r.
    working r.
    Wrightington wrist r.
    zygomatic arch r.

radiographic
    r. cephalometer
    r. density

radiography
    cephalometric r.
    direct digital r. (DDR)
    lateral head extraoral r.
    mental extraoral r.
    Waters extraoral r.

radiolucency
    apical r.

radiolucent
    r. lesion
    r. line

radiolunate
    r. angle
    r. arthrodesis
    r. joint

radionecrosis

radiopacity

radiopaque
    r. lesion
    r. mass
    r. skull

radioscapholunate ligament

radiotherapy

radiotransparent

radioulnar
    dorsal r. ligament
    palmar r. ligament
    r. subluxation
    r. synostosis

radius
    r. fossa
    donor r. fracture

radix *pl.* radices
    r. dentis
    r. facialis
    r. linguae
    r. longa ganglii ciliaris
    r. nasi
    r. nasociliaris
    r. nervi facialis
    r. unguis

Radovan
    R. breast implant
    R. subcutaneous tissue ex-
      pander
    R. tissue expander
    R. tissue expander tip

RAFF
    rectus abdominis free flap

Ragnell
    R. dissecting scissors
    R. double-ended retractor
    R. retractor
    R. undermining scissors
    R.-Kilner scissors

raised
    r. border
    r. skin flap

rake
    r. retractor

RAM
    radar absorbent material
    rectus abdominis musculo-
      cutaneous
        RAM flap
    rectus abdominis myocuta-
      neous
        RAM flap

Ramirez manipulator

rampart
    maxillary r.

ramping
    palatal r.

Ramsey Hunt syndrome

ramus *pl.* rami
    ascending r. of the mandible
    rami buccales
    r. of jaw
    mandibular r.

Randall
    R. operation
    R.-Tennison operation

random
    r. fasciocutaneous flap
    r. flap
    r. pattern blood supply
    r. pattern flap
    r.-pattern, palmar-based flap
    r. temporoparietal fascial flap

Raney clip

range
    maximum frequency r.

range of motion (ROM)
    active r. o. m. (AROM)
    mandibular r. o. m.
    r. o. m. of the wrist

ranine
    r. artery
    r. vein
    r. vein plexus

Ranke angle

ranula

Ranvier
    R. nodes
    nodes of R.
    R. tactile disks

raphe
    lateral canthal r.

raphe *(continued)*
    lateral palpebral r.
    linear r.
    lingual r.
    longitudinal r.
    longitudinal r. of tongue
    median longitudinal r.
    midpalatine r.
    palatine r.
    palpebral r.
    pharyngeal r.
    pterygomandibular r.
    supraumbilical r.
    vertical r.

rapid
    r. maxillary expansion
    r. palatal expansion device
    r. slide test

Rapp-Hodgkin syndrome

rash
    atopic dermatitis r.
    black currant r.
    brown-tail r.
    ecchymotic r.
    generalized maculopapular r.
    hemorrhagic r.
    lupus erythematosus–like r.
    macular r.
    maculopapular r.
    malar butterfly r.
    papulovesicular r.
    "slapped cheek" r.
    varicelliform r.
    wandering r.

rasp
    Aufricht glabellar r.
    Aufricht-Lipsett nasal r.
    Aufricht nasal r.
    Barsky nasal r.
    Berne nasal r.
    Brawley frontal sinus r.
    bone r.
    Converse r.
    Cottle r.
    Cottle-MacKenty elevator r.
    diamond nasal r.

rasp *(continued)*
    Fischer nasal r.
    Fomon nasal r.
    Israel nasal r.
    Joseph nasal r.
    Lamont nasal r.
    Leurs nasal r.
    Lorenz-Rees nasal r.
    Maliniac nasal r.
    Maltz r.
    Maltz-Anderson nasal r.
    Maltz-Lipsett nasal r.
    Parkes r.
    Peet nasal r.
    Stenstrom r.
    Wiener nasal r.

raspatory
    Barsky cleft palate r.
    Converse r.

raspberry tongue

rasping
    bony r.

rate
    r. of maturation
    tear clearance r.

ratio
    calorie-to-nitrogen r.
    carpal height r.
    Holdaway r.

Ravenna syndrome

Ravitch technique for reconstruction

ray
    roentgen r.

RBM implant

reabsorption

reaction
    allergic r. *(type I–IV)*
    allograft r.
    anaphylactic r.
    anaphylactoid r.
    antigen-antibody r.
    autoimmune r.
    epicutaneous r.

reaction *(continued)*
    fibroblastic r.
    foreign body r.
    graft-versus-host r.
    granulomatous r.
    granulomatous inflammatory r.
    homograft r.
    idiosyncratic allergic r.
    immunity r.
    inflammation r.
    intradermal r.
    manic r.
    marked localized r.
    photoallergic r.
    systemic r.
    vascular r.
    vasomotor r.
    wheal-and-flare r.
    white-graft r.

reactive
    r. angioendotheliomatosis
    r. hyperostosis
    r. ossification

reactivity
    tissue r.

Read facial curet

Reagan test

realignment rhinoplasty

reanimation
    facial r.

reassignment
    gender r.

reattachment

rebalancing
    tendon r.

recalcification

receding lower jaw

receptor
    epidermal growth factor r.
    juxtacapillary r.

recess
    Arlt r.

recess *(continued)*
    bony sphenoethmoidal r.
    facial r.
    frontal r.
    infundibuliform r.
    laryngopharyngeal r.
    nasal r.
    r. of nasopharynx
    palatine r.
    parotid r.
    pharyngeal r.
    prestyloid r.
    Rosenmüller r.
    sphenoethmoidal r.
    zygomatic r.

recipient
    r. bed
    r. site
    universal r.
    r. vessel

reciprocal
    r. innervation

Recklinghausen *(variant* von Recklinghausen)
    canals of R.
    central R. disease, type II
    R. disease
    R. neurofibromatosis

recoil
    elastic r.

recombinant
    r. human bone morphogenetic protein (rhBMP-2)
    r. human growth hormone (rhGH)
    r. human insulin-like growth factor (rhIGF)

reconstruction
    abdominal wall r.
    alar r.
    alloplastic r.
    areolar r.
    auricular r.
    autogenous r.
    axiolingual (AL) r.

reconstruction *(continued)*
    bell flap nipple r.
    bilateral internal mammary artery (BIMA) r.
    Blom-Singer vocal r.
    bone r.
    bony r.
    box top technique of nipple r.
    breast r.
    breast mound r.
    Brent eyebrow r.
    buccal mucosa graft for urethra r.
    burn r.
    buttress r.
    chest wall r.
    cleft lip nasal r.
    columellar r.
    composite mandibular r.
    conjunctival cul-de-sac r.
    cosmetic r.
    costochondral graft r.
    costochondral graft mandibular ramus r.
    craniofacial r.
    Cutler-Beard r.
    dermal pouch r.
    digital nerve r.
    double-paddle peroneal tissue transfer r.
    ear r.
    epiglottic r.
    esthetic breast r.
    expanded two-flap method for microtia r.
    exstrophy r.
    extensor tendon r.
    external genitalia r.
    eyelid r.
    facial r.
    facial artery musculomucosal flap r.
    facial paralysis r. with free muscle transfer
    facial paralysis r. with gracilis free muscle transfer

reconstruction *(continued)*

    facial paralysis r. with pectoralis minor muscle transfer

    facial paralysis r. with rectus abdominis muscle transfer

    finger r.

    forehead r.

    four-bone SLAC (scapholunate advanced collapse) wrist r.

    free bone r.

    free fillet extremity flap for r.

    free flap r.

    free gracilis muscle r.

    free tissue transfer r.

    functional r.

    Goldman nasal tip r.

    gracilis myocutaneous vaginal r.

    hair-bearing r.

    head and neck r.

    r. of heel and plantar area

    Hughes eye r.

    implant/flap r.

    internal mammary artery pedicled fasciocutaneous island flap r. of breast

    Istanbul flap for phallic r.

    Landolt eyelid r.

    laryngotracheal r. (LTR)

    latissimus dorsi breast r.

    lip r.

    lip and vermilion r.

    long bone r.

    mandibular r.

    mandibular functional r.

    r. of maxillectomy and midfacial defects

    maxillofacial r.

    microsurgical breast r.

    microtia r.

    microvascular r.

    Mladick ear r.

    modified autogenous latissimus breast r.

    morphofunctional vulvar r.

reconstruction *(continued)*

    multistaged r.

    nasal septa r.

    neoglottic r.

    neurovascular infrahyoid island flap for tongue r.

    nipple-areolar r.

    no-bone r.

    orbital rim r.

    orofacial r.

    oromandibular r.

    osteochondral r.

    osteoplastic r.

    palate r.

    paraumbilical perforator adiposal flap r. of breast

    peg latissimus dorsi flap breast r.

    penile r.

    perineal r.

    phallic r.

    pharyngocsophageal r.

    postmastectomy r.

    prosthetic r.

    pulley r.

    radial artery r.

    radial forearm free flap r.

    Ravitch technique for r.

    r. plates

    reversed island flaps for forefoot r.

    reverse ulnar hypothenar flap finger r.

    scalp r.

    secondary ear r.

    segmental bone and cartilage r.

    sensitive free flap r.

    septal r.

    sequential bilateral breast r.

    single internal mammary artery r. (SIMA)

    single-stage r.

    SLAC (scapholunate advanced collapse) r.

    SLAC (scapholunate advanced collapse) wrist r.

reconstruction *(continued)*
  sliding osteotomy in mandibular r.
  soft tissue r.
  soft tissue expansion r.
  soleus-fibula free transfer r. of lower limb
  staged r.
  staged breast r.
  Steffanoff ear r.
  subpectoral r.
  sural island flap for foot and ankle r.
  Tagliacozzi nasal r.
  TAL breast r.
  Tanzer auricle r.
  Thom flap laryngeal r.
  thumb r.
  total autogenous latissimus breast r.
  TRAM flap breast r.
  transmandibular r.
  transverse rectus abdominis musculocutaneous flap breast r.
  tunneled supraclavicular island flap for head and neck r.
  urethral r.
  vaginal r.
  vaginoperineal r.
  vulvovaginal r.
  Wookey pharyngoesophageal r.
  Zisser-Madden method of upper lip r.

reconstructive rhinoplasty

recontouring
  occlusal r.

record
  centric interocclusal r.
  centric maxillomandibular r.
  centric occluding relation r.
  eccentric interocclusal r.
  eccentric maxillomandibular r.
  face-bow r.

record *(continued)*
  interocclusal r.
  jaw relation r.
  maxillomandibular r.
  occluding centric relation r.
  profile r.
  protrusive interocclusal r.
  terminal jaw relation r.
  three-dimensional r.

recovery
  creep r.

recrudescent

recruitment
  incomplete r.

rectus
  r. abdominis flap
  r. abdominis free flap (RAFF)
  r. abdominis muscle
  r. abdominis muscle sheath
  r. abdominis musculocutaneous (RAM) flap
  r. abdominis myocutaneous (RAM) flap
  r. abdominis sheath
  r. capitis muscle
  r. fascia
  r. femoris fasciocutaneous flap
  r. femoris flap
  r. femoris muscle
  r. femoris musculocutaneous flap
  inferior r. muscle
  lateral r. capitis
  lateral r. muscle
  medial r. muscle
  r. sheath
  r. sheath hematoma
  superior r. muscle
  r. turnover flap

recurrent
  r. aphthous ulcer
  r. basal cell carcinoma
  r. cutaneous abscess
  r. ganglion
  r. laryngeal nerve (RLN)

recurrent *(continued)*
    r. pleomorphic adenoma
    r. squamous cell carcinoma
    r. ulcer
RED
    rigid external distraction
        RED system rigid ex-
        ternal distractor
red
    r. granulation
    r. nodule
    r. papule
    r. Robinson catheter
    r. rubber catheter
    r. zone of lip
redecussate
reduction
    r.-advancement genioplasty
    alar base r.
    Arie-Pitanguy breast r.
    r.-augmentation procedure
    breast r.
    calf r.
    caudal septal r.
    closed r.
    closed r. and internal fixa-
        tion
    conchal r.
    Frechet extended scalp r.
    r. genioplasty
    r. and internal fixation
    jowl r. lipectomy
    Lejour breast r.
    r. of lower palpebral bulge
    r. mammaplasty
    open r.
    open r. and internal fixa-
        tion (ORIF)
    scalp r.
    septal r.
    T-breast r.
    tuberosity r.
    volumetric fat r.
    Wiener breast r.
    Wise pattern in breast r.
redundancy
    eyelid r.

redundant
    r. abdominal apron
    r. skin
    r. tissue
    r. upper lid skin folds
reeducation
    muscle r.
Rees
    R. face-lift scissors
Reese
    R. dermatome
    R. ptosis knife
    R. ptosis operation
reepithelialization
reepithelialized
reexploration
reexposure
referred
    r. pain
    r. sensation
refill
    capillary r.
reflected skin flap
reflection
    mucobuccal r.
    r. of scalp
reflex
    abdominal r.
    accommodation r.
    acousticopalpebral r.
    asymmetric r's
    auricular r.
    auriculopalpebral r.
    auropalpebral r.
    Barkman r.
    basal joint r.
    Bekhterev-Mendel (Bech-
        terew-Mendel) r.
    brachioradial r.
    carotid sinus r.
    cephalic r's
    cephalopalpebral r.

reflex *(continued)*
  chin r.
  consensual r.
  crossed r.
  delayed r.
  dorsum pedis r.
  esophagosalivary r.
  faucial r.
  flexion r.
  flexion-extension r.
  Hennebert r.
  ipsilateral r.
  Jacobson r.
  jaw r.
  Kisch r.
  knee-jerk r.
  laryngeal r.
  laryngospastic r.
  latent r.
  lip r.
  mandibular r.
  masseter r.
  Mayer r.
  metacarpothenar r.
  middle ear muscle r.
  Moro r.
  myotatic r.
  nasal r.
  nasomental r.
  nose bridge–lid r.
  nose-eye r.
  orbicularis oculi r.
  palatal r.
  palatine r.
  palmar r.
  palmomental r.
  paradoxical r.
  pharyngeal r.
  radial r.
  Roger r.
  Starling r.
  stretch r.
  styloradial r.
  supinator longus r.
  supraorbital r.
  r. sympathetic dystrophy
    (RSD)
  thumb r.
  trigeminal-facial nerve r.

reflex *(continued)*
  trigeminofacial r.
  Trömner r.
  vestibulo-ocular r.
  withdrawal r.
  zygomatic r.

regeneration
  aberrant r.
  axonal r.
  bony r.
  guided bone r.
  guided tissue r.

regimen
  burn wound r.
  Washington r.

regio *pl.* regiones
  regiones abdominis
  r. buccalis
  r. carpalis anterior
  r. carpalis posterior
  regiones fasciales
  r. frontalis capitis
  r. inframammaria
  r. infraorbitalis
  r. mammaria
  r. mentalis
  r. nasalis
  r. oralis
  r. orbitalis
  r. submaxillaris
  r. submentalis
  regiones volares digitorum
    manus
  r. zygomatica

region
  abdominal r.
  auricular r.
  axillary r.
  basilar r.
  buccal r.
  facial r's
  femoral artery–saphenous
    bulb r.
  frontal r.
  frontoparietal r.
  glabellar r.
  inframammary r.

region *(continued)*
    infraorbital r.
    jugulodigastric r.
    labial r.
    laryngeal r.
    lower clival r.
    malar-zygomatic r.
    mammary r.
    mastoid r.
    mental r.
    mylohyoid r.
    nuchal r.
    occipital r.
    orbital r.
    palpebral r.
    parasymphyseal r.
    parietotemporal r.
    parotideomasseteric r.
    pterygomaxillary r.
    sphenopetroclival r.
    sternocleidomastoid r.
    subauricular r.
    submaxillary r.
    submental r.
    superior palpebral r.
    supraclavicular r.
    supraorbital r.
    temporal r.
    vestibular r.
    volar r's of fingers
    volar r. of hand
    zygomatic r.
    zygomaticofrontal r.
    zygomaticomaxillary r.

regional
    r. anesthesia
    r. block anesthesia
    r. excision
    r. flap
    r. lymph node
    r. muscle transfer
    r. node involvement
    r. perfusion

registration
    functional occlusal r.
    maxillomandibular r.
    occlusal r.

Regnault abdominoplasty

rehabilitation
    mouth r.
    occlusal r.
    oromandibular r.
    osseointegrated implant r.

Rehne
    R. skin graft knife
    R.-Delorme plication

Reid
    R. baseline
    R. classification for mutilat-
        ing injuries *(groups 1–6)*

Reilly granulations

reimplantation
    r. of extremity
    r. of fingertip

Reinke edema

reinnervate

reinnervation

reinsertion
    ligament r.
    maxillary removal and r.

Reissner membrane

rejection
    allograft r.
    chronic allograft r.
    graft r.
    white graft r.

rejuvenation
    complete facial r.
    facial r.
    midfacial r.
    r. surgery
    upper face r.

relation
    acentric r.
    acquired eccentric jaw r.
    alar-columella r.
    buccolingual r.
    centric r.
    centric jaw r.
    centric occluding r.

relation *(continued)*
 dynamic r.
 eccentric jaw r.
 intermaxillary r.
 jaw r.
 jaw-to-jaw r.
 lateral r.
 mandibular centric r.
 maxillomandibular r.
 median jaw r.
 median retruded r.
 median retruded jaw r.
 occlusal r.
 occlusal jaw r.
 posterior border jaw r.
 protrusive jaw r.
 rest jaw r.
 retruded jaw r.
 ridge r.
 statis r.
 unstrained jaw r.
 working bite r.

relationship
 abnormal occlusal r.
 bimaxillary r.
 cephalometric r.
 occlusal r.
 overbite/overjet r.
 scaphopisocapitate (SPC) r.
 upper tooth to upper lip r.

relator
 orthognathic occlusal r.

relaxant
 muscle r.

relaxation
 skin r.

relaxed skin tension lines
 (RSTL)

release
 Agee carpal tunnel r.
 carpal tunnel r. (CTR)
 chordee r.
 endoscopic carpal tunnel r.
  (ECTR)
 galea-frontalis-occipitalis r.
 Guyon canal r.

release *(continued)*
 laryngeal r.
 open carpal tunnel r.
  (OCTR)
 periosteal r.
 retroorbicularis fat pad r.
 retroorbicularis ocular fat
  pad r.
 single-portal endocarpal
  tunnel r.
 Skoog r. of Dupuytren contracture
 syndactyly r.

releasing incision

relief incision

relocation
 r. of anterior septum to
  midline
 Barsky alar cartilage r.
 Brown and McDowell alar
  cartilage r.
 Erich alar cartilage r.
 Humby alar cartilage r.
 septal r.

remodeling
 adaptive temporomandibu-
  lar joint r.
 bilateral forehead r.
 bilateral fronto-orbital r.
 bone r.
 r. of collagen
 frontocranial r.
 fronto-orbital r.
 peripheral temporomandibular joint r.
 progressive temporoman-
  dibular joint r.
 r. phase of wound healing
 supraorbital r.
 temporomandibular joint r.
 tissue r.

removal
 corrugator r.
 foreign body r.
 intracapsular tumor r.
 laser hair r.
 maxillary r. and reinsertion

removal *(continued)*
    medial-to-lateral tumor r.
    tattoo r.

remover
    anterior band r. (ABR)

Rendu-Osler-Weber syndrome

rent
    mucosal r.

reoperation
    bilateral coronal synosto-
      sis r.
    metopic synostosis r.
    sagittal synostosis r.

repair
    Alsus-Knapp eyelid r.
    r. of alveolar ridge defect
    Ammon eyelid r.
    anatomic r.
    apertognathia r.
    Arlt epicanthus r.
    Arlt eyelid r.
    Axhausen cleft lip r.
    Barsky cleft lip r.
    Bauer-Tondra-Trusler cleft
      lip r.
    Bauer-Trusler-Tondra cleft
      lip r.
    blepharoptosis r.
    Brand tendon r.
    calvarial r.
    cleft lip r.
    cleft palate r.
    columellar r.
    commissure r.
    dog-ear r.
    epineurial r.
    flexor tendon r.
    four-flap cleft palate r.
    Hagedorn-Le Mesurier
      method of cleft lip r.
    Langenbeck r.
    Le Mesurier r.
    Millard bilateral cleft lip r.
    Millard rotation-advance-
      ment unilateral cleft lip r.
    Mirault-Blair-Brown
      method of cleft lip r.

repair *(continued)*
    rectus turnover r.
    Rose cleft lip r.
    Rose-Thompson r.
    rotation-advancement cleft
      lip r.
    shoelace-type r.
    Skoog cleft lip r.
    staged abdominal r. (STAR)
    syndactyly r.
    Tennison-Randall cleft lip r.
    Tennison-Randall triangular
      flap r.
    tension-free r.
    tissue r.
    two-flap palatoplasty r.
    unilateral Millard r.
    Veau cleft lip r.
    Veau-Wardill-Kilner r.
    Veau-Wardill-Kilner cleft
      palate r.
    Verdan tendon r.
    von Langenbeck r.
    von Langenbeck method r.
    von Langenbeck perios-
      teal r.
    V-Y r.
    V-Y r. of cheek deficit
    V-Y pushback cleft palate r.
    V-Y retroposition cleft pal-
      ate r.
    Wardill-Kilner V-Y palatal r.
    Wiener eyelid r.
    Wynn cleft lip r.

reperfusion injury

replacement
    allograft joint r.
    hard tissue r. (HTR)
    joint r.
    mucosal patch r.

Replace system tapered im-
    plant

replantation
    digital r.
    ear r.
    finger r.
    hand r.

replantation *(continued)*
  heterotopic r.
  microsurgical ear r.
  scalp r.
  transmetacarpal r.

repositioning
  auricular r.
  jaw r.
  bony r.
  muscle r.
  W-Y palatal r.

requirement
  caloric r's for burn patients

rerouting
  facial nerve r.

resection
  abdominoperineal r.
  bone r.
  corrugator muscle r.
  craniofacial r.
  epidermoid r.
  marginal mandibular r.
  Mohs r.
  oncologic mandibular r.
  platysma r.
  radical subtotal r.
  rhinoplasty and submu-
    cous r.
  segmental r.
  septal r.
  skull base tumor r.
  soft tissue r.
  submucosal r.
  submucous r. (SMR)
  submucous r. and rhino-
    plasty
  total upper lip r.
  Wagner skull r.
  wedge r.
  Weir r. of the alar base

resection-arthrodesis

residual
  r. scarring

resin
  activated r.

resin *(continued)*
  macrofilled r.

resorbable
  r. bilayer collagen mem-
    brane
  r. copolymer PGA/PLLA-
    Lactosorb miniplate fixa-
    tion system
  r. plate and screw
  r. rigid fixation

resorcinol

resorption
  bone r.
  central r.
  compensatory bone r.
  frontal r.
  frontal bone r.
  graft r.
  horizontal r.
  massive r.
  progressive condylar r.
    (PCR)
  subchondral bony r.

respiration
  abdominal-diaphragmatic r.
  assisted r.
  laryngeal r.

resplit

resplitting of the earlobe

response
  autoimmune r.
  biphasic r.
  cell-mediated immune r.
  histiocytic r.
  immune r.
  inflammatory r.
  maladaptive r.
  middle latency r. (MLR)
  somatosensory r.

Resposable Spacemaker surgical balloon dissector

rest
  congenital cartilaginous r.
    of the neck (CCRN)

rest *(continued)*
    epithelial r.
    Malassez epithelial r.

Reston foam dressing

restoration
    esthetic r.
    implant r.
    IMZ-type r.
    intermediate r.
    maxillary r.
    metallic r.

Restore
    R. bone implant
    R. RBM implant

restriction
    mandibular r.

restructuring
    facial r.

resurfacing
    Achilles tendon r.
    island adipofascial flap in
        Achilles tendon r.
    laser r.
    skin r.

retainer
    matrix r.
    multiple r.

retardation
    growth r.
    maxillary r.
    mental r.

retention
    mechanical r.
    micromechanical r.

Rethi incision

reticular
    r. dermis
    r. lesion
    r. pattern

reticuloendothelial

reticuloendothelioma

reticuloendotheliosis

reticulogranuloma

reticuloid
    actinic r.

reticulosis
    disseminated pagetoid r.
    lipomelanic r.
    malignant r.
    malignant midline r.

reticulum
    r. cell sarcoma
    granular r.

retinaculotome
    Paine carpal tunnel r.

retinaculum *pl.* retinacula
    retinacula cutis
    extensor r.
    flexor r.
    inferior extensor r.
    r. tendinum

retinoic acid

retraction
    lid r.
    mandibular r.
    maxillary incisor r.
    midlamellar cicatricial r.

retractor
    alar r.
    Alexander-Ballen orbital r.
    Alter lip r.
    angled vein r.
    Army-Navy r.
    Aston nasal r.
    Aston submental r.
    Aufricht r.
    Aufricht nasal r.
    Austin r.
    baby Senn-Miller r.
    Barraquer lid r.
    Barsky r.
    Barsky nasal r.
    Bauer r.
    Berens r.
    Berens mastectomy r.

retractor *(continued)*
    Berens mastectomy skin
       flap r.
    Bergman wound r.
    Bernstein nasal r.
    Biggs mammaplasty r.
    Black r.
    Blair-Brown r.
    Blakesley uvula r.
    Brinker tissue r.
    Bristow-Bankart soft tis-
       sue r.
    Brown-Burr modified Gil-
       lies r.
    buttonhook nerve r.
    Cairns r.
    Callahan r.
    Campbell r.
    Castallo lid r.
    Castroviejo r.
    cat's paw r.
    cheek r.
    cheek and tongue r.
    Collins-Mayo r.
    Converse r.
    Converse alar r.
    Converse blade r.
    Converse double-ended r.
    Converse nasal r.
    Conway lid r.
    corrugated forehead r.
    Cottle alar r.
    Cottle-Joseph r.
    Cottle knife guide and r.
    Cottle-Neivert r.
    Cottle pronged r.
    Cottle soft palate r.
    Cottle thumb hook r.
    Cottle upper lateral r.
    Crile r.
    Crowe-Davis mouth r.
    Cushing nerve r.
    dacryocystorhinostomy r.
    David-Baker eyelid r.
    Deaver r.
    de la Plaza transconjuncti-
       val r.
    Desmarres lid r.
    Devine-Millard-Aufricht r.

retractor *(continued)*
    Dingman flexible r.
    Dingman zygoma hook r.
    Elschnig lid r.
    Emory EndoPlastic r.
    Endotrac r.
    ESI light-weight, narrow
       mammaplasty r.
    ESI long, narrow mamma-
       plasty r.
    ESI narrow mammaplasty r.
    extraoral sigmoid notch r.
    face-lift r.
    flexible neck rake r.
    Fomon nasal r.
    Fomon nostril r.
    Freeman face-lift r.
    Freer skin r.
    Freer submucous r.
    Gabarro r.
    Gifford r.
    Goldstein r.
    Gooch r.
    Gradle eyelid r.
    Groenholm lid r.
    Hajek r.
    Hajek lip r.
    Hardy lip r.
    Haslinger r.
    Heiss r.
    Hillis r.
    Hoen r.
    Holzheimer r.
    Hurd pillar r.
    Jaeger r.
    Jaffe r.
    Jansen r.
    Jansen-Gifford r.
    Johnson cheek r.
    Keizer r.
    Kirby r.
    Kleinert-Ragnell r.
    Knapp lacrimal sac r.
    lacrimal r.
    Latrobe r.
    Levy articulating r.
    lid r.
    lip r.
    Love nerve r.

retractor *(continued)*
  Lukens r.
  Maliniac r.
  mandibular body r.
  Martin r.
  Meyerding finger r.
  Meyerding skin hook and r.
  middle fossa r.
  Millard thimble r.
  Minnesota r.
  modified submental r.,
    flared tip
  Moorehead r.
  Moorehead cheek r.
  Muldoon r.
  multiprong rake r.
  nasal r.
  nasopharyngeal r.
  Neivert knife guide and r.
  nerve r.
  Oliver r.
  one-piece lip r.
  orbicular r.
  orbital r.
  palate r.
  periareolar r.
  Pierce cheek r.
  Proctor r.
  Ragnell r.
  Ragnell double-ended r.
  rake r.
  rigid neck rake r.
  Schepens orbital r.
  Scoville nerve r.
  Seldin r.
  self-retaining r.
  Senn r.
  Senn-Dingman r.
  Senn-Miller r.
  serrefine r.
  Sewall r.
  Shearer lip r.
  sigmoid notch r.
  Sistrunk r.
  Sistrunk band r.
  skin flap r.
  Sluder r.
  Sluder palate r.
  soft palate r.

retractor *(continued)*
  Stevenson r.
  Stille cheek r.
  submucous r.
  Tebbetts ribbon r.
  Terino facial implant r.
  three-pronged r.
  vein r.
  Viboch iliac graft r.
  Walden-Aufricht nasal r.
  Walker r.
  Weitlaner r.
  Wills r.

retraining
  neuromuscular r.

retransplant

retroareolar mass

retroauricular
  r. artery
  r. free flap
  r. incision
  r. lymph node
  r. sulcus
  r. vein

retrobulbar hemorrhage

retrobuccal

retrodisplaced maxillae

retrodisplacement
  conchal r.

retrofacial

retrogenia

retrognathia
  inferior r.
  mandibular r.
  maxillary r.
  superior maxillary r.

retrognathic
  r. mandible
  r. profile

retrognathism
  bird-face r.
  mandibular r.
  mandibular r./retrusion

retrograde
    r. dissection
    r.-flow flap
    r. perfused fasciocutaneous
      flap
    r. venous drainage

retrolingual

retromammary

retromandibular
    r. fossa
    r. triangle
    r. vein

retromastoid

retromaxillary prognathism

retromolar pad

retromylohyoid
    r. eminence
    r. space

retronasal

retroorbicularis ocular fat
  (ROOF)
    r. o. f. pad excision
    r. o. f. pad release

retroparotid

retropharyngeal
    r. abscess
    r. edema
    r. lymph node
    r. node
    r. space

retroposition
    mandibular r.
    maxillary r.

retropulsion
    globe r.

retroseptal
    r. space
    r. transconjunctival ap-
      proach

retrosigmoid
    r. approach

retrosigmoid (continued)
    r. vesicular neurectomy

retrosinus

retrotarsal
    r. fold

retrotragal incision

retrozygomatic space

retruded
    r. centric
    r. jaw relation
    r. mandible
    r. position

retrusion
    mandibular r.
    mandibular retrognathism/
      r.
    maxillary r.
    midfacial r.

Retzius
    lines of R.

Reuse Expanda-graft dermatome

revascularization

revascularize

revascularized bone graft

Reverdin
    R. epidermal free graft
    R. graft
    R. method
    R. needle
    R. operation
    R. osteotomy
    R. skin graft

reverse
    r. Barton fracture
    r. Bennett fracture
    r. digital artery flap
    r. digital artery island flap
    r. dorsal digital island flap
    r. facial osteotomy
    r. flow island flap
    r. flow vascularization
    r. Karapandzic flap

reverse *(continued)*
  r. Kingsley splint
  r. medial arm flap
  r. muscle flap
  r. Robert view radiograph
  r. U-flap
  r. ulnar hypothenar flap finger reconstruction
reversed
  r. digital artery flap
  r. dorsal digital flap
  r. extensor digitorum muscle island flap
  r. extensor digitorum muscle island flap procedure
  r. fasciosubcutaneous flap
  r. island flaps for forefoot reconstruction
  r. pedicle flap
revised
  r. Salzburg lag screw system
  r. wound margins
  r. Würzburg mandibular reconstruction system
revision
  r. and débridement
  free flap for burn scar r.
  fusiform skin r.
  r. of graft
  r. rhinoplasty
  scar r.
  W-plasty r.
  Z-plasty r.
Revolution micropigmentation handpiece
Reynolds
  R. dissecting scissors
  R. and Horton alar cartilage technique
RF
  rheumatoid factor
rhabdomyoma
rhabdomyosarcoma
rhagades

rhagadiform
rhBMP-2
  recombinant human bone morphogenetic protein
rhegmatogenous
rheostosis
rheumatic
  r. fever
  r. nodule
rheumatism
  Besnier r.
  chronic articular r.
  Heberden r.
  MacLeod capsular r.
  muscular r.
  nodose r.
  osseous r.
  palindromic r.
  subacute r.
rheumatoid
  r. arthritis (RA)
  r. clawing
  r. factor (RF)
  r. nodulosis
  r. osteoarthritis
  r. sialadenitis
rhGH
  recombinant human growth hormone
rhIGF
  recombinant human insulin-like growth factor
rhinion
rhinitis
  atrophic r.
  foreign body r.
  gangrenous r.
  r. medicamentosa
  vasomotor r.
Rhino
  R. Rocket nasal packing
  R. Triangle brace
rhinocanthectomy

rhinocephaly

rhinocheiloplasty

rhinocleisis

rhinodacryolith

rhinodymia

rhinokyphectomy

rhinokyphosis

rhinolith

rhinolithiasis

rhinologic surgeon

rhinomanometry
anterior active mask r.

rhinometry
acoustic r.

rhinonecrosis

rhinophycomycosis

rhinophyma

rhinoplasty
adjunctive r.
Bardach cleft r.
Carpue r.
cleft r.
closed r.
conservative subtraction-
addition r. (CSAR)
cosmetic r.
Cottle r.
r. diamond bur
endonasal r.
esthetic r.
extended open-tip r.
functional r.
r. implant
Indian r.
Italian r.
Joseph r.
minimal r.
open r.
open sky r.
posttraumatic r.

rhinoplasty *(continued)*
realignment r.
reconstructive r.
revision r.
r. scissors
secondary r.
r. and submucous resec-
tion
submucous resection
and r.
tagliacotian r.
tip r.

rhinorrhaphy

rhinorrhagia

rhinorrhea
cerebrospinal r.
cerebrospinal fluid (CSF) r.
gustatory r.
halo test for cerebrospinal
fluid (CSF) r.

rhinoscleroma

rhinoscopy
anterior r.
median r.

rhinoseptoplasty

rhinosinusitis
chronic hypertrophic r.
hyperplastic r.

rhinotomy

rhomboid
r. aponeurosis
r. flap
r. glossitis
r. swelling
r. transposition flap

rhytid
forehead r's
glabellar r's
horizontal r's
minor r's
periocular r's
superficial r's
transverse r's

rhytid *(continued)*
   vertical lateral glabellar r's

rhytidectomy
   cervicofacial r.
   complex superficial muscu-
      loaponeurotic system r.
   composite r.
   deep-plane r.
   extended posterior r.
   full-thickness skin r.
   platysma r.
   SASMAS suspension r.
   r. scissors
   SMAS (superficial muscu-
      loaponeurotic system) r.
   SMILE (subperiosteal mini-
      mally invasive laser endo-
      scopic) r.
   subcutaneous r.
   subperiosteal minimally in-
      vasive laser endoscopic
      (SMILE) r.
   sub-SMAS r.
   superficial plane r.
   superficial SMAS r.

rhytidoplasty
   endoscopic forehead-
      brow r.

rhytidosis

rib
   cervical r.

Rica
   R. nasal septal speculum
   R. rongeur

Richey condyle marker

rictus

Ridell operation

ridge
   alveolar r.
   anatomic r.
   bicoronal r.
   bony r.
   buccal r.
   buccal cervical r.

ridge *(continued)*
   buccal triangular r. (BTR)
   center of r.
   digastric r.
   epidermal r's
   epithelial r.
   external oblique r.
   infraorbital r. of maxilla
   internal occipital r.
   interpapillary r's
   key r.
   linguocervical r.
   linguogingival r.
   longitudinal r. of hard pal-
      ate
   mammary r.
   mandibular r.
   r. of mandibular neck
   marginal r.
   mental r.
   mylohyoid r.
   nasal r.
   orbitozygomaticomalar
      bone r.
   palatine r.
   Passavant r.
   petrosal r.
   pterygoid r. of sphenoid
      bone
   residual r.
   rete r's
   sphenoidal r.
   sublingual r.
   superior petrosal r.
   supraorbital r.
   transverse palatine r.
   vomerine r.
   zygomaxillare r.

Riedel
   R. frontal ethmoidectomy
   R. struma

Riehl
   R. melanoderma
   R. melanosis

RIF
   rigid internal fixation

rigid
  r. external distraction
    (RED)
  r. internal fixation (RIF)
  r. lag screw fixation
  r. plate fixation

rigidity
  clasp-knife r.
  cogwheel r.
  hemiplegic r.

rim
  alar r.
  fronto-orbital r.
  helical r.
  infraorbital r.
  mandible r.
  orbital r.
  piriform r.
  superior orbital r.
  supraorbital r.

rima *pl.* rimae
  r. glottidis
  intercartilaginous r.
  r. oris
  r. palpebrarum
  r. vocalis

ring
  r. avulsion injury
  Bickel r.
  blepharostat r.
  r. block
  cricoid r.
  lymphoid r.
  palatopharyngeal r.
  signet r. sign on x-ray
  r. ulcer
  umbilical r.
  Valtrac anastomosis r.
  Waldeyer throat r.
  Waldeyer tonsillar r.

Riolan
  R. bones
  R. bouquet
  R. nosegay

ripple deformity

Risdon
  R. approach
  R. extraoral incision
  modified R. approach
  R. pretragal incision
  R. wire

risorius
  r. muscle
  musculus r.

risus
  r. caninus
  r. sardonicus

Ritchie cleft palate tenaculum

Rivinus
  R. canals
  R. ducts
  R. gland
  R. membrane
  R. notch

rivus
  r. lacrimalis

road burn

Roaf syndrome

ROAM
  roaming optical access
    multiscope

roaming optical access multiscope

Robert
  reverse R. view radiograph
  R. view radiograph

Robin
  Pierre R. sequence
  R. sequence
  R. syndrome

Robinow
  R. dwarfism
  R. mesomelic dysplasia
  R. syndrome

Robinson
  R. catheter
  red R. catheter

Robinson *(continued)*
    R. vein graft

Robles cutting point cannula

Rochester method

rod
    condyle r.
    fixation r.
    Hydroflex penile implant r.
    Meckel r.
    Silastic r.
    silicone flexor r.

rodeo thumb

roentgen
    r. absorbed dose (rad)
    r. ray
    r. therapy

roentgenogram
    cephalometric r.
    jughandle r.
    lateral oblique jaw r.
    lateral ramus r.
    lateral skull r.
    maxillary sinus r.
    panoramic r.
    scout r.
    submental vertex r.
    Towne projection r.
    transcranial r.
    Waters view r.

roentgenograph

roentgenography
    sectional r.
    serial r.
    spot-film r.

Roger
    R. reflex
    R. syndrome

Roger Anderson
    R. A. facial fracture appliance
    R. A. pin
    R. A. pin fixation appliance

Rolando fracture

roll
    dorsal back r.
    lumbar r.

Romaña sign

Romberg
    R. disease
    R. facial deformity
    facial hemiatrophy of R.
    R. hemiatrophy
    R. hemifacial atrophy
    R. sign
    R. spasm
    R. syndrome
    R. trophoneurosis

rongeur
    Adson r.
    Bacon r.
    Bane r.
    Belz r.
    Boies-Lombard mastoid r.
    bone-biting r.
    Callahan r.
    Callahan lacrimal r.
    Campbell nerve r.
    Citelli sphenoid r.
    Converse r.
    Converse-Lange r.
    Converse nasal r.
    Converse nasal root r.
    Cottle-Kazanjian r.
    Cottle nasal-biting r.
    Dean r.
    Defourmental nasal r.
    end-biting r.
    Goldman-Kazanjian r.
    Hajek-Koffler sphenoidal r.
    Husk r.
    Ivy r.
    Kerrison r.
    Lange-Converse nasal
        root r.
    Leksell r.
    Lombard-Boies r.
    Mead r.
    Mollison r.
    Rica r.
    round-nosed r.

rongeur *(continued)*
  Rowland nasal r.
  Ruskin r.
  Simplex mastoid r.
  SMIC r.
  Whiting r.

rongeur forceps
  Adson r. f.
  Bacon r. f.
  Cottle-Jansen r. f.
  Defourmental r. f.
  Hudson r. f.
  oral r. f.

ROOF
  retroorbicularis ocular fat

roof
  r. of mouth
  r. of the nail fold
  orbital r.
  r. of skull

Rookey sign

Roos test

root
  facial r.
  facial nerve r.
  intra-alveolar r.
  lingual r.
  motor r's of submandibular
    ganglion
  motor r. of trigeminal
    nerve
  nasal r.
  palatal r.
  palatine r.
  sensory r. of trigeminal
    nerve
  r. of tongue

rope
  r. flap
  r. graft

Ropes test

ropy
  r. mass

ropy *(continued)*
  r. saliva
  r. tumor

rosacea
  acne r.
  corticosteroid r.
  granulomatous r.
  hypertrophic r.

Rose
  R. cleft lip repair
  R. position
  R.-Thompson repair

Rosenberg gynecomastia dissection instrument

Rosenburg operation

Rosenmüller
  R. cavity
  R. fossa
  R. recess
  R. valve

rostral

rostrum *pl.* rostra
  sphenoidal r.

rotation
  caudal r.
  center of r.
  center of r. of wrist
  r. flap
  Mallet scale shoulder external r.
  r. osteotomy
  r. of philtrum
  skin flap r.
  tip r.

rotation-advancement
  r.-a. flap
  r.-a. method

rotational
  r. deformity
  r. deformity of finger

rotationplasty
  hip r.

rotatory subluxation of scaphoid (RSS)

Rothmund
R. syndrome
R.-Thomson syndrome

rotundum
foramen r.

rounding
lip r.

round-nosed rongeur

Roux method

row
proximal carpal r.

Rowe disimpacting forceps

Rowland nasal rongeur

RSD
reflex sympathetic dystrophy

RSS
rotatory subluxation of scaphoid

RSTL
relaxed skin tension lines

rubber
silicone r.

Rubens
R. flap
R. free flap for breast reconstruction

Rubin
R. blade
R. bone planer
R. cartilage planer
R. nasal chisel
R. nasofrontal osteotome

Rubin *(continued)*
R. osteotomy
R. septal morcellizer

Rubinstein-Taybi syndrome

rubor
skin r.

ruby laser

rudimentary

Ruffini
R. corpuscles
R. papillary endings

ruga *pl.* rugae
r. palatina
palatine r.

rugal folds

rugose

rugous

rule
morphographemic r.
r. of nines formula for percentage of body surface burned
Wallace r. of nines

run-around
r. abscess
r. infection

rupia
r. escharotica

rupture
attrition r. of extensor tendon
intracapsular r.
tendon r.

Ruskin rongeur

S
S-flap
S-plasty
S-shaped scar

sabre
coup de s.
en coup de s.

sac
endolymphatic s.
Hilton s.
lacrimal s.
nasal s.
tear s.

sacciform

saccular
s. cyst
s. duct
s. fossa
s. nerve

saccule
laryngeal s. of Hilton
s. of larynx

sacculoutricular duct

sacculus *pl.* sacculi
s. endolymphaticus
s. lacrimalis
s. laryngis

saccus *pl.* sacci

Sachs skull bur

sac-vein decompression

saddle
s. arch
s. defect
s. deformity
s. joint
s. nose
s. nose defect
s. nose deformity
s.-shaped arch

Saemisch ulcer

Saethre
S.-Chotzen craniosynosto-
sis
S.-Chotzen syndrome

SAF-Clens chronic wound
cleanser

SAF-Gel hydrogel dressing

Safian nasal splint

Sage-Clark cheilectomy

sagittal
s. axis
s. craniectomy
s. fontanelle
s. furrow
s. incisure
s. mandibular movement
s. orientation
s. plane
s. projection
s. ramus osteotomy
s. section
s. sinus
s. splitting of mandible
s. split mandibular osteotomy
s. split osteotomy (SSO)
s. split ramus osteotomy
(SSRO)
s. suture
s. suture line
s. suture synostosis
s. synostosis reoperation

sail of cartilage

SAL
suction-assisted lipectomy

salabrasion

salicylic acid

salient

saline
s. breast implant
s. dressing
s.-filled expander

saline *(continued)*
    s. implant exchange
    s. irrigation

saliva
    artificial s.
    chorda s.
    ganglionic s.
    lingual s.
    parotid s.
    ropy s.
    sublingual s.
    submandibular s.
    submaxillary s.
    sympathetic s.

salivary
    s. calculus
    s. fistula
    s. gland virus disease
    s. lipoma
    s. lithiasis
    s. neoplasm
    s. stone
    s. tube

salivary duct
    s. d. carcinoma (SDC)
    s. d. cyst
    s. d. obstruction

salivary gland
    s. g. alveolus
    s. g. aplasia
    s. g. capsule
    s. g. carcinoma (SGC)
    s. g. cyst
    s. g. enlargement
    s. g. mass
    s. g. neoplasm
    s. g. pleomorphic adenoma
    s. g. retention cyst
    sublingual s. g.
    submandibular s. g.
    submaxillary s. g.
    s. g. tumor
    s. g. virus disease

salivate

salivolithiasis

salmon patch

salpingemphraxis

salpingopalatine
    s. fold
    s. membrane

salpingopharyngeal
    s. fold
    s. membrane
    s. muscle

salpingopharyngeus muscle

salt
    mineral s.

Salter
    S. incremental lines
    S.-Harris classification of
      epiphyseal fractures *(I–V)*

salvage
    knee s.
    s. laryngectomy
    limb s.
    s. mastectomy
    s. technique

Salyer modification of Obwegeser mandibular osteotomy

Salzburg
    revised S. lag screw system

SAM
    short arm motion
      SAM protocol

S.A.M.
    subcutaneous augmenta-
      tion material
      S.A.M. facial implant

Samonara palatoplasty

Sampson cyst

sandpaper dermabrader

sandwich
    s. epicranial flap
    s. flap

sandwich *(continued)*
    s.-type splint

Sanfilippo
    mucopolysaccharidosis
        type III S. A (MPS-IIIA)
    mucopolysaccharidosis
        type III S. B (MPS-IIIB)
    mucopolysaccharidosis
        type III S. C (MPS-IIIC)

sanguineous
    s. drainage
    s. exudate
    s. fluid
    s. inflammation

sanguineus
    nevus s.

sanguinopurulent

Santorini
    S. canal
    S. cartilage
    S. concha
    concha S.
    S. fissures
    incisura S.
    S. muscle
    papilla of S.
    S. tubercle
    S. vein

saphenous
    s. artery
    s. bulb
    s. nerve
    s. vein interposition graft

SAPHO
    synovitis, acne, pustulosis,
        hyperostosis, osteitis
            SAPHO syndrome

Sappey
    S. fibers
    S. ligament
    S. plexus

Sapphire 2000 micropigmenta-
    tion handpiece

sarcoid
    s. arthritis

sarcoid *(continued)*
    Boeck s.
    s. sialadenitis
    Spiegler-Fendt s.

sarcoidosis
    cutaneous s.

sarcoma *pl.* sarcomas, sarco-
    mata
    Abernethy s.
    adipose s.
    alveolar soft part s. (ASPS)
    ameloblastic s.
    chondroblastic s.
    chondrogenic s.
    clear cell s.
    craniofacial osteogenic s.
    endothelial s.
    epithelial s. (ES)
    epithelioid s.
    Ewing s.
    fascial s.
    fibroblastic s.
    fibrogenic s.
    idiopathic multiple hemor-
        rhagic s.
    idiopathic multiple pig-
        mented hemorrhagic s.
    intraoral Kaposi s.
    juxtacortical osteogenic s.
    Kaposi s.
    Kaposi s. of mastoid
    melanotic s.
    mesenchymal s.
    multiple benign s.
    multiple idiopathic hemor-
        rhagic s.
    neurogenic s.
    osteogenic s.
    osteoid s.
    pseudo-Kaposi s.
    reticulum cell s.
    round cell s.
    serocystic s.
    synovial s.
    telangiectatic osteogenic s.

sarcomatosis
    s. cutis

sarcomatous

Sargenti method

Sargon implant

SA-RPE
  surgical-assisted rapid palatal expansion

sartorius
  s. flap
  s. muscle

SAS
  synthetic absorbable suture
    Ethicon SAS

SASMA
  skin-adipose superficial musculoaponeurotic (system)
    SASMA face-lift

SASMAS
  skin-adipose superficial musculoaponeurotic system
    SASMAS suspension rhytidectomy

Satchmo syndrome

satellite
  s. abscess
  s. lesion
  s. nodule

saucerize
  s. a cyst

saucerization

saucer-shaped erosion

sausage
  s. digit
  s. finger
  s. toe

sausaging of vein

Sauve-Kapandji procedure

Savin operation

saw
  Adams s.

saw *(continued)*
  bayonet s.
  Bosworth-Joseph nasal s.
  Bosworth nasal s.
  Clerf laryngeal s.
  Converse s.
  Converse nasal s.
  Cottle-Joseph s.
  Cottle nasal s.
  Cottle Universal nasal s.
  diamond wafering s.
  Farrior-Joseph nasal s.
  Gigli s.
  Gigli wire s.
  gold s.
  intranasal s.
  Isomet low speed s.
  Isomet Plus precision s.
  Joseph s.
  Joseph-Maltz s.
  Lamont s.
  Langenbeck s.
  laryngeal s.
  Lell laryngofissure s.
  Maltz s.
  rhinoplasty s.
  separating s.
  Slaughter s.
  Stille-Joseph s.

Sayoc operation

sc
  subcutaneous

scabbard trachea

scaffold
  biodegradable polymer s.

scaffolding
  cartilage s.
  three-dimensional biocompatible s.

scala media

scalded-skin syndrome

scale
  Abbreviated Injury S.
  Glasgow Coma S.
  House-Brackmann facial weakness s.

scale *(continued)*
>modified Mallet s.
>Mohs hardness s.
>pityriasis-type s.
>Pressure Ulcer S. for Healing (PUSH) Tool
>psoriatic-type s.
>Sessing pressure ulcer assessment s.
>Shea s.
>Shea pressure ulcer assessment s.

scalenus
>s. anterior muscle
>s. medius muscle
>s. posterior muscle

scalene
>s. adenopathy
>s. lesion
>s. lymph node biopsy

scaler
>anterior s.
>deep s.
>McCall s.

scaling
>deep s.
>electrosurgical s.
>s. lesion
>s. skin-colored lesion

scalloping
>s. of lower lid

scalp
>dissecting cellulitis of s.
>expanded free s. flap
>s. expansion
>s. extension
>Frechet extended s. reduction
>s. lift
>locally invasive congenital cellular blue nevus of s.
>s. muscle
>pilar tumor of s.
>s. reconstruction
>s. reduction
>s. replantation

scalp *(continued)*
>s. sickle flap
>s. tissue expansion

scalpel
>s. blade
>electrosurgical s.
>Endotron-Lipectron ultrasonic s.
>lid s.
>Lipectron ultrasonic s.
>ultrasonic s.

scalping
>s. flap
>s. flap of Converse
>postauricular and retroauricular s. (PARAS)

scan
>axial computed tomography s.
>coronal computed tomography s.
>CT s.
>MRI s.
>radioisotope s.
>technetium bone s.
>three-dimensional computed tomography s's

scanner
>color flow Doppler s.
>Cencit facial s.
>scintillation s.
>Silktouch CO_2 Flash S.

scanning
>scintillation s.

Scanpor tape

scapha

scaphion

scaphocapitate
>s. articulations
>s. fusion
>s. syndrome

scaphocephalic
>s. deformity

scaphocephalous

scaphocephaly

scaphoconchal angle

scaphohydrocephaly

scaphoid
  elliptical s. fossa
  s. fossa
  s. fat pad
  s. fracture
  humpback deformity of s.
  s. nonunion
  occult s. fracture
  rotatory subluxation of s.
    (RSS)
  s. shift
  s. tubercle

scaphoid-capitate
  s.-c. arthrodesis
  s.-c. fusion

scaphoid-trapezium-trapezoid
  (STT) joint

scapholunate
  s. advanced collapse
    (SLAC)
  s. angle
  s. articulation
  s. disruption
  s. dissociation
  s. gap
  s. instability
  s. joint space
  s. motion

scaphopisocapitate (SPC)
  s. relationship

scaphotrapezoid

scaphotrapeziotrapezoid (STT)
  joint

scapula pl. scapulae
  s. crest pedicled bone graft
  s. free flap

scapular
  s. blade
  s. flap
  s. flap transfer

scapular (continued)
  s. island flap
  s. island flap technique
  s. osteocutaneous flap

scar
  areolar s.
  argon laser–induced s's
  atrophic s.
  atrophic acne s.
  atrophic facial acne s.
  atrophic white s.
  cigarette-paper s's
  circumareolar s.
  contracting s.
  s. contracture
  s. fibroblast
  s. formation
  fusiform s.
  hypertrophic s.
  hypertrophic burn s.
  icepick-type s.
  immature s.
  inferior longitudinal s.
  infra-areolar s.
  infrabrow s.
  inframammary s.
  inverted T s.
  keloid s.
  lateral s.
  s. massage
  osteopetrotic s.
  papyraceous s.
  parenchymal s.
  periareolar s.
  preauricular s.
  radial s.
  s. tissue
  S-shaped s.
  thickened s.
  T-shaped s.
  U-shaped s.
  vertical s.
  well-healed s.
  Y-shaped s.

scarabrasion

Scar Fx lightweight silicone
  sheeting

scarf nevus

scarification

Scarpa
   S. adipofascial flap
   canals of S.
   S. fascia
   S. foramen

scarring
   s. alopecia
   cigarette-paper s.
   hypertrophic s.
   keloidal s.
   residual s.

SCC
   squamous cell carcinoma
      oral SCC

SCCHN
   squamous cell carcinoma
      of head and neck

Schacher ganglion

Schamberg
   S. dermatitis
   S. progressive pigmented
      purpuric dermatosis

Schanzioni craniotomy forceps

Schatten mammaplasty

Schatzki syndrome

Schaumann
   S. bodies
   S. syndrome

Scheibe malformation

Scheie
   mucopolysaccharidosis
      type I S. (MPS-IS)

schema *pl.* schemata

Schepens orbital retractor

Schimek operation

Schimmelbusch disease

Schinzel acrocallosal syndrome

Schirmer
   S. tear test

Schirmer *(continued)*
   S. test

schistocoelia

schistoglossia

schistomelia

schistoprosopia

Schmidt syndrome

Schmincke-Regaud lymphoepithelial carcinoma

Schmithhuisen sphenoid punch

schneiderian
   s. carcinoma
   inverted s. papilloma
   s. membrane
   s. respiratory membrane

Schnitman skin hook

Schönbein operation

Schreger lines

Schrötter catheter

Schrudde
   S. aspirative lipoplasty
   S. curet technique

Schuchardt-Pfeifer operation

Schuknecht classification of
   congenital aural atresia

Schultze
   S. cells
   S. membrane

Schwalbe corpuscle

Schwann
   S. cell
   sheath of S.
   S. tumor

schwannoma
   granular cell s.
   malignant s.
   mixed type parapharyn-
      geal s.

Schwartz
   S. syndrome

Schwartz *(continued)*
    S. test

Schartzmann maneuver

Schweninger
    S.-Buzzi anetoderma

Sciatic Function Index

SCID
    severe combined immuno-
      deficiency

scintigram
    technetium s.

scintillation scanning

scintimammography (SMM)

scintiscanner

scirrhous

scissors
    Abeli tenotomy s.
    angled s.
    AROSupercut s.
    ASSI Super-Cut s.
    Aston face-lift s.
    Aufricht s.
    Baltimore nasal s.
    Barsky nasal s.
    Becker s.
    Becker septal s.
    Beckman nasal s.
    Biro dermal nevus s.
    s.-bite crossbite
    Bonn miniature iris s.
    Brophy s.
    Brophy plastic surgery s.
    Brun plastic surgery s.
    bulldog nasal s.
    Caplan nasal bone s.
    Castanares face-lift s.
    Castroviejo s.
    Castroviejo tenotomy s.
    Converse s.
    Converse nasal tip s.
    Converse plastic surgery s.
    Cottle bulldog nasal s.
    Cottle dorsal s.
    Cottle dressing s.

scissors *(continued)*
    Cottle heavy septal s.
    Cottle nasal s.
    craniotomy s.
    Davis rhytidectomy s.
    Dean s.
    Diamond-Edge Supercut s.
    dissecting s.
    Douglas nasal s.
    face-lift s.
    facial plastic surgery s.
    Fomon dorsal s.
    Fomon face-lift s.
    Fomon lower lateral s.
    Fomon saber-back s.
    Fomon upper lateral s.
    Fox s.
    Freeman rhytidectomy s.
    ganglion s.
    Gillies s.
    Goldman septal s.
    Goldman-Fox wound dé-
      bridement s.
    Gorney face-lift s.
    Gorney rhytidectomy s.
    Gorney septal s.
    Gorney turbinate s.
    Gradle s.
    Heath suture s.
    Heath wire-cutting s.
    Heyman nasal s.
    Hoskins-Westcott tenoto-
      my s.
    Huger diamond-back na-
      sal s.
    iris s.
    Jameson face-lift s.
    Joseph nasal s.
    Joseph serrated s.
    Kaye face-lift s.
    Kazanjian nasal cutting s.
    Kleinert-Kutz tenotomy s.
    Knight nasal s.
    LaGrange s.
    Lakeside nasal s.
    Laschal s.
    Littauer dissecting s.
    Littauer Junior suture s.
    Littauer stitch s.

scissors *(continued)*
 Littauer suture s.
 Littler suture carrying s.
 MacKenty s.
 Mayo s.
 McReynolds pterygium s.
 Metzenbaum s.
 micro-mosquito curved s.
 micro-mosquito straight s.
 Miltex blepharoplasty s.
 Miltex saber-back rhytidec-
    tomy s.
 Miltex stitch s.
 Miltex undermining s.
 Northbent suture s.
 O'Brien stitch s.
 plastic surgery s.
 PowerStar bipolar s.
 pterygium s.
 Quimby s.
 Ragnell dissecting s.
 Ragnell undermining s.
 Ragnell-Kilner s.
 Rees face-lift s.
 Reynolds dissecting s.
 rhinoplasty s.
 saber-back s.
 septal s.
 serrated s.
 serrated iris s.
 Shortbent s.
 Shortbent suture s.
 sickle s.
 Sistrunk s.
 Sistrunk dissecting s.
 Southbent s.
 Spencer stitch s.
 StaySharp face-lift Super-
    Cut s.
 Stevens tenotomy s.
 Stille dissecting s.
 Stille Super Cut s.
 Storz stitch s.
 straight s.
 Super-Cut s.
 superior radial tenotomy s.
 suture s.
 suture wire-cutting s.
 Taylor dural s.

scissors *(continued)*
 tenotomy s.
 thin-shaft nasal s.
 tissue s.
 utility s.
 Werb rhinostomy s.
 Wescott stitch s.
 Wilmer conjunctival and
    utility s.
 wire-cutting suture s.

sclera *pl.* sclerae
 blue s.

scleral
 s. shield
 s. show

sclerema

scleritis
 diffuse s.
 nodular s.

sclerodactyly

scleroderma
 circumscribed s.
 diffuse s.
 generalized s.
 linear s.
 localized s.
 systemic s.

sclerodermalike
 s. eruption
 s. skin thickening

sclerodermatous

sclerodermoid

ScleroLaser
 Candela S.

scleroplasty

ScleroPlus
 S. HP
 S. LongPulse dye laser sys-
    tem

sclerosing
 s. agent
 s. hemangioma
 s. injection

sclerosing *(continued)*
 s. lipogranulomatosis
 s. lymphangitis
 s. mastoiditis
 s. osteitis
 s. substance

sclerosis
 amyotrophic lateral s.
  (ALS)
 diffuse systemic s.
 miliary s.
 multiple s.
 muscular s.
 progressive systemic s.
 venous s.

sclerostenosis

sclerotherapy
 endoscopic variceal s.
  (EVS)
 tetracycline hydrochlo-
  ride s.

scoliosis

score
 Gustilo fracture s.
 Japan Facial S.
 OMENS (orbit, mandible,
  ear, cranial nerves, and
  soft tissue) s.

scored alar mucocartilaginous
 flap

scoring
 cartilage s.
 Gustilo s. for open frac-
  tures *(types II, IIIA, IIIB,
  IIIC)*
 House-Brackmann s.

Scott chronic wound care system

scout film

Scoville
 S. curved nerve hook
 S. nerve retractor

screw
 ACE bone s.
 ACE cortical bone s.

screw *(continued)*
 adjustable s.
 alar s.
 anchoring s.
 Asnis 2 guided s.
 axial anchor s.
 bicortical superior bor-
  der s.
 carpal scaphoid s.
 cortical anchoring s.
 fixation s.
 Henderson lag s.
 Herbert s.
 Herbert-Whipple s.
 implant s.
 Implant Innovations titanium s.
 Implant Support Systems titanium s.
 lag s.
 Leibinger Micro Plus s.
 Leibinger Mini-Würzburg s.
 Leibinger Würzburg s.
 Luhr Vitallium s.
 mandibular angle fracture
  intraoral open reduc-
  tion s.
 monocortical s.
 pretapped synthes lag s.
 resorbable plate and s.
 s.-retained prosthesis
 self-tapping bone s.
 self-tapping Leibinger lag s.
 Sherman bone s.
 Sherman molybdenum s.
 Sherman plate and s's
 Sherman Vitallium s.
 TiMesh emergency s.
 Vitallium s.

screwdriver
 Sherman s.

Screw-Vent implant

scrofuloderma

scrofulous rhinitis

scroll ear

scrotal
 s. compartment

scrotal *(continued)*
    s. elephantiasis
    s. hemangioma
    s. tongue

scrotoplasty

scrotum

sculpting
    body s.

sculpture
    body s.

sculpturing
    abdominal s.

Scultetus
    S. bandage
    S. binder

scurf

scutiform

scutular

scutum

SDC
    salivary duct carcinoma

Sea-Clens wound cleanser

seal
    palatal s.
    velopharyngeal s.

sealant
    fibrin s.

seam
    epithelial s.

SeaSorb alginate wound dress-
    ing

sebaceous
    s. adenoma
    s. carcinoma
    s. cyst
    s. gland
    s. hyperplasia
    s. lymphadenoma
    s. metaplasia
    s. nevus

sebaceous *(continued)*
    s. skin

sebaceum
    adenoma s.

Sebbin
    S. ultrasound-assisted lipo-
        plasty machine
    S. ultrasound device

Sebileau hollow

seborrhea
    s. adiposa
    s. capitis
    concrete s.
    s. congestiva
    eczematoid s.
    s. furfuracea
    s. nigra
    s. oleosa
    s. sicca

seborrheic
    s. dermatitis
    s. keratosis
    s. verruca

sebum
    cutaneous s.
    s. cutaneum
    s. palpebrale

Seckel
    S. bird-headed dwarf
    S. dwarfism
    S. syndrome

second
    s. toe wraparound flap
    s. intention wound closure

secondary
    s. closure of wound
    s. ear reconstruction
    s. infection
    s. lesion
    s. occlusal traumatism
    s. palate
    s. rhinoplasty
    s. sequestrum
    s. sutures
    s. telangiectasia

secondary *(continued)*
   s. wound closure

second-line drug

second-look
   s.-l. biopsy
   s.-l. procedure

secretion
   nasopharyngeal s.
   viscid s.
   viscous s.

secretory
   s. duct
   s. nerve

section
   attached cranial s.
   detached cranial s.
   frozen s.
   sagittal s.
   serial s.
   tangential s.

Secur-Its silicone cushion mat

Seddon
   S. classification for nerve
      injuries *(types 1–3)*
   S. nerve graft

Sédillot operation

Seeligmüller sign

segment
   basilar s.
   cleft maxillary s.
   labyrinthine s.

segmental
   s. alveolar osteotomy
   s. bone defect
   s. graft
   s. fracture
   s. gracilis muscle trans-
      plantation
   s. loss of helix
   s. mandibulectomy
   s. microvascular transfers
   s. neurofibromatosis
   s. perforators
   s. resection

segmental *(continued)*
   s. vitiligo

Seiler
   S. cartilage
   S. MC-M900 surgical micro-
      scope

Seldin retractor

selective
   s. anesthesia
   s. neck dissection (SND)
   s. photothermolysis

self-tapping
   s.-t. bone screw
   s.-t. Leibinger lag screw

sella
   empty s.
   dorsum s.
   s.-nasion–B point
   s.-nasion (S-N) plane
   s.-nasion-subspinale angle
      (SNA, S-N-A)
   s.-nasion-supramentale an-
      gle (SNB, S-N-B)
   s. turcica

sellar

Sellick maneuver

semicartilaginous

semicircular ducts

semicompressive dressing

semicrista
   s. incisiva

semidecussation

semi-Fowler position

semilunar
   s. bone
   s. cartilage
   s. conjunctival fold
   s. fibrocartilage
   s. flap
   s. fold

semimembranous muscle

semiocclusive dressing

semiopen dressing

semipermeable
  s. dressing
  s. membrane dressing

semipermanent retention

semipressure dressing

semirecumbent position

semirigid fixation

Semken
  S. dressing forceps
  S. tissue forceps
  S.-Taylor forceps

Semmes
  S.-Weinstein monofilament
    (SWMF)
  S.-Weinstein monofilament
    test
  S.-Weinstein nylon monofil-
    ament (SWMF)

Senear
  S.-Usher disease
  S.-Usher syndrome

senile
  s. angioma
  s. atrophoderma
  s. elastosis
  s. fibroma
  s. hemangioma
  s. keratoderma
  s. keratoma
  s. keratosis
  s. lentigo
  s. melanoderma
  s. sebaceous hyperplasia
  s. skin
  s. wart

senilis
  alopecia s.
  arcus s.
  keratosis s.
  lentigo s.
  pruritus s.
  verruca s.

Senn
  S. bone plate
  S. retractor
  S.-Dingman retractor
  baby S.-Miller retractor
  S.-Miller retractor

sensate
  s. cutaneous flap
  s. flap
  s. medial plantar free flap
  s. pedicled neoclitoro-
    plasty

sensation
  graft s.
  laryngopharyngeal s.
  referred s.

sensor
  MicroMirror gold s.

sensory
  s. deficit
  s. impairment
  s. loss
  s. nerve
  s. pathway

sentence
  matrix s.

sentinel
  s. lymph node
  s. skin paddle

separation
  jaw s.
  mechanical tooth s.
  pterygomaxillary s.
  septal s.

separator
  mechanical s.

sepsis
  joint s.
  s. lenta
  s. syndrome

septate

septal
  s. artery

septal *(continued)*
  s. cartilage
  s. chisel
  s. chondromucosal graft
  s. defect
  s. deformity
  s. deviation
  s. displacement
  s. elevator
  s. fracture
  s. hematoma
  s. intranasal lining flap
  locked s. displacement
  s. mucoperichondrium
  s. mucosa
  s. necrosis
  s. overlap
  s. panniculitis
  s. perforation
  s. posterior nasal artery
  s. reconstruction
  s. reduction
  s. ridge forceps
  s. scissors
  s. separation
  s. space
  s. speculum
  s. splint
  s. straightener
  telescoping s. fracture

septation
  bony s.

septectomy

septic
  s. arthritis
  s. dactylitis
  s. joint
  s. metastasis
  s. process
  s. shock
  s. wound

septicemia
  bacterial s.
  cryptogenic s.
  streptococcal s.

septodermoplasty

septomarginal

septonasal

septoplasty
  endoscopic sphenoeth-
    moidectomy with s.
  frontal sinus s.

septorhinoplasty
  esthetic s.

septostomy

septum *pl.* septa
  alveolar s.
  s. alveoli
  anterior s.
  bony s.
  bony nasal s.
  cartilaginous s.
  caudal s.
  collagen s.
  deviated s.
  deviated nasal s.
  s. of frontal sinuses
  hypothenar s.
  interalveolar s.
  s. interalveolaria maxillae
  interradicular s.
  Körner s.
  lingual s.
  membranous s.
  s. mobile nasi
  nasal s.
  s. nasi
  s. nasi osseum
  oblique s.
  orbital s.
  s. orbitale
  pharyngeal s.
  sinus s.
  s. sinuum frontalium
  s. sinuum sphenoidalium
  sphenoidal sinus s.
  s. of sphenoidal sinuses
  tarsus orbital s.
  s. of tongue

sequela
  abdominal s.

sequence
  deformation s.

sequence *(continued)*
    disruption s.
    malformation s.
    Pierre Robin s.
    Robin s.
    SLAC (scapholunate advanced collapse) s.

sequential
    s. bilateral breast reconstruction
    s. free flaps
    s. graft

sequestration
    s. cyst
    s. dermoid

sequestrectomy

sequestrotomy

sequestrum *pl.* sequestra
    bone s.
    primary s.
    secondary s.
    tertiary s.

serial
    s. cephalometric x-rays
    s. excisions of skin lesion
    s. expansion
    s. scar excisions
    s. scar injections

series
    panoramic s.

serofibrinous

seroma
    s. formation
    wound s.

seromembranous

seromucous

seropositive

seropurulent

serosanguineous

serous
    s. acinus

serous *(continued)*
    s. alveolus
    s. cystadenoma
    s. exudate
    s. fluid
    s. gland
    s. inflammation
    s. tumor

serpiginosa
    elastosis perforans s.
    zona s.

serpiginosum
    angioma s.

serpiginous
    s. ulcer

serrated
    s. curet
    s. forceps
    s. knife
    s. scissors
    s. sutures

serratus
    s. anterior
    s. anterior flap
    s. anterior muscle
    s. anterior muscle flap
    s. posterior inferior muscle
    s. posterior superior muscle

serrefine forceps

Serres
    S. angle
    S. glands

serum *pl.* sera
    antiepithelial s.
    antilymphocytic s.
    s. complement (*C1–C9*)
    s. complement level
    s. hepatitis (SH)

Serre operation

serrefine
    Blair s.
    s. clamp

serrefine *(continued)*
    s. forceps
    s. retractor

sessile
    s. adenoma
    s. lesion
    s. swelling

Sessing pressure ulcer assess-
    ment scale

set
    Molina mandibular distrac-
        tor s.
    Tebbetts rhinoplasty s.

setback

Setopress high-compression
    bandage

setting sun sign

severe combined immunodefi-
    ciency (SCID)

Sewall retractor

Sewell internal mammary im-
    plantation

sex
    s. conversion
    morphological s.
    s. reassignment surgery

Sézary
    S. erythroderma
    S. syndrome

S-flap

SFP
    synostotic frontal plagio-
        cephaly

SFS
    superficial fascial system

SGBI
    silicone gel–filled breast
        implant

SGC
    salivary gland carcinoma

SGMI
    silicone gel–filled mam-
        mary implant

SH
    serum hepatitis

shadow
    calcific s.
    s. density
    metallic-dense s.
    ring s.

shaft
    s. of bone
    hair s.
    s. of phalanx

Shah nasal splint

shampoo
    GraftCyte post-surgical s.

shape
    ear s.
    fleur-de-lis s.
    keyhole s.
    s. memory clamp
    signet ring s. of scaphoid

shaped
    funnel-s.
    s. glandular flap
    s. random pattern flap

shaping
    s. of breast
    cartilage s.

sharing
    nerve s.
    nipple s.

Shark-tip cannula

sharp
    s. dissection

Sharpey fibers

Sharplan
    S. argon laser
    S. CO_2 laser
    S. Erbium SilkLaser

Sharplan *(continued)*
    S. FeatherTouch SilkLaser
    S. laser
    S. Laser 710 Acuspot
    S. SilkTouch flashscan surgical laser

SharpLase Nd:YAG laser

sharply circumscribed nodule

Sharpoint
    S. blade
    S. crescent blade
    S. microsurgical knife
    S. V-lance blade

Sharptome
    S. crescent blade
    S. microblade

shave
    s. biopsy
    s. excision
    superficial upper lateral s.

Shea
    S. pressure ulcer assessment scale
    S. scale

Shearer lip retractor

shearing edge

sheath
    anterior s.
    carotid s.
    check-valve s.
    epithelial s.
    fascial s.
    fiberoptic s.
    fibrous s.
    flexor s.
    flexor tendon s.
    Huxley s.
    myelin s.
    nerve s.
    Neumann s.
    periosteum s.
    rectus s.
    rectus abdominis s.
    rectus abdominis muscle s.
    s. of Schwann

sheath *(continued)*
    synovial s.
    tendon s.
    vascular s.
    venous s.

shedding
    virus s.

sheet
    barrier s.
    Biobrane s.
    s. graft
    in vitro–grown palatal mucosa s.
    keratinous s.
    s's of nevus cells
    Prolene mesh s.
    Sil-K silicone s.

sheeting
    Cica-Care silicone gel s.
    Epi-Derm silicone gel s.
    New Beginnings GelShapes silicone gel s.
    Scar Fx lightweight silicone s.

shelf
    buccal s.
    implant s.
    palatal s.
    palatine s.

shell
    s. earmold
    implant elastomer s.
    Terino malar s.

shelled out

Sherman
    S. bone plate
    S. bone screw
    S. molybdenum screw
    S. plate
    S. plate and screws
    S. screwdriver
    S. Vitallium screw

shield
    Barraquer eye s.

shield *(continued)*
  binocular s.
  Buller eye s.
  Carapace disposable face s.
  Cox II ocular laser s.
  Durette external laser s.
  Fox aluminum eye s.
  laser s.
  lead s.
  lingual s.
  metal scleral s.
  protective eye s.
  scleral s.
  Stevanovsky metal eye s.
  Trelles metal scleral s.
  s.-type graft

shift
  scaphoid s.

shifter
  suture shape s.

shingles

Shirley wound drain

shock
  allergic s.
  anaphylactic s.
  anaphylactoid s.
  anesthetic s.
  break s.
  burn s.
  cardiogenic s.
  electric s.
  hematogenic s.
  hemorrhagic s.
  hypovolemic s.
  septic s.

shoelace
  s. suture
  s. technique
  s.-type repair

short
  s. arc motion (SAM) proto-
    col
  s.-arm thumb spica cast
  s. extensor muscle

short *(continued)*
  s. face syndrome
  s. flexor muscle
  s. gut syndrome
  s. mandible
  s. radial extensor muscle
  s. scar technique

Shortbent
  S. scissors
  S. suture scissors

shortening
  radial s.
  tendon s.
  s. of tendon

shot-feel

shoulder
  drop s.
  s. flap
  s. of furrow
  linguogingival s.
  s. impingement syndrome
  s. of rhytid

show
  conchal s.
  scleral s.

Shrapnell membrane

shunt
  arteriovenous s.
  capillary bed s.
  endolymphatic-subarach-
    noid s.
  tracheopharyngeal s.
  ventriculoperitoneal s.

Shur-Clens wound cleanser

Shur-Strip wound closure tape

shutter flap

sialadenitis
  acute submandibular s.
  allergic s.
  bacterial s.
  chronic s.
  epithelioid-cell s.
  granulomatous s.

sialadenitis *(continued)*
  myoepithelial s.
  obstructive s.
  postirradiation s.
  rheumatoid s.
  sarcoid s.
  submandibular chronic
    sclerosing s.
  suppurative s.
  viral s.

sialadenography

sialadenoncus

sialadenosis
  metabolic s.

sialoadenectomy

sialoadenotomy

sialodochoplasty
  parotid s.

sialography

sialolith

sialolithotomy

sialometaplasia
  necrotizing s.

sialorrhea

sialoschesis

sialostenosis

sialosyrinx

sicca
  keratoconjunctivitis s.
  laryngitis s.
  pharyngitis s.
  rhinitis s.

sickle
  s. blade
  s. flap
  s. scissors

sideburn
  displaced s.

sideroderma

siderosis

sieve graft

sieving
  mandibular s.

sigmoid
  s. notch
  s. sinus
  s. sulcus

sign
  accessory s.
  Agee s.
  Aufrecht s.
  Auspitz s.
  Battle s.
  Beevor s.
  Bekhterev (Bechterew) s.
  Bezold s.
  Biermer s.
  Blumberg s.
  Bozzolo s.
  Bunnell s.
  Brickner s.
  Burton s.
  Buschke-Ollendorf s.
  Charcot s.
  chin-retraction s.
  Darier s.
  David Letterman s.
  dimple s.
  Dupuytren s.
  Ewing s.
  Finkelstein s.
  focalizing s's
  Frank s.
  Froment s.
  Gerhardt s.
  Griesinger s.
  hair collar s.
  Heyring s.
  Hutchinson s.
  impingement s.
  lemon s.
  Leser-Trélat s.
  Linburg s.
  linguine s.
  lipstick s.
  Macewen s.
  melanoma warning s.

sign *(continued)*
    navicular fat stripe s.
    Obagi s.
    oil drop change s.
    Parrot s.
    Payr s.
    Phalen s.
    prodromic s.
    Quant s.
    Romaña s.
    Romberg s.
    Rookey s.
    sail s.
    seat belt s.
    setting sun s.
    signet ring s.
    Seeligmüller s.
    signet ring s.
    signet ring s. on x-ray
    spilled teacup s.
    stepladder s.
    target s.
    tenting s.
    Terry nail s.
    Terry-Thomas s.
    Tinel s.
    Wartenberg s.
    wet leather s.
SignaDRESS dressing
signet ring
    s. r. sign
    s. r. sign on x-ray
    s. r. shape of scaphoid
Sigvaris compression stockings
Silastic
    S. allograft
    S. chin implant
    S. chin prosthesis
    S. finger implant
    S. foam dressing
    S. gel dressing
    S. HP tissue expander
    S. implant
    S. mammary prosthesis
    S. otoplasty prosthesis
    S. penile implant
    S. penile prosthesis

Silastic *(continued)*
    S. rhinoplasty implant
    S. rod
    S. silicone rubber implant
    S. strap
    S. subdermal implant
    S. testicular implant
    S. toe implant
Silhouette endoscopic laser
silica-carbon layer
silicone
    s. adhesive
    Biocell textured s.
    s. bleed
    s. deposition
    s. dressing
    s. elastomer
    s. epistaxis catheter
    s.-filled implant
    s.-filled mammary implant
    s. flexor rod
    s. gel
    s. gel bleed
    s. gel breast implant
    s. gel–filled breast implant (SGBI)
    s. gel–filled mammary implant (SGMI)
    s. gel–filled mammary implant explanation surgery
    s. gel implant
    s. gel prosthesis
    s. granuloma
    s. injection
    s. leakage
    s. lip augmentation
    s. lubricant
    s. mastitis
    s. nasal strut implant
    s. rubber
    s. synovitis
    s. textured mammary implant
    s.-treated surgical silk sutures
    s.-treated wound
    s. tube
Silima breast prosthesis

silk
s. interrupted mattress suture
s. pop-off suture
s. stay suture
s. suture

SilkLaser
S. aesthetic CO_2 laser
EpiTouch Ruby S.
FeatherTouch S.
Sharplan Erbium S.
Sharplan FeatherTouch S.

Sil-K silicone sheet

Silktouch
S. CO_2 Flash Scanner
S. laser

sill
s. length
nasal s.
nostril s.

silo
Prolene mesh s.

Silon
S.-TSR wound dressing
S. wound dressing

Siloskin dressing

SilqueClenz skin cleanser

Siltex mammary implant

Silverlon wound packing strips

SIMA
single internal mammary
artery reconstruction

Simmonds
S. disease
S. syndrome

Simon
S. cheiloplasty
S. colpocleisis
S. operation

Simonart band

Simons classification of malocclusion

simple
s. anchorage
s. angioma
s. apertognathia
s. bone cyst
s. dislocation
s. flaring suture
s. lentigo
s. mandibular distraction
s. mastectomy
s. running suture
s. skull fracture
s. sinusotomy

simplex
acne s.
angioma s.
disseminated herpes s.
epidermolysis s.
epidermolysis bullosa s.
erythema s.
herpes s.
lentigo s.
lymphangioma superficium s.
verruca s.

Simplex mastoid rongeur

Simpson splint

simultaneous free flaps

Singapore
modified S. flap

singer
s's nodes
s's nodules

single
s. cortical bone onlay
s. fracture
s. internal mammary artery
reconstruction (SIMA)

single-chambered saline implant

single-hatching undermining

single-lumen cannula

single-pedicle flap

single-portal endocarpal tunnel
  release

single-stage
  s.-s. débridement
  s.-s. reconstruction

sinistral

sinodural angle

sinonasal
  s. melanoma
  s. papilloma
  s. tract

sinus
  accessory s's of nose
  air s.
  alveolar s.
  Arlt s.
  barber's pilonidal s.
  basilar s.
  bony frontal s.
  bony maxillary s.
  bony sphenoidal s.
  branchial s.
  branchial cleft s.
  Breschet s.
  carotid s.
  cavernous s.
  s. chisel
  s. closure
  s. cranialization
  cutaneous s.
  dermal s.
  ethmoidal s.
  first branchial cleft s.
  frontal s.
  inferior petrosal s.
  s. irrigation
  lacteal s.
  lactiferous s.
  laryngeal s.
  lateral s.
  s. lift osteotome
  s. line
  lunate s. of radius

sinus (continued)
  lunate s. of ulna
  Luschka s.
  Maier s.
  mastoid s.
  maxillary s.
  middle s's
  s. of Morgagni
  s. mucocele
  s. of nail
  opacified frontal s.
  Palfyn s.
  paranasal s.
  piriform s.
  posterior s's
  preauricular s.
  right frontal s.
  sagittal s.
  sigmoid s.
  sphenoidal s.
  sphenoparietal s.
  tarsal s.
  s. thrombophlebitis
  s. thrombosis
  s. tract
  s. tract cyst
  s. unguis
  wide sigmoid s.

sinusectomy
  branchial cleft s.

sinusitis
  acute frontal s.
  acute maxillary s.
  chronic frontal s.
  chronic maxillary s.
  chronic paranasal s.
  ethmoidal s.
  frontal s.
  isolated sphenoid s.
  maxillary s.
  osteoblastic s.
  sphenoidal s.
  vacuum s.

sinusoid

sinusoidal

sinusoscopy
  maxillary s.

sinusotomy
 endoscopic intranasal frontal s.
 simple s.

SinuSpacer turbinate stent

Sipple syndrome

SIPS
 sympathetically indepen-
  dent pain syndrome

sirenomelia

Sisson-Cottle septal speculum

Sistrunk
 S. band retractor
 S. dissecting scissors
 S. operation
 S. procedure
 S. retractor
 S. scissors

site
 donor s.
 fibula donor s.
 immunocompetent s.
 pedicled enteric donor s.
 pedicle flap donor s.
 pooling s.
 recipient s.

size
 donor s.

sizer
 Whitaker malar s.

Sjögren syndrome

skate
 s. flap
 s. graft

skeletal
 s. deformity
 s. disproportion
 s. distraction
 s. fixation
 s. hypertrophy
 s. maturation
 s. occlusion

skeletal *(continued)*
 s. open bite
 s. overgrowth
 s. pin fixation
 s. stabilization

skeleton
 axial s.
 cephalic s.
 s. earmold
 extralaryngeal s.
 s. hand
 osseocartilaginous craniofacial s.

skeletonize

skier
 s's tear
 s's thumb

skin
 ablated s.
 s.-adipose superficial musculoaponeurotic system
  (SASMA)
 alligator s.
 s. atrophy
 s. barrier
 biologic creep of s.
 s. brassiere
 s. breakdown
 buttonholing of s.
 circumferential tearing of s.
 combination s.
 Composite Cultured S.
  (CCS)
 s. creep
 deciduous s.
 s. depigmentation
 devitalized s.
 s. edge necrosis
 s. edges approximated
 s. envelope
 s. eruption
 s.-colored lesion
 s. exfoliation
 s. expansion
 farmer's s.
 fish s.
 flaccid s.

skin *(continued)*
   s. flap
   s. flap retractor
   s. flap rotation
   s. flap rotation technique
   glabrous s.
   golfer's s.
   s. graft
   s. graft expander mesh
   s. graft hook
   s. grafting
   s. graft mesh
   granulomatous slack s.
   hanging s.
   harvesting s.
   heavy s.
   India rubber s.
   inherent extensibility of s.
   Integra artificial s.
   s. integrity
   s. involvement
   s. island
   juxtabrow s.
   lax s.
   s. lesion
   s. lesion artifact
   loose s.
   s. maceration
   s. markings
   mechanical creep of s.
   s. mesh
   s./muscle flap blepharo-
     plasty
   s. necrosis
   new s.
   s. peel
   piebald s.
   porcupine s.
   primary macular atrophy
     of s.
   primary neuroendocrine
     carcinoma of the s.
   redundant s.
   s. relaxation
   residual s.
   s. resurfacing
   s. rubor
   sailor's s.
   sebaceous s.

skin *(continued)*
   senile s.
   shagreen s.
   slack s.
   sloughing of s.
   s.-sparing mastectomy
   striate atrophy of s.
   s.-subcutaneous dissection
     with SMAS manipulation
   suborbicularis s.
   s. substitute
   s. tag
   thickened s.
   tissue-cultured s.
   s. turgor
   viscoelastic property of s.
   s. wheal

skin care product
   Aesthetica C topical vita-
     min C s. c. p.
   Aqua Glycolic s. c. p.

skinfold
   s. calipers

skin paddle
   boomerang-shaped s. p.
   crescentic-shaped s. p.
   elliptical transverse s. p.
   fleur-de-lis–shaped s. p.
   horizontal-shaped s. p.
   musculocutaneous flap
     s. p.
   sentinel s. p.
   Y-shaped s. p.

Skinlight erbium:YAG (yttrium-
aluminum-garnet) laser

Skinscan

Skin Skribe pen

SkinTech medical tattooing device

SkinTegrity hydrogel dressing

skip
   s. areas
   s. lesion
   s. metastasis

Skoog
    S. cleft lip repair
    S. fasciectomy
    S. incision in palmar fas-
        ciectomy
    S. mammaplasty
    S. method
    modified S. technique
    S. nasal chisel
    S. release of Dupuytren
        contracture

skull
    s. base
    s. base chordoma
    s. base suture
    s. base tumor resection
    cloverleaf s.
    hot cross bun s.
    lacuna s.
    maplike s.
    natiform s.
    s., occiput, mandibular im-
        mobilization (SOMI)
        brace
    s., occiput, mandibular im-
        mobilization (SOMI) or-
        thosis
    radiopaque s.
    steeple s.
    tower s.
    trilobed s.
    trilobed cloverleaf s.
    West lacuna s.
    West-Engstler s.

skullcap

skyrocket capillary ectasia

Skytron operating bed

SLAC
    scapholunate advanced
        collapse
            SLAC destruction
            four-bone SLAC wrist
                reconstruction
            midcarpal SLAC
            SLAC pattern of degen-
                erative change

SLAC (continued)
        SLAC reconstruction
        SLAC sequence
        SLAC wrist
        SLAC wrist reconstruc-
            tion

slag burn

SLAM
    simultaneous LATRAM and
        mastectomy

slapped
    "s. cheek" appearance
    "s. cheek" rash
    "s. face" appearance

Slaughter saw

sleeve
    delivery assistance s.
    mucoperichondrial s's
    s. graft

slice graft

sliding
    epidermal s.
    s. flap
    s. genioplasty
    s. inlay bone graft
    s. oblique osteotomy
    s. skin flap technique

sling
    cervicofacial s.
    facial s.
    fascial s.
    fascial s. for facial paralysis
    hand cock-up s.
    s. ligation
    mandibular s.
    muscle s.
    pterygomasseteric s.
    static s.
    sublimis s.
    suspension s.
    s. suture
    temporalis s.

slip
    medial s.

slipped strut

SLN
  superior laryngeal nerve
slope
  mandibular anteroposte-
  rior ridge s.

slope-shouldered lesion

slough

sloughing
  s. of skin
  s. ulcer

slow
  s. maxillary expansion
  s. palatal expander

slow-twitch
  s.-t. fatigue-resistant skeletal muscle
  s.-t. fibers

SLS Chromos long pulse ruby
  laser system

Sluder
  S. neuralgia
  S. palate retractor
  S. retractor
  S. sphenoidal hook
  S. sphenoidal speculum

slumping

Sly
  mucopolysaccharidosis
  type VII S. (MPS-VII)

Small
  S.-Carrion penile implant
  material
  S.-Carrion Silastic rod for
  penile implant

small
  s.-bore cannula
  s. cell carcinoma
  s. cell neuroendocrine carcinoma
  s. incisional biopsy
  s. joint arthrodesis
  s. joint arthroplasty

small (continued)
  s. joint fusion
  s. vessel anastomosis
  s. vessel vasculitis

SMAS
  superficial musculoaponeu-
  rotic system
  SMAS complex
  SMAS deep-plane face-
  lift
  SMAS face-lift tech-
  nique
  SMAS fascia
  SMAS imbrication face-
  lift
  SMAS lift
  SMAS manipulation
  SMAS-platysma deep-
  tissue face-lift
  SMAS-platysma face-lift
  SMAS-platysma flap
  SMAS plication
  SMAS plication face-lift
  SMAS plication proce-
  dure
  SMAS rhytidectomy
  sub-SMAS rhytidec-
  tomy
  superficial SMAS rhyti-
  dectomy
  SMAS tissue

smasectomy
  lateral s.

SMEI
  SMEI ultrasound-assisted
  lipoplasty machine
  SMEI ultrasound device

SMIC
  SMIC nasal speculum
  SMIC rongeur

SMILE
  subperiosteal minimally invasive laser endoscopic
  SMILE face-lift
  SMILE rhytidectomy

smile
  canine s.

smile *(continued)*
    Mona Lisa s.

Smirmaul eyelid speculum

Smith
    S. eyelid operation
    S. fracture
    S. lid-retracting hook
    S. orbital floor implant
    space of S.
    S.-Lemli-Opitz syndrome
    S.-Riley syndrome

SMM
    scintimammography

smoker
    s's cancer
    s's lines
    s's palate
    s's patch
    s's tongue

smooth
    s. lesion
    s. muscle
    s. skin-colored lesion

SMPS
    sympathetically maintained
        pain syndrome

SMR
    submucous resection

S-N
    sella-nasion
        S-N plane

SNA, S-N-A
    sella-nasion-subspinale an-
        gle

snapping finger

SNB, S-N-B
    sella-nasion-supramentale
        angle

SND
    selective neck dissection

Sneddon-Wilkinson disease

Snellen
    S. forceps
    S. ptosis operation

SN-N
    sternal notch to nipple

Snoopy breast

snuffbox
    anatomic s.

socia parotidis

Soemmering
    S. ligament
    S. muscle
    S. spot

Sof-Gel palm shield splint

SOFS
    superior orbital fissure syn-
        drome

SofSorb absorptive dressing

soft
    s. cartilage
    s. cleft palate
    s. lesion
    s. papilloma
    s. triangle of the nose
    s. ulcer
    s. wart

SoftCloth absorptive dressing

SoftForm facial implant

SoftLight laser

Soft N Dry Merocel sponge

soft palate
    s. p. cleft
    s. p. paralysis
    pillar of s. p.
    posterior nasal spine to
        s. p. (PNSP)
    s. p. retractor
    s. p. tip

Softscan

soft tissue
    s. t. augmentation
    s. t. calcification

soft tissue *(continued)*
   s. t. contracture
   s. t. curettage
   s. t. cyst
   s. t. deformity
   s. t. dehiscence
   s. t. elevator
   s. t. expander
   s. t. hypoplasia
   s. t. mass
   s. t. nocardiosis
   s. t. reconstruction
   s. t. resection
   s. t. shaving cannula
   s. t. thickness
   s. t. tumor
   s. t. undercut
   s. t. window
   vascularized s. t.

software
   Dentofacial Planner s.
   Materialise computer-aided
     design s.
   MedMorph III s.

Sof-Wick
   S. drain
   S. dressing
   S. sponge

solar
   s. cheilitis
   s. dermatitis
   s. elastosis
   s. keratosis
   s. lentigo
   s. urticaria

soleus
   s.-fibula free transfer recon-
     struction of lower limb
   s. flap
   s. muscle

solitary
   s. bone cyst
   s. keratoacanthoma
   s. lesion
   s. neurofibroma
   s. nodule
   s. simple lymphangioma

SoloSite
   S. nonsterile hydrogel
   S. wound gel

solution
   bacitracin s.
   bacteriostatic s.
   balanced salt s. (BSS)
   Burow s.
   Dakin s.
   Jessner s.
   Microfil s.

Solvang graft

somatoschisis

SOMI
   sternal-occipital-mandibu-
     lar immobilizer
     SOMI brace
     SOMI orthosis

somite
   mesodermal s.

Sommers compression dressing

Song and Song method

Sonnenschein nasal speculum

Sono-stat Plus EMG machine

SOOF
   suborbicularis oculi fat

sore
   canker s.
   desert s.
   fungating s.
   hard s.
   ischial pressure s.
   mixed s.
   Naga s.
   Oriental s.
   summer s.
   tropical s.
   veldt s.

Sorensen reusable canister

Sorrin operation

Sourdille
   S. keratoplasty

Sourdille *(continued)*
    S. ptosis operation

Southbent scissors

sound
    adventitious breath s's
    coarse breath s.
    cracked-pot s.

space
    air s.
    anatomical dead s.
    s. of body of mandible
    bregmatic s.
    buccal s.
    buccinator s.
    buccopharyngeal s.
    carotid s.
    cartilage s.
    Chassaignac s.
    dead s.
    deep s.
    digastric s.
    s. of Donders
    dorsal subaponeurotic s.
    embrasure s.
    epicerebral s.
    fascial s.
    free way s.
    geniohyoid s.
    haversian s's
    Henke s.
    hypothenar s.
    iliocostal s.
    infraglottic s.
    infraorbital s.
    infratemporal s.
    interalveolar s.
    interarytenoid s.
    intercellular s.
    intercostal s.
    interocclusal rest s.
    interorbital s.
    interradicular s.
    joint s.
    lateral pharyngeal s.
    lattice s.
    Lesgaft s.
    lymph s.

space *(continued)*
    mandibular s.
    masseteric s.
    masseter-mandibuloptery-
        goid s.
    mediastinal s.
    midpalmar s.
    Nance leeway s.
    palmar s.
    parapharyngeal s.
    Parona s.
    parotid s.
    peripharyngeal s.
    pharyngomaxillary s.
    pneumatic s.
    postzygomatic s.
    pterygomandibular s.
    quadrangular s.
    quadrilateral s.
    retromylohyoid s.
    retropharyngeal s.
    retroseptal s.
    retrozygomatic s.
    scapholunate joint s.
    septal s.
    s. of Smith
    sphenomaxillary s.
    sphenopalatine s.
    subepicranial s.
    subfascial palmar s.
    subfascial web s.
    subgaleal s.
    sublingual s.
    submandibular s.
    submaxillary s.
    submental s.
    subumbilical s.
    suprahyoid s.
    suprasternal s.
    thenar s.
    thenar web s.
    thumb-index web s.
    thyrohyal s.
    Trautmann triangular s.
    web s.
    zygomaticotemporal s.

spacer
    C-bar web-s.

spacing
    excessive s.
    s. material

spade fingers

Spaeth
    S. facial nerve block
    S. ptosis operation

spaghetti fat grafting technique

spasm
    Bell s.
    chin s.
    clonic s.
    diffuse esophageal s.
    facial s.
    fixed s.
    glottic s.
    hemifacial s.
    intention s.
    laryngeal s.
    masticatory s.
    mixed s.
    Romberg s.
    vasomotor s.

spasmodic

spasmus
    s. glottidis

spasticity

spatula
    s. foot
    Freer nasal s.
    s. tip cannula

spatulated
    ASSI breast dissector s.

Spaulding classification

SPC
    scaphopisocapitate
        SPC relationship

Spectra-System implant

Spectrum
    S. K1 laser
    S. ruby laser

speckled
    s. lentiginous nevus
    s. leukoplakia

specimen
    nontraumatized full-thick-
        ness s.

spectrum *pl.* spectra, spec-
    trums

speculum *pl.* specula
    Alfonso eyelid s.
    Allen-Heffernan nasal s.
    Aufricht septal s.
    Beckman-Colver nasal s.
    Beckman nasal s.
    Bionix disposable nasal s.
    Bosworth nasal wire s.
    Callahan modification s.
    Chevalier Jackson larynge-
        al s.
    Coakley nasal s.
    Converse nasal s.
    Cottle nasal s.
    Cushing-Landolt trans-
        sphenoidal s.
    Desmarres eye s.
    Downes nasal s.
    Duplay-Lynch nasal s.
    flat-bladed nasal s.
    Forbes esophageal s.
    Gerzog nasal s.
    Hajek-Tieck nasal s.
    Halle nasal s.
    Halle-Tieck nasal s.
    Hartmann nasal s.
    Ingals nasal s.
    Jaffe eyelid s.
    Killian-Halle nasal s.
    Killian nasal s.
    Merz-Vienna nasal s.
    Mosher nasal s.
    nasal s.
    nasopharyngeal s.
    Rica nasal septal s.
    septal s.
    Sisson-Cottle septal s.
    Sluder sphenoidal s.

speculum *(continued)*
    SMIC nasal s.
    Smirmaul eyelid s.
    Sonnenschein nasal s.
    Storz nasal s.
    Storz septal s.
    Thudichum nasal s.
    Tieck nasal s.
    transsphenoidal s.
    Vienna nasal s.
    Vienns Britetrac nasal s.
    Yankauer nasopharyn-
        geal s.

Spee
    curve of S.
    curve of von S.

speech
    mimic s.

speech-motor function

Spence
    axillary tail of S.
    tail of S.

Spencer stitch scissors

SPF
    sun protection factor

sphacelation

sphacelism

sphaceloderma

sphacelous

sphacelus

sphenobasilar

sphenocephaly

sphenoethmoidal
    s. recess
    s. suture

sphenoethmoidectomy
    endoscopic s. with septo-
        plasty

sphenofrontal
    s. suture
    s. suture line

sphenoid
    s. bone
    s. dysplasia
    greater wing of s. bone
    lateral wall of s. bone
    lesser wing of s. bone
    s. process

sphenoidal
    s. bur
    s. concha
    s. cyst
    s. fissure
    s. fontanelle
    s. nasal conchae
    s. ostium
    s. process
    s. ridge
    s. rostrum
    s. sinus
    s. sinusitis
    s. sinus septum
    s. spine
    s. turbinate bones
    s. wing

sphenoidale

sphenoidectomy
    frontoethmoidal s.

sphenoiditis

sphenoidostomy

sphenoidotomy

sphenomandibular ligament

sphenomalar

sphenomaxillary
    s. fissure
    s. ganglion
    s. suture

spheno-occipital
    s. encephalocele
    s. suture
    s. synchondrosis

sphenopagus

sphenopalatine
    s. artery

sphenopalatine *(continued)*
   s. branch of internal maxillary artery
   s. canal
   s. fissure
   s. foramen
   s. ganglion
   s. nerve
   s. neuralgia
   s. notch of palatine bone
   s. space

sphenoparietal
   s. suture
   s. suture line

sphenopetroclival region

sphenopetrosal
   s. fissure
   s. suture

sphenosquamosal

sphenosquamous
   s. suture

sphenotemporal
   s. suture

sphenotresia

sphenoturbinal

sphenovomerine
   s. suture

sphenozygomatic
   s. suture

spherical
   s. contracture
   s. form of occlusion

sphincter
   anatomical s.
   annular s.
   artificial s.
   esophageal s.
   s. of eye
   eyelid s.
   functional s.
   myovascular s.
   ostial s.
   palatopharyngeal s.

sphincter *(continued)*
   pharyngoesophageal s.
   s. pharyngoplasty
   precapillary s.

sphincterectomy

sphincteroplasty

spiculated
   s. calcification
   s. lesion

spicule
   bone s.

spider
   s. angioma
   arterial s.
   s.-burst
   s. finger
   s. hemangioma
   s. mole
   s. nevus
   s. telangiectasia
   s. telangiectasis
   s. varicosity
   vascular s.
   s. vein

Spiegler
   S.-Fendt pseudolymphoma
   S.-Fendt sarcoid

Spigelius line

spina *pl.* spinae
   s. angularis
   s. bifida anterior
   s. bifida cystica
   s. bifida occulta
   s. frontalis
   s. helicis
   s. meatus
   s. mentalis
   s. nasalis anterior maxillae
   s. nasalis ossis frontalis
   s. nasalis ossis palatini
   occult s. bifida
   s. ossis sphenoidalis
   spinae palatinae
   s. suprameatum
   s. ventosa

spinal
  s. accessory chain lymph
    node
  s. accessory nerve
  s. tract of trigeminal nerve

spindle
  s. cell
  s. cell carcinoma
  s. cell hemangioendothe-
    lioma
  s. cell lipoma
  muscle s.
  s. cell tumor

spine
  alar s.
  angular s.
  anterior nasal s. (ANS)
  anterior nasal s. of maxilla
  anterior superior iliac s.
  basilar s.
  Civinini s.
  cleft s.
  ethmoidal s. of Macalister
  greater tympanic s.
  s. of helix
  Henle s.
  horny s.
  iliac s.
  mandibular s.
  s. of maxilla
  meatal s.
  mental s.
  nasal s. of frontal bone
  nasal s. of palatine bone
  palatine s's
  pharyngeal s.
  posterior nasal s.
  posterior nasal s. to soft
    palate (PNSP)
  sphenoidal s.
  s. of sphenoid bone
  Spix s.
  suprameatal s.

spinning
  marginal s.

spiradenoma
  cylindromatous s.

spiradenoma (continued)
  eccrine s.

spiral
  s. artery
  s. band of Gosset
  s. computed tomography
  s. flap
  s. fracture
  s. ligament
  s. vein

Spitz nevus

Spix spine

splanchnocranium

S-plasty

splayed
  s. alar cartilage
  s. arteries
  s. facial nerve

splenius
  s. capitis
  s. cervicis

splint
  acrylic ear s.
  AirFlex carpal tunnel s.
  airplane s.
  air s.
  Alumafoam nasal s.
  anchor s.
  Anderson s.
  Angle s.
  Aquaplast nasal s.
  Asch s.
  Asch nasal s.
  Atkins nasal s.
  baseball finger s.
  Bridgemaster nasal s.
  Brooke Army Hospital s.
  Brown nasal s.
  calibrated clubfoot s.
  canine-to-canine lingual s.
  cap s.
  Capner boutonnière s.
  Carter intranasal s.
  cast lingual s.
  Cawood nasal s.

splint *(continued)*
  coaptation s.
  compressive plastic s.
  Converse s.
  Denis Browne clubfoot s.
  Denver nasal s.
  Doyle nasal s.
  dynamic s.
  Erich maxillary s.
  Erich nasal s.
  Essig-type s.
  external nasal s.
  Formatray mandibular s.
  full occlusal s.
  functional s.
  Gilmer s.
  Goode nasal s.
  Gunning s.
  hand cock-up s.
  Haynes-Griffin mandibu-
    lar s.
  implant surgical s.
  interdental s.
  intranasal s.
  jaw s.
  Joint Jack finger s.
  joint spring s.
  Jones nasal s.
  Joseph nasal s.
  Joseph septal s.
  Kanavel cock-up s.
  Kazanjian s.
  Kazanjian nasal s.
  Kingsley s.
  Kirschner wire s.
  Kleinert dynamic traction s.
  labial s.
  labiolingual s.
  lingual s.
  Love nasal s.
  MacKay nasal s.
  mandibular s.
  Mayer nasal s.
  Neiman nasal s.
  occlusal s.
  O'Malley jaw fracture s.
  onlay s.
  polymethyl methacrylate
    ear s.

splint *(continued)*
  Porzett s.
  replant s.
  reverse Kingsley s.
  Safian nasal s.
  sandwich-type s.
  septal s.
  Shah nasal s.
  Simpson s.
  Sof-Gel palm shield s.
  Stader s.
  static s.
  Supramead nose s.
  synergistic wrist motion s.
  tenodesis s.
  thermoplastic extension
    pan s.
  turnbuckle functional posi-
    tion s.
  Ultraflex ankle dorsiflexion
    dynamic s.
  Versi-S.
  volar s.
  Xomed Doyle nasal air-
    way s.

splinter hemorrhage

splinting

split
  anterior cricoid s.
  s.-bone technique
  s. calvarial graft
  cricoid s.
  s. hand/s. foot malforma-
    tion
  mandibular s.
  palatal s.
  s. papule
  s. plate appliance
  s.-skin graft
  s.-thickness flap
  s.-thickness graft
  s.-thickness skin graft
    (STSG)

splitting
  sagittal s. of mandible

SPOA
  subperiosteal orbital ab-
    scess

spondylitis
  ankylosing s.
  Bekhterev (Bechterew) s.
  s. ossificans ligamentosa
  posttraumatic s.
  psoriatic s.

spondylolysis
  cervical s.

sponge
  absorbable gelatin s.
  Bernay s.
  fibrin s.
  Mediskin hemostatic s.
  nasal tampon s.
  Naso-Tamp nasal packing s.
  Soft N Dry Merocel s.
  Sof-Wick s.

spongiosis

spongy bone

spontanea
  dactylolysis s.

spontaneous
  s. gangrene of newborn
  s. fracture
  s. pseudoscar

spoon
  scaphoid s. handle
  s.-shaped hand
  sharp s.
  Volkmann s.

spot
  aberrant mongolian s.
  blue s.
  café au lait s's
  Campbell De Morgan s's
  cayenne pepper s.
  cherry s.
  cotton-wool s.
  De Morgan s's
  Filatov s.
  Fordyce s's
  Forschheimer s's

spot (continued)
  Graefe s.
  Janeway s.
  Koplik s's
  liver s.
  mongolian s.
  mulberry s.
  rose s.
  ruby s.
  saccular s.
  sacral s.
  Soemmering s.
  spongy s.
  tendinous s.
  Trousseau s.
  white s.

sprain
  temporomandibular joint s.

spread-and-cut technique

spreader
  Wakai s.

spring
  Coffin s.

spur
  s. crusher
  nasal s.
  septum s.
  vascular s.
  vomerine s.

SQ
  subcuticular

squama pl. squamae
  frontal bone s.
  mental s.
  occipital s.
  perpendicular s.
  temporal s.

squamocolumnar junction

squamofrontal

squamomastoid suture

squamoparietal suture

squamosomastoid suture

squamosoparietal suture

squamososphenoid suture

squamosphenoid suture

squamotemporal

squamotympanic fissure

squamous
s. bone
s. cell carcinoma (SCC)
s. cell carcinoma of head
and neck (SCCHN)
s. cell carcinoma–inhibi-
tory factor (SSCIF)
s. cell papilloma
s. cell pseudoepithelioma
s. epithelial ingrowth
s. epithelium
s. odontogenic tumor
s. papilloma
s. suture
s. suture lines
s. suture of cranium

square-shouldered lesion

Squeeze-Mark surgical marker

SSCIF
squamous cell carcinoma–
inhibitory factor

S-shaped scar

SSL
subtotal supraglottic laryngectomy

SSO
sagittal split osteotomy

SSRO
sagittal split ramus osteotomy

stability
occlusal s.

stabilization
columellar s.
columellar subluxation s.
coronoradicular s.
jaw s.
skeletal s.

Stacke mastoidectomy

Stader splint

Stafne bone cyst

stage
desmolytic s.
maturative s.
morphogenic s.

staged
s. abdominal repair (STAR)
s. genioplasty
s. muscle transfer
s. procedure
s. reconstruction

staging
American Joint Committee
on Cancer (AJCC) s.
Haagensen s. of breast carcinoma
intraoperative tumor s.
Papineau bone graft s.
(stages I–III)
TNM tumor s.
Viegas s. for lunotriquetral
instability

Stahl ear

Stahr gland

stain
Brown-Brenn s.
hypertrophic port-wine s.
immunofluorescent s.
immunoperoxidase s.
Masson trichrome s.
metallic s.
port-wine s.

staircase technique for lip reconstruction

stairstep deformity

stalk
umbilical s.

Stallard
S. dissector
S. flap operation

stand
Mayo s.

standards
cephalometric s.

stapes
    monopodal ankylotic s.

staphylectomy

staphylion

staphyloderma

staphylodialysis

staphyloncus

staphylopharyngorrhaphy

staphyloplasty

staphyloplegia

staphyloptosis

staphylorrhaphy

staphyloschisis

staphylotome

staphylotomy

staple
    Bio-Absorbable s.
    s. bone plate
    Ellison fixation s.
    skin s.
    titanium mandibular s.

stapler
    Appose skin s.
    Concorde disposable
        skin s.
    Graftac-S skin s.
    Proximate disposable
        skin s.

STAR
    staged abdominal repair

Starling reflex

STAR*LOCK
    STAR*LOCK multi-purpose
        submergible threaded im-
        plant
    STAR*LOCK Press-Fit cylin-
        der implant

stasis
    s. dermatitis
    s. eczema
    s. edema
    s. vascular ulcer

Sta-Tic impression material

Stat-Temp II liquid crystal tem-
    perature monitor

Status-X machine

staurion

StaySharp face-lift Super-Cut
    scissors

stay suture

STE
    subperiosteal tissue ex-
        pander

steal
    lateral crural s. (LCS)

steatocystoma multiplex

steatogenous

steatoma

steatomery

steatopygia

Steele classification of intra-ar-
    ticular fractures (types I–III)

steeple flap

Steffanoff ear reconstruction

Steiger joint

Stein
    S. cheiloplasty
    S.-Abbe lip flap
    S.-Kazanjian lower lip flap

Steindler flexorplasty

Steinmann
    S. calibration pin
    S. fixation pin
    S. pin with ball bearing
    S. pin with Crowe pilot
        point

stellate
    s. abscess
    s. block anesthesia
    s. fracture
    s. ganglion
    s. ganglion block
    s. pattern
    s. pseudoscar

stellectomy

stenion

Stener lesion

stenobregmatic

stenocephalous

stenocephaly

stenocrotaphia

stenosed

stenosing tenosynovitis

stenosis *pl.* stenoses
    acquired nasopharyngeal s.
    choanal s.
    cicatricial s.
    granulation s.
    glottic s.
    high-flow arterial s.
    hypopharyngeal s.
    iatrogenic nasal s.
    laryngeal s.
    laryngotracheal s.
    meatal s.
    nasal s.
    nasopharyngeal s.
    piriform aperture s.
    subglottic s.
    supraglottic s.
    tracheal s.

stenostenosis

stenostomia

stenotic cleft

Stensen
    S. canal
    S. duct

Stensen *(continued)*
    S. duct caruncle
    S. foramen
    S. plexus

Stenstrom
    S. alar cartilage technique
    S. foot flap
    S. otoplasty
    S. rasp
    S. technique
    S. technique in otoplasty

Stent
    S. graft
    S. mass
    S. skin graft technique

stent
    Aboulker s.
    antihemorrhagic s.
    Doyle II silicone s.
    Dumon silicone s.
    Gianturco expanding metal-
        lic s.
    Gianturco-Rösch Z-s.
    labial s.
    laryngeal s.
    maxillary s.
    methyl methacrylate ear s.
    occlusal s.
    ostiomeatal s.
    Palmaz s.
    SinuSpacer turbinate s.
    trismus s.
    Wallstent expanding metal-
        lic s.

stenting

stephanion

stepladder
    s. incision
    s. sign
    s. technique for lip recon-
        struction

step-off
    bone s. at zygomaticofron-
        tal suture

sterile
    s. abscess

sterile *(continued)*
  s. compression dressing
  s. field
  s. field barrier
  s. pustule

sterilization
  defined s.

Steri-Strip skin closure

Steri-Stripped incision

Steritapes closure

sternal
  s. angle
  s. cleft
  s. notch to nipple (SN-N)

sternectomy

sternoclavicular
  s. joint
  s. junction
  s. notch

sternocleidomastoid
  s. fascia
  s. flap
  s. muscle
  s. musculocutaneous flap
  s. myocutaneous flap
  s. vein

sternocostal

sternomastoid

sternoschisis

sternothyroid
  s. muscle
  s. muscle flap laryngo-
    plasty

sternotomy
  s. dehiscence
  s. wound

sternum
  cleft s.
  s. turnover procedure

stertor
  hen-cluck s.

Stevanovsky metal eye shield

Stevens
  S. hook
  S. tenotomy scissors
  S.-Johnson syndrome

Stevenson retractor

Stewart-Treves syndrome

stick
  mouth s.

Stickler
  S. disease
  S. syndrome

stigma *pl.* stigmas, stigmata
  Giuffrida-Ruggieri s.
  nasolabial s.

Stille
  S. cheek retractor
  S. conchotome
  S. dissecting scissors
  S. Super Cut scissors
  S.-Joseph saw

Stillman
  S. cleft
  S. method

stimulator
  electric nerve s.
  Hilger facial nerve s.

stitch
  alar suspension s.
  dermoepidermal Gillies s.
  figure-of-eight s.
  Frost s.
  key s.
  mattress s.
  Prolene s.
  quilting s.
  s. scissors
  subperiosteal pulling s.

S&T Lalonde hook forceps

stocking
  Jobst s's
  s. nevus

stocking *(continued)*
Sigvaris compression s's
support s's
venous pressure gradient
support s's (VPGSS)

Stoerk blennorrhea

stoma *pl.* stomas, stomata

stomatitis
angular s.
aphthous s.
fusospirochetal s.
gangrenous s.
membranous s.
mercurial s.
mycotic s.
s. medicamentosa
necrotizing ulcerative s.
s. nicotina
nicotine s.
s. papulosa
s. traumatica
ulcerative s.
vesicular s.
Vincent s.
viral vesicular s.

stomatodynia

stomatodysodia

stomatoglossitis

stomatognathic

stomatomalacia

stomatonecrosis

stomatonoma

stomatoplasty

stomatorrhagia

stomatoschisis

stomion

stomoschisis

stone
intraglandular s.
salivary s.
skin s's

stork bite

storm
thyroid s.

Storz
S. microserrefine
S. nasal speculum
S. nasopharyngeal biopsy
forceps
S. septal speculum
S. stitch scissors
S.-Hopkins laryngoscope

Stout continuous wiring

strabismus

straight
s. mosquito hemostat
s. scissors
s. tubular graft

straightener
Asch septal s.
Cottle-Walsham s.
Cottle-Walsham septal s.
septal s.
Walsham s.

strain
mechanical s.

Straith
S. chin implant
S. nasal implant
S. nasal splint kit
S. otoplasty
S. profilometer
S. Z-plasty

strand
epithelial s.

strap
API universal foam chin s.
breast s.
Circumpress chin s.
lingual s.
s. muscle
palatal s.
Press Lift chin s.
Silastic s.

strap *(continued)*
    supinator s.

strategy
    ankle s.

stratified squamous epithelium

stratum *pl.* strata
    s. basale
    s. basale epidermidis
    s. corneum epidermidis
    s. disjunctum
    s. functionale
    s. germinativum epidermidis
    s. granulosum
    s. granulosum epidermidis
    s. intermedium
    s. lucidum epidermidis
    s. malpighii
    s. spinosum epidermidis
    s. subcutaneum
    superior s.

Strauss syndrome

strawberry
    s. angioma
    s. birthmark
    s. hemangioma
    s. nevus
    s. tumor

streak
    pigmented linear s.

streblodactyly

streblomicrodactyly

strength
    compressive s.
    edge s.
    wet s.
    wound tensile s.

streptococcus
    anaerobic s.

streptomicrodactyly

stress
    maximal s.

stretch marks

stretcher
    Brandy scalp s. I, rear closure
    Brandy scalp s. II, front closure
    Küttner wound s.

stria *pl.* striae
    striae of abdomen
    s. alba
    s. albicans
    s. atrophica
    striae of breasts
    striae cutis distensae
    striae gravidarum
    s. nasi transversa
    striae of pregnancy
    s. rubra
    s. spinosa
    striae scleroatrophy
    striae of thighs
    Wickham striae

striated

striation

stricture
    annular s.
    bridle s.
    cicatricial s.
    contractile s.
    ductal s.
    esophageal s.
    functional s.
    impassable s.
    impermeable s.
    organic s.
    recurrent s.
    spasmodic s.
    urethral s.

stricturoplasty

stricturotome

stridor
    congenital laryngeal s.
    s. dentium
    laryngeal s.

string
    intermediate s.

strip
> bacitracin s's
> Cover-Strip wound clo-
>> sure s.
> demineralized flexible lami-
>> nar bone s.
> fascial s.
> fascia lata s.
> flexible laminar bone s.
> Gore-Tex s's
> Mylar s.
> Nu-Hope skin barrier s.
> Pacific Coast flexible lami-
>> nar bone s.
> Silverlon wound packing
>> s's
> tear s's
> Ultimatics flexible laminar
>> bone s.

stripper
> cartilage s.
> endonerve s.
> fascia s.
> LaVeen helical s.
> rib s.
> tendon s.
> vein s.

stripping
> vein s.

stroma *pl.* stromata
> myxochondroid s.
> myxoid s.
> s. of thyroid gland

stromal desmoplasia

Strombeck technique for reduction mammaplasty

structure
> bipenniform s.
> deep s.
> implant s.
> supporting s.

struma
> s. aberranta
> cast iron s.
> ligneous s.
> s. lymphomatosa

struma *(continued)*
> s. maligna
> s. nodosa
> Riedel s.
> substernal s.

strut
> Anderson nasal s.
> columellar s.
> dorsal s.
> implant substructure s.
> slipped s.
> substernal metallic s.
> Teflon s.

Struyken conchotome

STSG
> split-thickness skin graft

STT
> scaphoid-trapezium-trape-
>> zoid
>>> STT joint
> scaphotrapeziotrapezoid
>>> STT joint

stuck finger

study
> baseline s.
> immunohistochemical s.

stump
> nerve s.

Sturge-Weber syndrome

stuttering
> laryngeal s.

styloglossus muscle

stylohyoid
> s. ligament
> s. muscle
> s. nerve
> s. syndrome

styloid
> s. bone
> s. process

styloiditis

stylomandibular
> s. artery

stylomandibular *(continued)*
  s. ligament
  s. membrane
  s. tunnel

stylomastoid
  s. artery
  s. foramen
  s. vein

stylomaxillary

stylopharyngeal
  s. muscle
  s. nerve

stylostaphyline

subantral
  s. augmentation

subareolar

subaurale

subauricular

subcapsular flap

subchondral
  s. bony resorption
  s. cyst

subciliary
  s. approach
  s. incision

subclavian
  s. flap technique
  s. steal syndrome

subcostal muscle

subcutaneous (sc, SQ)
  s. adipose tissue
  s. angiolipoma
  s. augmentation material
    (S.A.M.)
  s. calcification
  s. fascia
  s. fat
  s. fat lines
  s. fat necrosis
  s. granulomatous nodule
  s. implantation
  s. laterodigital reverse flap

subcutaneous *(continued)*
  s. lipoma
  s. mastectomy
  s. musculoaponeurotic sys-
    tem
  s. necrotizing infection
  s. neuroma
  s. nodule
  s. pedicled flap
  s. rhytidectomy
  s. suture
  s. temporofacial face-lift
  s. temporomalar face-lift
  s. tenotomy
  s. tissue
  s. tunneling device
  s. turnover flap

subcuticular
  s. fat
  s. pull-out suture
  s. suture
  s. wire

subdermal
  s. graft
  s. implant
  s. layer
  s. nasal tissue

subepicranial space

subepidermal
  s. abscess
  s. collagen
  s. nodular fibrosis
  s. vesiculation

subepithelial
  s. connective tissue graft
  s. membrane
  s. nerve plexus

subfascial carpal tunnel decompression

subgaleal
  s. dissection
  s. elevation
  s. fascia
  s. flap
  s. plane
  s. space

subglenoid
s. dislocation

subglossitis

subglottic
s. forceps
s. hemangioma
s. squamous cell carcinoma
s. stenosis

subjacent

subjugal

sublabial
s. adhesion
s. approach
s. incision
s. transsphenoidal approach

sublamina densa

sublingual
s. artery
s. caruncle
s. crescent
s. cyst
s. duct
s. fibrogranuloma
s. fold
s. fossa
s. gland
s. hematoma
s. mucosa
s. nerve
s. obstruction
s. papilla
s. ridge
s. salivary gland
s. space
s. sulcus
s. ulcer
s. vein

sublingualis
plica s.

sublinguitis

subluxation
radioulnar s.

subluxation *(continued)*
rotatory s. of scaphoid (RSS)
temporomandibular joint s.

submalar

submammary
s. crease
s. dissector
s. incision

submandibular
s. augmentation
s. chronic sclerosing sialadenitis
s. duct
s. fossa
s. ganglion
s. gland
s. lymph node
s. nerve
s. obstruction
s. salivary gland
s. space
s. triangle
s. trigone

submandibulectomy

submasseteric

submaxilla

submaxillary
s. cellulitis
s. duct
s. fossa
s. ganglion
s. lymph node
s. nerve
s. salivary gland
s. space
s. triangle

submaxillitis

submedial

submental
s. approach
s. artery
s. artery flap
s. fat pad

submental *(continued)*
s. fistula
s. hematoma
s. incision
s. island flap
s. liposuction
s. lymph node
s. region
s. space
s. space abscess
s. triangle
s. vein
s. vertex roentgenogram

submentocervical view

submentonian dermo-fatty flap

submentoplasty

submentovertical axial projection

submitted
s. for biopsy
s. for frozen section
s. for microsection

submucosa

submucosal
s. connective tissue
s. dissection
s. gland hypertrophy
s. hemorrhage
s. implant
s. resection
s. vascular pattern
s. venous plexus
s. vessels

submucous
s. chisel
s. cleft
s. cleft palate
s. dissection
s. dissector
s. fibrosis
s. layer
s. membrane
s. resection (SMR)
s. resection and rhino-
    plasty

submucous *(continued)*
s. retractor

submuscular
s. aponeurotic system
s. implant
s. pocket

subnasal

subnasale

subnasion

suboccipital
s. approach
s. craniectomy
s. decompression
s. plexus
s. triangle

suboccipitobregmatic diameter

suborbicularis
s. oculi fat (SOOF)
s. skin

suborbital

subpectoral
s. augmentation
s. implant
s. reconstruction
s.-subserratus muscle im-
    plantation

subperiosteal
s. abscess
s. abscess of frontal sinus
s. approach
s. brow lift
s. dissection
s. elevation
s. face-lift
s. implant
s. malar cheek lift
s. mid-face lift
s. minimally invasive face-
    lift
s. minimally invasive laser
    endoscopic (SMILE) face-
    lift
s. minimally invasive laser
    endoscopic (SMILE) rhyti-
    dectomy

subperiosteal *(continued)*
 s. orbital abscess (SPOA)
 s. pulling stitch
 s. tissue expander (STE)
 s. vomerine-ethmoidal
  plane

subpharyngeal

subplatysmal
 s. face-lift technique
 s. fat
 s. plane

subpontic hyperostosis

subscaphocephaly

subscapular
 s. artery
 s. flap
 s. system free flap

sub-SMAS (superficial musculoaponeurotic system) rhytidectomy

subserosa

subserous fascia

subspinale

substance
 intercellular s.
 sclerosing s.

substantia *pl.* substantiae
 s. compacta
 s. compacta ossium
 s. corticalis
 s. spongiosa
 s. trabecularis

substitute
 Biobrane experimental
  skin s. (AlloMatrix injectable putty bone graft substitute)
 bone graft s.
 skin s.
 unilaminar skin s.

substructure
 neck implant s.

subsuperficial musculoaponeurotic system (sub-SMAS) rhytidectomy

subtarsal

subtotal
 s. cleft palate
 s. excision
 s. glossectomy
 s. laryngectomy
 s. supraglottic laryngectomy (SSL)
 s. thyroidectomy

subungual
 s. abscess
 s. exostosis
 s. hematoma
 s. hyperkeratosis
 s. keratoacanthoma (SUKA)
 s. melanoma
 s. squamous cell carcinoma

succinate dehydrogenase

succinic dehydrogenase

Sucquet
 S. anastomosis
 S. canals
 S.-Hoyer anastomosis
 S.-Hoyer canals

suction
 Adson s.
 s. aspiration
 s. aspirator
 s. cannula
 s. drainage
 s. extraction
 s. forceps
 s. lipectomy
 s. system
 s. tip
 s. tube
 wound incision and s.

suction-assisted
 s.-a. lipectomy (SAL)
 s.-a. lipocontouring
 s.-a. lipolysis

suctioning
  malar bag s.

Sugita microsurgical table

SUKA
  subungual keratoacan-
    thoma

sulcal epithelium

sulciform

sulcus *pl.* sulci
  alveolobuccal s.
  alveololabial s.
  alveololingual s.
  s. anthelicis transversus
  s. auriculae anterior
  s. auriculae posterior
  buccal s.
  carotid s.
  s. cruris helicis
  sulci cutis
  s. ethmoidalis
  ethmoidal s. of Gegenbaur
  ethmoidal s. of nasal bone
  gingivobuccal s.
  gingivolabial s.
  gingivolingual s.
  s. gluteus
  greater palatine s. of max-
    illa
  s. for greater palatine
    nerve
  greater palatine s. of pala-
    tine bone
  s. hamuli pterygoidei
  implant gingival s.
  infraorbital s.
  infraorbital s. of maxilla
  infrapalpebral s.
  intergluteal s.
  labial s.
  labial-buccal s.
  labiodental s.
  labiomarginal s.
  lacrimal s. of lacrimal bone
  lacrimal s. of maxilla
  lingual s.

sulcus *(continued)*
  lip s.
  mandibular s.
  s. of mandibular neck
  s. of mastoid canaliculus
  s. matricis unguis
  median lingual s.
  mentolabial s.
  mylohyoid s.
  mylohyoid s. of mandible
  s. of nasal process of max-
    illa
  nasolabial s.
  occlusal s.
  s. olfactorius nasi
  olfactory s. of nose
  palatine s.
  palatine sulci of maxilla
  palatovaginal s.
  paraglenoid s.
  paralingual s.
  periconchal s.
  petrosal s.
  postauricular s.
  preauricular s.
  prejowl s.
  s. of pterygoid hamulus
  s. pterygopalatinus
  retroauricular s.
  sigmoid s.
  sublingual s.
  s. spinosus
  supratarsal s.
  temporal s.
  tonsillolingual s.
  vomeral s.
  vomerovaginal s.
  s. of wrist

sump
  Argyle silicone Salem s.

Sunderland classification for
  nerve injuries *(grades I–V)*

sunken-eye appearance

sunken-in face

sun protection factor (SPF)

super-absorptive polymer
dressing

Super-Cut
  S. blade
  S. scissors

superficial
  s. abdominal fascia
  s. abrasion
  s. angioma
  s. basal cell carcinoma
  s. basal cell epithelioma
  s. bleeders
  s. brachial flap
  s. circumflex iliac artery
  s. circumflex iliac vein
  s. dermis
  s. facial fascia
  s. fascia
  s. fascial system (SFS)
  s. granulomatous pyo-
    derma
  s. hemangioma
  s. implant
  s. liposculpture
  s. malignant melanoma
  s. musculoaponeurotic sys-
    tem (SMAS)
  s. palmar arch
  s. palmar branch of radial
    artery
  s. parotidectomy
  s. parotid node
  s. perineal fascia
  s. plane rhytidectomy
  s. radial nerve
  s. spreading melanoma
  s. suture
  s. temporal artery
  s. temporal crest
  s. temporal fascia
  s. temporal vein
  s. ulceration
  s. upper lateral shave
  s. varicosity
  s. vein
  s. wound

superior
  s. alveolar artery
  s. alveolar nerve
  ankyloglossia s.
  s. auricular artery
  s. auricular muscle
  s. cantholysis
  s. constrictor muscle
  s. constrictor pharyngeal
    muscle
  s. crus of antihelix
  s. dermal pedicle
  s. epigastric artery
  s. gluteal flap
  s. labial artery
  s. lacrimal gland
  s. laryngeal artery
  s. laryngeal nerve (SLN)
  s. laryngeal vein
  s. laryngotomy
  s. lip
  s. longitudinal muscle of
    tongue
  s. maxilla
  s. maxillary bone
  s. maxillary foramen
  s. maxillary nerve
  s. maxillary retrognathia
  s. nasal concha
  s. nasal nerve
  s. orbital fissure
  s. orbital fissure syndrome
    (SOFS)
  s. orbital rim
  s. palpebral region
  s. palpebral vein
  s. parathyroid gland
  s. petrosal ridge
  s. pharyngeal artery
  s. pharyngeal constrictor
  s. stratum
  s. surface of horizontal
    plate of palatine bone
  s. tarsal muscle
  s. thyroid artery
  s. thyroid gland
  s. thyroid notch

superior *(continued)*
  s. thyroid vein
  s. turbinate

superiorly based
  s. b. Dardour lateral flap
  s. b. Nataf lateral flap

superjacent

superinfection

supernumerary
  s. auricle
  s. digit
  s. limb
  s. nipple
  s. tendon

superolateral
  s. aspect
  s. surface of maxilla

superomedial

superstructure
  implant surgical splint s.

supervascularization

supinated oblique view on x-ray

supination

supinator
  s. longus reflex
  s. muscle
  s. strap

supply
  random pattern blood s.

support
  alveolar s.
  cartilaginous s.
  chin s.
  Dale oxygen cannula s.
  Dale ventilator tubing s.
  excessive lip s.
  facial s.
  fixed s.
  insufficient lip s.
  mammary s.
  multiple abutment s.
  orbital s.
  s. ridge

support *(continued)*
  s. stockings

supporting
  s. bone
  s. cell
  s. structure
  s. tissue

suppuration

suppurative
  s. inflammation
  s. osteomyelitis
  s. tenosynovitis

supra-alar pinching

supra-auricular

suprabasal clefting

suprabuccal

supraciliary
  s. canal
  s. incision

supraclavicular
  s. adenopathy
  s. fossa
  s. lymph node

supracricoid
  s. laryngectomy

supraglenoid

supraglottic
  s. carcinoma
  s. closure
  s. laryngectomy
  s. larynx
  s. squamous cell carcinoma
  s. stenosis

supraglottoplasty

suprahyoid
  s. epiglottitis
  s. muscle
  s. neck dissection
  s. node
  s. space

supralaryngeal tension

supramammary

supramandibular

supramastoid

supramaxilla

supramaxillary

Supramead nose splint

supramental

supramentale

Supramid
S. mesh implant
S. polyamide mesh

supranasal

supraocclusion

supraomohyoid
s. neck dissection

supraorbital
s. air cell
s. artery
s. bar
s. bandeau
s. canal
s. ethmoid
s. foramen
s. nerve
s. notch
s. plate
s. remodeling
s. ridge
s. rim

supraperichondrial dissection

supraperiosteal
s. flap
s. implant

suprascapular
s. nerve compression
s. nerve entrapment

suprasternal
s. fascia
s. notch

supratarsal sulcus

supratemporal

supratip
s. deformity
s. fullness

supratonsillar fossa

supratragal notch

supratrochlear
s. artery
s. nerve

supraumbilical
s. incision
s. raphe

supreme
s. nasal concha
s. turbinate bone

Suraci zygoma hook elevator

sural
s. artery flap
s. island flap for foot and
ankle reconstruction
s. nerve cable graft
s. nerve entrapment

Sure-Closure
S.-C. skin closure system
S.-C. skin stretching system

Sureseal pressure bandage

surface
alveolar s. of mandible
alveolar s. of maxilla
anterior s. of maxilla
articular s. of mandibular
fossa
bosselated s.
corneal s.
distal s.
dorsal condylar s.
facial s. of maxilla
implant-bearing s.
inferior s.
inferior s. of tongue
infratemporal s. of maxilla
labial s.
lateral s. of zygomatic bone

surface *(continued)*
   lingual s.
   malar s. of zygomatic bone
   maxillary s.
   maxillary s. of great wing
   maxillary s. of perpendicu-
      lar plate of palatine bone
   medial s.
   medial s. of maxilla
   occlusal s.
   oral s.
   palatine s.
   posterior s. of maxilla
   superior s. of horizontal
      plate of palatine bone
   superolateral s. of maxilla
   temporal s. of frontal bone
   temporal s. of zygomatic
      bone
   vermilion s. of lip
   working occlusal s.

Surgamid polyamide suture material

surgeon
   nonoculoplastic s.
   oral s.
   rhinologic s.

surgery
   access flap in osseous s.
   aesthetic s.
   body-contour s.
   Bosker TMI s.
   breast-conserving s.
   conchal s.
   conservation s.
   cosmetic s.
   cranial base s.
   craniofacial s.
   craniomaxillofacial s.
   dentofacial s.
   double jaw s.
   ear s.
   ectopic parts s.
   endoscopic s.
   endoscopic sinus s.
   esthetic s.
   helical s.

surgery *(continued)*
   laryngeal framework s.
   laser s.
   levator aponeurosis s.
   mandibular s.
   Marzola hair restoration s.
   maxillary s.
   maxillofacial s.
   microlaryngeal s.
   microvascular s.
   Mohs s.
   Mohs micrographic s.
      (MMS)
   Mohs micrographic s. by
      fixed-tissue technique
   mucogingival s.
   oral s.
   oral and maxillofacial s.
      (OMS)
   orthognathic s.
   osseous s.
   reconstructive s.
   rejuvenation s.
   second-look s.
   sex reassignment s.
   silicone gel–filled mam-
      mary implant explana-
      tion s.
   spare parts s.
   suspension microlaryn-
      geal s.
   transsexual s.

Surgibone

Surgica K6 laser

surgical-assisted rapid palatal
   expansion (SA-RPE)

Surgicel
   S. gauze

Surgiguide template

Surgipulse XJ 150 CO_2 laser

Surgitek
   S. Flexi-Flate II penile im-
      plant
   S. mammary implant
   S. T-Span tissue expander

Surgitron
  S. ultrasound-assisted lipo-
    plasty machine
  S. 3000 ultrasound device

surrogate host

survival
  allograft s.
  neuronal s.

suspension
  s. anastomosis
  anterior s. of hyoid bone
  balanced s.
  fascial s.
  frontalis s.
  s. microlaryngeal surgery
  nasal valve s.
  s. power
  s. sling
  s. vector

suspensory ligament

Sutton
  S. disease
  S. nevus
  S. ulcer

sutura *pl.* suturae

suture (*a fibrous joint of the*
  skull)
  anterior palatine s.
  arcuate s.
  basilar s.
  bilateral coronal s.
  biparietal s.
  bony s.
  bregmamastoid s.
  bregmatomastoid s.
  coronal s.
  cranial s's
  cranial vault s.
  cutaneous s. of palate
  dentate s.
  ethmoidolacrimal s.
  ethmoidomaxillary s.
  false s.
  flat s.

suture (*continued*)
  frontal s.
  frontoethmoidal s.
  frontolacrimal s.
  frontomalar s.
  frontomaxillary s.
  frontonasal s.
  frontoparietal s.
  frontosphenoid s.
  frontozygomatic s.
  s. of Goethe
  harmonic s.
  incisive s.
  infraorbital s.
  interendognathic s.
  intermaxillary s.
  intermediate s.
  internasal s.
  interparietal s.
  jugal s.
  lacrimoconchal s.
  lacrimoethmoidal s.
  lacrimomaxillary s.
  lacrimoturbinal s.
  lambdoid s.
  longitudinal s.
  longitudinal s. of palate
  malomaxillary s.
  mastoid s.
  mastoid-conchal s.
  median palatine s.
  metopic s.
  nasal s.
  nasofrontal s.
  nasomaxillary s.
  neurocentral s.
  occipital s.
  occipitomastoid s.
  occipitoparietal s.
  occipitosphenoidal s.
  overlapping s.
  palatine s.
  palatoethmoid s.
  palatoethmoidal s.
  palatomaxillary s.
  parietal s.
  parietomastoid s.
  parietooccipital s.

suture *(continued)*
    petrobasilar s.
    petroclival s.
    petrosphenobasilar s.
    petrosphenooccipital s. of
      Gruber
    petrosquamous s.
    petrotympanic s.
    plane s.
    premaxillary s.
    rhabdoid s.
    sagittal s.
    serrated s.
    skull base s.
    sphenoethmoidal s.
    sphenofrontal s.
    sphenomalar s.
    sphenomaxillary s.
    spheno-occipital s.
    spheno-orbital s.
    sphenoparietal s.
    sphenopetrosal s.
    sphenosquamous s.
    sphenotemporal s.
    sphenovomerine s.
    sphenozygomatic s.
    squamomastoid s.
    squamoparietal s.
    squamosomastoid s.
    squamosoparietal s.
    squamososphenoid s.
    squamosphenoid s.
    squamous s.
    squamous s. of cranium
    synostotic s.
    temporal s.
    temporomalar s.
    temporozygomatic s.
    transverse palatine s.
    transverse s. of Krause
    unilateral coronal s.
    zygomaticofrontal s.
    zygomaticomaxillary s.
    zygomaticosphenoidal s.
    zygomaticotemporal s.

suture *(a material for closing wounds)*
    absorbable s's

suture *(continued)*
    adjustable external s.
    alar cinch s's
    alternating s's
    anchor s.
    anchoring s.
    apposition s's
    approximation s's
    arterial silk s.
    atraumatic s's
    atraumatic braided silk s's
    atraumatic chromic s's
    basal bunching s's
    basting s.
    Bell s.
    black braided s.
    black silk s.
    black twisted s.
    blanket s's
    bolster s's
    Bondek absorbable s.
    braided s's
    braided Vicryl s.
    Bunnell s.
    buried s's
    button s's
    cable wire s's
    capitonnage s's
    catgut s. (CGS)
    chromic s's
    chromic catgut s's
    chromic catgut mattress
      s's
    chromicized catgut s's
    cinch s.
    coaptation s's
    coated s.
    coated Vicryl s.
    coated Vicryl Rapide s.
    cobbler's s's
    collagen s's
    collagen absorbable s.
    conchomastoidal s's
    conchoscaphal s's
    continuous s's
    continuous running s's
    Cottony-Dacron s.
    deep suspension s.

suture *(continued)*
    Dexon s.
    doubly armed s's
    end-on mattress s's
    Ethicon s.
    Ethilon s.
    everting interrupted s's
    eyelid crease s.
    far-and-near s's
    figure-of-eight s's
    Frost s.
    Gaillard-Arlt s's
    Giampapa s.
    Gillies horizontal dermal s.
    glover's s's
    Gore-Tex s.
    Halsted s.
    Halsted mattress s's
    harelip s.
    hemostatic s.
    horizontal mattress s.
    implanted s's
    interrupted s's
    intracuticular s's
    intracuticular running s's
    intradermal s's
    intradermal mattress s's
    intradermal polyglactic
       acid s.
    intradermic s's
    intrafascicular s.
    large-caliber nonabsorba-
       ble s.
    Le Dentu s.
    Le Fort s.
    mattress s's
    Maxon s.
    Mersilene s.
    modified Frost s.
    Monocryl s.
    monofilament s.
    monofilament nylon s.
    Mustardé s.
    nerve s's
    nonabsorbable s's
    nonabsorbable mattress s.
    Nurolon s.
    nylon s's

suture *(continued)*
    over-and-over s's
    Palfyn s.
    Pancoast s.
    Paré s.
    PDS s.
    perineurial s.
    plastic s's
    Polydek s.
    polyglactic acid s.
    polydioxanone s. (PDS)
    Prolene s.
    pull-out s's
    purse string s's
    quilted s's
    relaxation s's
    retention s's
    secondary s's
    serrated s's
    shoelace s.
    silicone-treated surgical
       silk s's
    silk s.
    silk interrupted mattress s.
    silk pop-off s.
    silk stay s.
    simple flaring s.
    simple running s.
    spiral s's
    stay s.
    subcutaneous s.
    subcuticular s.
    subcuticular pull-out s.
    superficial s.
    swaged s.
    synthetic absorbable s.
       (SAS)
    tacking s's
    tantalum wire monofila-
       ment s.
    tendon s's
    tension s's
    Tevdek s.
    through-and-through reab-
       sorbable s.
    transfixation s.
    transverse palatal s.
    uninterrupted s's

suture *(continued)*
 Vicryl s.
 Vicryl Rapide absorbable s.
 wire s's

sutured-in-place, shield-shaped
 tip graft

SutureStrip Plus wound closure

sutrectomy

Suzanne gland

swab
 antibiotic-soaked s's

swag
 drapery s. of cheek

swage

swaged
 s. needle
 s. suture

swan neck deformity

sweat gland
 apocrine s. g's
 eccrine s. g's
 s. g. carcinoma

swelling
 boggy s.
 fugitive s.
 fusiform s.
 periarticular soft tissue s.
 rhomboid s.
 sessile s.

swimmer's ear

Swiss Therapy eye mask

switch flap

SWMF
 Semmes-Weinstein nylon
  monofilament

sycosis
 s. frambesiformis
 lupoid s.
 s. nuchae necrotisans
 s. tarsi

Sydney crease

symblepharon
 anterior s.
 posterior s.
 total s.

symblepharopterygium

symbrachydactyly

symmelia

symmetry
 breast s.
 facial s.
 philtral s.

sympathectomy
 surgical s.

sympathetic
 s. ganglion
 s. nerve fibers
 s. nervous system
 reflex s. dystrophy (RSD)
 spinal s. chain

sympathetically
 s. independent pain syn-
  drome (SIPS)
 s. maintained pain syn-
  drome (SMPS)

sympatholysis

symphalangism
 syndromic s.
 true s.

symphyseal

symphysial

symphysion

symphysis *pl.* symphyses
 s. mandibulae
 s. menti

symphysodactyly

symptom
 Bekhterev (Bechterew) s.
 Bezold s.
 cardinal s.
 concomitant s.

symptom *(continued)*
  equivocal s.
  esophagosalivary s.
  Griesinger s.
  Macewen s.
  pathognomonic s.
  prodromal s.
  Wartenberg s.

symptomatic

synchilia

synchondrosis *pl.* synchon-
  droses
  anterior intraoccipital s.
  s. arycorniculata
  carpal s.
  congenital s.
  congenital carpal s.
  s's of cranium
  intercarpal joint s.
  intersphenoidal s.
  occipitosphenoidal s.
  petro-occipital s.
  posterior intraoccipital s.
  s's of skull
  spheno-occipital s.
  sphenopetrosal s.

syncope
  laryngeal s.

syndactyly
  complete s.
  complicated s.
  double s.
  incomplete s.
  partial s.
  simple s.
  single s.
  symmetric s.
  triple s.

syndrome
  Aarskog-Scott s.
  acrofacial s.
  acute radiation s.
  adherence s.
  Adie s.
  afferent loop s.
  aglossia-adactylia s.
  Aicardi s.

syndrome *(continued)*
  Albright s.
  Albright-Hadorn s.
  Albright-McCune-Stern-
    berg s.
  Alezzandrini s.
  Andermann s.
  androgen insensitivity s.
  angio-osteohypertrophy s.
  ankyloglossia superior s.
  Apert s.
  Ascher s.
  auriculotemporal nerve s.
  Avellis s.
  Baller-Gerold s.
  Barrett s.
  Bogorad s.
  Bardet-Biedl s.
  basal cell nevus s.
  Bazex s.
  Beckwith s.
  Beckwith-Wiedemann s.
  Benjamin s.
  Berndorfer s.
  Binder s.
  Birt-Hogg-Dubé s.
  Bloch-Sulzberger s.
  Bloom s.
  blue rubber bleb nevus s.
  Boerhaave s.
  Bogorad s.
  Bonnet-Dechaume-Blanc s.
  Böök s.
  Brissaud-Marie s.
  Brown s.
  Caffey s.
  caput ulnae s.
  carpal tunnel s. (CTS)
  Carpenter s. (CTS)
  cat cry s.
  cavernous sinus s.
  cephalopolysyndactyly s.
  cerebellopontine angle s.
  cerebrocostomandibular s.
    (CCMS)
  cheilitis-glossitis-gingivi-
    tis s.
  Charlin s.
  chronic pain s.

syndrome *(continued)*
- cleft palate and lateral synechia s. (CPLS)
- Cobb s.
- Coffin-Lowry s.
- Coffin-Siris s.
- Cogan s.
- compartment s.
- complex regional pain s's (CRPS)
- congenital alveolar synechia s.
- constriction ring s.
- Crandall s.
- craniofacial s's
- cri du chat s.
- s. of crocodile tears
- Crouzon s.
- cubital tunnel s.
- Dejerine s.
- dentopulmonary s.
- de Quervain s.
- DiGeorge s.
- disseminated form Albright s.
- dorsal wrist s. (DWS)
- dry eye s.
- Eagle-Barrett s.
- Ehlers-Danlos s.
- Ellis-van Creveld s.
- familial atypical multiple mole melanoma s. (FAMMM)
- fetal alcohol s.
- fetal face s.
- fetal hydantoin s.
- fibular tunnel s.
- Franceschetti s.
- Franceschetti-Jadassohn s.
- Franke s.
- Fraser s.
- Freeman-Sheldon s.
- fetal valproate s.
- Garcin s.
- Gianotti-Crosti s.
- Giedion s.
- Godtfredsen s.
- Goeminne s.

syndrome *(continued)*
- Goldenhar s.
- Goltz s.
- Gorlin s.
- Gorlin-Chaudhry-Moss s.
- Gougerot-Sjögren s.
- Greig s.
- Greig cephalopolysyndactyly s.
- Guyon canal s.
- Haber s.
- Hajdu-Cheney s.
- Hallermann-Streiff s.
- Hallermann-Streiff-François s.
- Hanhart s.
- heart and hand s.
- Hejdu-Cheney s.
- Holt-Oram s.
- Horner s.
- Hunt s.
- Hunter s.
- Hurler s.
- Hurler-Scheie s.
- Hutchinson-Gilford s.
- hypoglossia-hypodactylia s.
- hypoglossia-hypodactyly s.
- hypothenar hammer s.
- immotile cilia s.
- Jackson s.
- jugular foramen s.
- Kallmann s.
- Kanner s.
- Kartagener s.
- Kasabach-Merritt s.
- kleeblattschädel s.
- Klinefelter s.
- Klippel-Trénaunay s.
- Laband s.
- lacrimoauriculodentodigital s.
- Lambert-Eaton myasthenic s.
- Landry-Guillain-Barré s.
- Leri-Weill s.
- Larsen s.
- long face s.
- 3M s.

syndrome *(continued)*
  McCune-Albright s.
  MacKenzie s.
  Maffucci s.
  Mallory-Weiss s.
  Mannerfelt s.
  Marfan s.
  Marshall s.
  Mayer-Rokitansky s.
  Mayer-Rokitansky-Küster-
    Hauser s. (MRKHS)
  median cleft face s.
  Meige s.
  Melkersson s.
  Melkersson-Rosenthal s.
  Meniere s.
  Meyenburg-Altherr-Uehlin-
    ger s.
  middle fossa s.
  Mikulicz s.
  Miller-Fisher variant of
    Guillain-Barré s.
  minimal brain dysfunc-
    tion s.
  Möbius s.
  Mohr-Tranebjaerg s.
  mole melanoma s.
  Morquio s.
  MPD s.
  mucocutaneous lymph
    node s.
  multiple hamartoma s.
  myofascial pain s. (MPS)
  myofascial pain-dysfunc-
    tion s.
  Nager s.
  nerve compression s.
  neuropolyendocrine s.
  occipital condyle s.
  ocular–mucous mem-
    brane s.
  oculopharyngeal s.
  orbital compartment s.
  orofacial dysfunction s.
  Osler-Weber-Rendu s.
  Paget I s.
  Paget II s.
  Paine s.

syndrome *(continued)*
  Palant-Feingold-Berkman s.
  Papillon-Lefèvre s.
  Papillon-Léage and
    Psaume s.
  Parkes-Weber s.
  Parsonage Turner s.
  Pfeiffer s.
  Plummer-Wilson s.
  Poland s.
  pronator s.
  prune belly s.
  quadriga s.
  radial tunnel s.
  Ramsey Hunt s.
  Rapp-Hodgkin s.
  Ravenna s.
  Rendu-Osler-Weber s.
  Roaf s.
  Robin s.
  Robinow s.
  Roger s.
  Romberg s.
  Rothmund s.
  Rothmund-Thomson s.
  Rubinstein-Taybi s.
  Saethre-Chotzen s.
  Satchmo s.
  scalded-skin s.
  scaphocapitate s.
  Schatzki s.
  Schaumann s.
  Schinzel acrocallosal s.
  Schmidt s.
  Schwartz s.
  Seckel s.
  Senear-Usher s.
  sepsis s.
  Sézary s.
  short face s.
  short gut s.
  shoulder impingement s.
  Simmonds s.
  Sipple s.
  Sjögren s.
  Smith-Lemli-Opitz s.
  Smith-Riley s.
  Stevens-Johnson s.

syndrome *(continued)*
  Stewart-Treves s.
  Stickler s.
  Strauss s.
  Sturge-Weber s.
  stylohyoid s.
  subclavian steal s.
  superior orbital fissure s.
    (SOFS)
  sympathetically indepen-
    dent pain s. (SIPS)
  sympathetically maintained
    pain s. (SMPS)
  Tapia s.
  tarsal tunnel s.
  Teebi hypertelorism s.
  Teebi-Shalout s.
  temporomandibular joint
    (TMJ) s.
  temporomandibular joint
    pain-dysfunction s.
  Thompson s.
  thoracic outlet s.
  Treacher Collins s. (TCS)
  triad s.
  trichorhinophalangeal s.
  ulnar carpal abutment s.
  ulnar impaction s.
  Vail s.
  van Buchem s.
  van der Hoeve s.
  Van der Woude s.
  Veeneklaas s.
  velocardiofacial s.
  Vernet s.
  Waardenburg s.
  Waardenburg-Klein s.
  Wallenberg s.
  Weber-Cockayne s.
  Werner s.
  Weyers s.
  Weyers-Fülling s.
  Weyers-Thier s.
  whistling face s.
  Wildervanck s.
  Wildervanck-Smith s.
  Winchester s.
  Witkop-von Sallman s.
  Wolf-Hirschhorn s.

syndrome *(continued)*
  Wyburn-Mason s.
  Yunas-Varon s.

synechia *pl.* synechiae

synostosis *pl.* synostoses
  bicoronal s.
  bilateral coronal s.
  compensatory s.
  coronal s.
  cranial suture s.
  Crouzon syndromic s.
  metopic s.
  multiple-suture s.
  plagiocephaly without s.
  radioulnar s.
  sagittal s.
  sagittal suture s.
  single-suture s.
  syndromic s.
  tribasilar s.
  unicoronal s.
  unilambdoid s.
  unilateral coronal s.

synostotic
  s. frontal plagiocephaly
    (SFP)
  s. suture

synovial
  s. dissector
  s. proliferation

synovitis
  silicone s.
  villonodular s.

synpolydactyly

Synthes facial curet

synthesis
  collagen s.

synthetic absorbable suture
  (SAS)

syphilis
  meningovascular s.

syringe
  aspirating s.
  laryngeal s.

system
    Adolph Gasser camera s.
    All Access laser s.
    angled-vision lens s.
    AO/ASIF titanium craniofacial s.
    Aston cartilage reduction s.
    Becker vibrating cannula s.
    BioBarrier membrane guided tissue regeneration s.
    Bioplate screw fixation s.
    Bioquant histomorphometry s.
    Blade-Vent implant s.
    Boehringer Autovac autotransfusion s.
    bone tack s.
    Bosker TMI Reconstruction s.
    Bosker transmandibular reconstructive surgical s.
    Brånemark implant s.
    Breslow microstaging s. for malignant melanoma
    Calcitek drill s.
    carpal tunnel release s. (CTRS)
    Champy miniplate rigid fixation s.
    COM/MAND mandibular fixation s.
    computer-assisted neurosurgical navigational s. (CANS)
    Dall-Miles cable grip s.
    deep muscular aponeurotic s. (DMAS)
    dorsalis pedis-FDMA s.
    Dumbach mandibular reconstruction s.
    EpiLaser s.
    EpiLight hair removal s.
    EpiTouch Alex laser hair removal s.
    EpiTouch Ruby SilkLaser hair removal s.
    ethmoidal infundibular s.

system (continued)
    Facial Grading S. (FGS)
    Facial Grading S. voluntary movement (FGSM)
    FiberLase flexible beam delivery s. for CO_2 surgical lasers
    GelShapes scar management s.
    GentlePeel skin exfoliation s.
    Glogau s. of skin evaluation
    Haid Universal bone plate s.
    Hall mandibular implant s.
    haversian s.
    Herbert alphanumeric classification s. for scaphoid fractures (types A1, A2, B1–4, C, D1, D2)
    Hoffman external fixation s.
    House-Brackmann s.
    Hunstad s. for tumescent anesthesia
    immune s.
    implant s.
    IMZ implant s.
    Innovation implant s.
    KTP/Nd:YAG XP surgical laser s.
    LactoSorb craniofacial plate fixation s.
    LaseAway ruby laser s.
    Leibinger plating s.
    Leibinger titanium Würzburg mandibular reconstruction s.
    Luhr maxillofacial fixation s.
    Luhr microfixation s.
    Magna-Site locating s.
    Mectra irrigation/aspiration s.
    Medtronics Sequestra 1000 autotransfusion s.
    Mentor Contour Genesis ultrasonic assisted lipoplasty s.
    MicroLux video camera s.

system *(continued)*
  Micro Plus plating s.
  Microsponge delivery s.
  Micro-Vent implant s.
  Mini-Würzburg Flexplates
    craniomaxillofacial plat-
    ing s.
  Mini-Würzburg standard
    craniomaxillofacial plat-
    ing s.
  Montgomery thyroplasty
    implant s.
  musculoaponeurotic s.
  Natural Profile abutment s.
  NovaPulse laser s.
  Obagi Nu-Derm s.
  Opmilas laser s.
  Permark micropigmenta-
    tion s.
  PhotoDerm T laser s.
  resorbable copolymer
    PGA/PLLA-Lactosorb
    miniplate fixation s.
  revised Salzburg lag
    screw s.
  revised Würzburg mandib-
    ular reconstruction s.
  ScleroPlus LongPulse dye
    laser s.
  Scott chronic wound
    care s.
  skin-adipose superficial
    musculoaponeurotic s.
    (SASMA)
  SLS Chromos long pulse
    ruby laser s.
  subcutaneous musculoapo-
    neurotic s.

system *(continued)*
  submuscular aponeurot-
    ic s.
  suction s.
  superficial fascial s. (SFS)
  superficial musculoaponeu-
    rotic s. (SMAS)
  Sure-Closure skin closure s.
  Sure-Closure skin stretch-
    ing s.
  sympathetic nervous s.
  Tebbetts EndoPlastic in-
    strument s.
  Therabite jaw motion reha-
    bilitation s.
  three-dimensional plating s.
  TiMesh craniomaxillofacial
    plating s.
  TiMesh rigid fixation bone
    plating s.
  titanium hollow-screw os-
    seointegrating reconstruc-
    tion plate (THORP) s.
  Verdan zone s.
  Visage Cosmetic Surgery S.
  Vitek-Kent hemi TMJ re-
    placement s.
  Vitek-Kent total TMJ re-
    placement s.
  Würzburg fracture s.
  Würzburg maxillofacial
    plating s.
  Würzburg plating s.
  Würzburg reconstruc-
    tion s.
  XPS Sculpture s.
  YagLazr s.

T
T-bar of Kazanjian
T-breast reduction
T-incision
inverted T-scar
T-shaped graft
T-shaped scar

tabatière anatomique

tabes dorsalis

table
t. bones of skull
inner t. of frontal bone
outer t. of frontal bone
Sugita microsurgical t.

tache
t's bleuâtres
t. cérébrale
t's laiteuses
t. noire
t. spinale

tack
ACE bone screw t.
biodegradable surgical t.
Graftac absorbable skin t.
titanium t.

tacking
t. sutures
tailor-t.

TAF
tumor angiogenic factor

tag
auricular t's
cutaneous t.
question t.
radioactive t.
skin t.

tagliacotian
t. operation
t. rhinoplasty

Tagliacozzi
T. flap
T. nasal reconstruction

tail
axillary t. of Spence
t. of breast
t. of helix
t. of Spence
velar t.

Taillefer valve

tailor
t.-tacking

Tait
T. flap
T. graft
T. perineoplasty

Takahashi
T. ethmoidal forceps
T. nasal forceps
T. nasal punch

take
t. of the graft

takedown
t. of adhesions
t. of anastomosis
fistula t.

TAL
total autogenous latissimus
TAL breast reconstruction

talar tendon

talipes

talipomanus

talonavicular

talus *pl.* tali

tamponade
nasal t.
postnasal balloon t.

tamponage
vaselinized nasal t.

Tan otoplasty

tangential
t. excision

tangential *(continued)*
  t. plane
  t. projection
  t. view

Tanner
  T. mesher
  T. mesh graft dermacarrier
  T.-Vandeput graft
  T.-Vandeput mesh derma-
    tome

tannic acid

Tansini breast amputation

Tansley operation

tantalum
  t. fixation
  t. mesh graft
  t. plate
  t. wire monofilament suture

Tanzer auricle reconstruction

tape
  Blenderm t.
  brow t.
  Dermicel t.
  Elastikon elastic t.
  Haelan t.
  Hy-T. surgical t.
  Medipore H surgical t.
  Micropore t.
  Scanpor t.
  Shur-Strip wound closure t.

tapetum *pl.* tapeta

Tapia syndrome

tapinocephaly

tapir
  bouche de t.

tardus
  nevus t.

tardy
  t. median palsy
  t. palsy

target
  t. lesion
  t. sign

tarsadenitis

tarsal
  t. canal
  t. cyst
  t. fold
  t. synostosis
  t. tunnel syndrome

tarsitis

tarsocheiloplasty

tarsoconjunctival flap

tarsomalacia

tarso-orbital

tarsophyma

tarsoplasty

tarsorrhaphy

tarsotomy

tarsus *pl.* tarsi
  bony t.
  t. inferior palpebrae
  t. orbital septum
  t. osseus
  t. superior palpebrae

Tatagiba line

tattoo
  decorative t.
  Derma-T. surgical t.
  eyeline t.
  nipple-areola t.
  t. removal
  traumatic t.
  vermilion-skin junction t.

Taylor
  T. dural scissors
  esthetic T. mandibular an-
    gle implant

T-bar of Kazanjian

T-breast reduction

TBSA
  total body surface area

TCA
  trichloroacetic acid
  TCA peel

TCB
  transconjunctival blepharoplasty

TCN
  terminal capillary network

TCS
  Treacher Collins syndrome

tear (*to pull apart, or something pulled apart*)
  degenerative t.
  horseshoe t.
  lunotriquetral t.
  lunotriquetral ligament t.
  perineal t.
  skier's t.
  traumatic t.
  triangular fibrocartilage complex (TFCC) t.
  triangular fibrocartilage complex (TFCC) meniscus t
  triquetral impingement ligament t. (TILT)

tear (*the watery secretion of the lacrimal gland*)
  t. clearance rate
  crocodile t's
  t. duct
  t. duct tube
  t. strips
  syndrome of crocodile t's

teardrop
  inverted t. areola deformity
  t. foramen
  t.-shaped breast implant
  t.-shaped nipple-areola complex

tearing
  circumferential t. of skin

Tebbetts
  T. EndoPlastic instrument system

Tebbetts (*continued*)
  T. rhinoplasty set
  T. ribbon retractor

technique
  angle bisection t.
  aseptic t.
  Baek musculocutaneous pedicle t.
  balanced force instrumentation t.
  Bernard-Burow t.
  bilobed skin flap t.
  Blaskovics eyelid shortening t.
  bone graft harvesting t.
  bulk pack t.
  Burow t.
  cap t.
  cartilage-breaking t.
  cartilage-molding t.
  cartilage-weakening t.
  channel shoulder pin t.
  chevron marking t.
  Chow t.
  Converse t.
  Conway t.
  cross-facial t.
  cut-as-you-go t.
  Cutler-Beard t.
  Delerm and Elbaz t.
  dermal brassiere t.
  dermal orbicular pennant t.
  dermal pedicle t.
  dermofat t.
  distal pedicle flap t.
  double pedicle t.
  elliptical excision t.
  epithelialization t.
  extended mesh t.
  extended supraplatysmal plane (ESP) face-lift t.
  fascial anchoring t.
  feathering t.
  four-flap Webster-Bernard t.
  galeal scoring t.
  Garceau tendon t.
  Giampapa suturing t.
  Gillies-Millard t.

technique *(continued)*
  Hartel t.
  Huber t.
  Ilizarov t.
  Illouz liposuction t.
  immediate extension t.
  incision-halving t.
  intact canal wall t.
  Karapandzic t.
  Kawamoto t.
  Kazanjian vestibuloplasty t.
  Kesselring curette t.
  Kuhnt-Szymanowski t.
  labiolingual t.
  lag screw t. of interfrag-
    mentary compression
  Lassus t.
  lid-loading t.
  lid-sharing t.
  lingual split-bone t.
  lipoinjection t.
  lipo layering t.
  McCraw t.
  McGoon t.
  McIndoe t.
  McSpadden endodontic t.
  mandibular-sparing t.
  maxillary sinus Foley cath-
    eter balloon placement t.
  Merendino t.
  Messerklinger t.
  microetching t.
  micrograft punctiform t.
  Millard forked flap t.
  modified anterior scoring t.
  modified Bernard-Burow t.
  modified Skoog t.
  Mohs fresh tissue chemo-
    surgery t.
  Mohs micrographic surgery
    by fixed-tissue t.
  mucoperiosteal flap t.
  mucosal relaxing incision t.
  multiplanar endoscopic fa-
    cial rejuvenation t.
  multiplanar upper facial re-
    juvenation t.
  Mustardé t.
  Muti t.

technique *(continued)*
  N2-Sargenti t.
  onlay t.
  open flap t.
  open harvesting t.
  Orticochea scalping t.
  Panas ptosis correction t.
  Papineau t.
  periareolar t.
  progressive tension suture
    t. in abdominoplasty
  Ravitch t. for reconstruc-
    tion
  Reynolds and Horton alar
    cartilage t.
  salvage t.
  scapular island flap t.
  Schrudde curet t.
  shoelace t.
  short scar t.
  skin flap rotation t.
  sliding skin flap t.
  SMAS (superficial muscu-
    loaponeurotic system)
    face-lift t.
  spaghetti fat grafting t.
  split-bone t.
  spread-and-cut t.
  staircase t. for lip recon-
    struction
  Stenstrom t.
  Stenstrom alar cartilage t.
  Stenstrom t. in otoplasty
  Stent skin graft t.
  stepladder t. for lip recon-
    struction
  Strombeck t. for reduction
    mammaplasty
  subclavian flap t.
  subperiosteal implant one-
    phase t.
  subplatysmal face-lift t.
  Teimourian and Adhan t.
  Teimourian curet t.
  tension-control suture t. in
    open rhinoplasty
  tissue-expansion t.
  tumescent t.
  two-flap palatoplasty t.

technique *(continued)*
  underlay fascia t.
  Van Beek-Zook t.
  Van Millingen eyelid repair t.
  V-Y advancement t.
  Wagner-Baldwin t.
  Wardill t.
  Weine t.
  Weir t.
  Weir pattern skin flap t.
  wet t.
  Zocchi ultrasound-assisted lipoplasty t.
  Z-plasty t.

technology
  Lifecore cutting advance t.

tectocephaly

tectonic

Teebi
  T. hypertelorism syndrome
  T.-Shalout syndrome

TefGen-FD
  T.-FD guided tissue regeneration membrane
  T.-FD plastic membrane

Teflon
  T. block
  T. graft
  T. implant
  T. material
  T. mesh implant
  T. orbital floor implant
  T. strut

Tegaderm
  T. dressing
  T. occlusive dressing
  T. semipermeable dressing
  T. transparent dressing

tegmen *pl.* tegmina
  t. cellulae
  t. cranii
  t. mastoideum

tegmental
  t. region

tegmental *(continued)*
  t. wall

tegmentum *pl.* tegmenta

Teimourian
  T. and Adhan technique
  T. aspirative lipoplasty
  T. curet technique

telangiectasia
  cephalo-oculocutaneous t.
  dermatomal superficial t.
  essential t.
  hemorrhagic t.
  hereditary hemorrhagic t.
  t. macularis eruptiva perstans (TMEP)
  nevoid t.
  oculocutaneous t.
  periungual t.
  secondary t.
  spider t.
  unilateral nevoid t.
  t. verrucosa

telangiectasis *pl.* telangiectases
  linear t's
  multiple hereditary hemorrhagic t's
  spider t.
  tortuous t.

telangiectatic
  t. erythema
  t. wart

telangiectaticum
  granuloma t.

telangiitis

telangioma

telangiosis

telecanthus

telephone ear

telescope
  angled t.
  Hopkins endoscopy t.

Telfa
  T. 4 × 4 bandage

Telfa *(continued)*
    T. dressing
    T. gauze
    T. island dressing
    T. pad
    T. plastic film dressing
    T. sterile adhesive pad

telorbitism

telorism

temperature
    maturing t.

temperature-dependent dermatosis

template
    implant t.
    McKissock keyhole areolar t.
    surgical t.
    Surgiguide t.
    tissue expander t.
    tissue sizer t.
    total toe t.

Templeton-Zim carpal tunnel projection

temporal
    t. arteritis
    t. artery
    t. bone
    t. canthus
    t. diploic vein
    t. facial nerve
    t. fascia
    t. fascial flap
    t. fossa
    t. giant cell arteritis
    t. island pedicle scalp flap
    t. lobe
    t. muscle
    t. muscle and fascia flap
    t. nerve
    t. plane
    t. process of mandible
    t. process of zygomatic bone
    t.-pterygomaxillary fossa

temporal *(continued)*
    t. region
    t. sulcus
    t. surface of frontal bone
    t. surface of zygomatic bone
    t. suture
    t. vein

temporalis
    t. fascia
    t. fascia graft
    t. flap
    linea t.
    t. muscle
    t. muscle–fascia transfer
    t. muscle flap
    t. muscle transposition
    t. sling
    t. superficialis fascia

temporary endodontic restorative material (TERM)

temporoauricular

temporofacial

temporofrontal

temporohyoid

temporomalar

temporomandibular
    t. arthralgia
    t. arthrosis
    t. articulation
    t. dysfunction (TMD)
    t. endoscopic lift
    t. ligament
    t. luxation
    t. neuralgia
    t. pain-dysfunction (TMPD)
    t. pain-dysfunction disorder (TMPD)

temporomandibular joint (TMJ)
    t. j. ankylosis
    t. j. articular eminence
    t. j. capsule
    t. j. click
    t. j. dislocation

temporomandibular joint *(continued)*
  t. j. dysfunction (TMD, TMJ)
  t. j. fossa
  t. j. hypermobility
  interarticular disk of t. j.
  t. j. osteoarthritis (TMJ-OA)
  t. j. pain-dysfunction syndrome
  t. j. radiograph
  t. j. remodeling
  t. j. sprain
  t. j. subluxation
  t. j. (TMJ) syndrome
  t. j. synovial fluid

temporomaxillary

temporo-occipital

temporoparietal
  t. fascia flap (TPFF)
  t. fascial flap (TPFF)

temporoparieto-occipital
  t. flap
  t. rotation flap

temporosphenoid

temporozygomatic

tenaculum
  Adair t.
  atraumatic t.
  breast t.
  Brophy t.
  cleft palate t.
  Cottle single-prong t.
  double-hook skin t.
  Joseph t.
  Lahey t.
  Miltex t. hook
  nasal t.
  Ritchie cleft palate t.
  White t.

tenderness
  focal t.

tendinitis
  calcific t.

tendinitis *(continued)*
  t. ossificans traumatica
  t. stenosans
  stenosing t.

tendinoplasty

tendinosuture

tendinous

tendo *pl.* tendines
  t. cricoesophageus
  t. oculi
  t. palpebrarum

tendolysis

tendon
  Achilles t.
  t. adhesions
  t. advancement
  attrition rupture of extensor t.
  common t.
  t. dislocation
  extensor carpi radialis longus (ECRL) t.
  extensor carpi ulnaris (ECU) t.
  extensor digiti minimi t.
  extensor digitorum communis t.
  extensor indicis proprius (EIP) t.
  extensor pollicis longus (EPL) t.
  flexor carpi radialis t.
  flexor carpi ulnaris t.
  flexor digitorum profundus (FDP) t.
  flexor digitorum superficialis (FDS) t.
  flexor pollicis longus (FPL) t.
  t. graft
  inferior crus of lateral canthal t.
  intermediate t.
  t. lengthening
  masseter t.

tendon *(continued)*
    medial canthal t.
    t. necrosis
    palmaris longus t.
    t. passer
    plantaris t.
    profundus t.
    proprius t.
    t. rebalancing
    t. rupture
    ruptured flexor t.
    t. sheath
    t. sheath irrigation
    t. shortening
    t. stripper
    superficialis t.
    supernumerary t.
    talar t.
    t. transfer
    t. transplantation
    t.-tunneling forceps
    Zinn t.

tendoplasty

tendosynovitis *(variant of* teno-synovitis)

tendotomy

tenectomy

Tennison
    T. cheiloplasty
    T. operation
    T. Z-plasty
    T.-Randall cleft lip repair
    T.-Randall triangular flap
        repair

tenodesis

tenolysis

tenomyoplasty

tenomyotomy

tenonectomy

tenontomyoplasty

tenontoplasty

tenophyte

tenoplasty

tenorrhaphy

tenostosis

tenosuspension

tenosynovectomy
    extensor t.

tenosynovitis
    adhesive t.
    coccidioidomycosis t.
    t. crepitans
    de Quervain t.
    flexor t.
    gonococcal flexor t.
    granulomatous t.
    t. hypertrophica
    localized nodular t.
    t. serosa chronica
    t. stenosans
    stenosing t.
    suppurative t.
    villonodular pigmented t.
    villous t.

tenotomy
    curb t.
    graduated t.
    t. scissors
    subcutaneous t.
    three-step t.

tenovaginitis

tension
    interfacial surface t.
    laryngeal t.
    t. skin lines
    supralaryngeal t.
    t. sutures

tension-control suture tech-nique in open rhinoplasty

tension-free
    t.-f. anastomosis
    t.-f. repair
    t.-f. scalp fixation

tensor
    t. fasciae latae
    t. fasciae latae flap

tensor *(continued)*
    t. fasciae latae muscle
    musculus t. fasciae latae
    t. veli palatini
    t. veli palatini muscle

Tenzel
    T. calipers
    T. double-end periosteal elevator
    T. periosteal elevator

teras *pl.* terata

teratogenic

teratoma *pl.* teratomata
    adult t.
    benign cystic t.
    cystic t.
    mature t.

teres
    t. major muscle
    t. minor
    t. minor muscle

Terino
    T. anatomical chin implant
    T. facial implant retractor
    T. implant
    T. malar shell

TERM
    temporary endodontic restorative material

terminal capillary network (TCN)

Terry
    T. line
    T. nail sign

Terry-Thomas sign

Tessier
    T. bone bender
    T. classification
    T. classification of craniofacial clefts (*Tessier numbers 0–14*)
    T. cleft
    T. cleft axis

Tessier *(continued)*
    T. craniofacial cleft
    T. craniofacial instrument
    T. craniofacial operation
    T. disimpaction device forceps
    T. dislodger
    T. elevator
    T. facial dysostosis operation
    T. osteomicrotome
    T. osteotome
    T. osteotomy
    T. type of frontal bone advancement

test
    Adson t.
    Allen t.
    ballottement t.
    capillary fragility t.
    capillary resistance t.
    carpal compression t.
    chi-square t.
    collagen skin t.
    collagen vascular serologic t.
    Cybex t.
    Deep T. of Articulation
    dorsal wrist syndrome t.
    finger extension t. (FET)
    Finochietto-Bunnell t.
    Fisher exact t.
    fluorescein instillation t.
    fluorescent antinuclear antibody t. (FANA)
    Haines-Zancolli t.
    halo t. for cerebrospinal fluid (CSF) leak
    halo t. for cerebrospinal fluid (CSF) rhinorrhea
    Kappa t.
    Kleinman t.
    lacrimation t.
    Linscheid t.
    lunotriquetral compression t.
    lunotriquetral shear t.
    Masquelet t.

test *(continued)*
  maximum stimulation t.
    (MST)
  median nerve compres-
    sion t.
  Metz recruitment t.
  Moberg pickup t.
  Mohs hardness t.
  monofilament t.
  motor control t.
  motor coordination t.
    (MCT)
  mucin clot t.
  Mueller t.
  nerve excitability t.
  ocular dysmetria t.
  qualitative melanin t.
  rapid slide t.
  Reagan t.
  Roos t.
  Ropes t.
  Schirmer t.
  Schirmer tear t.
  Schwartz t.
  Semmes-Weinstein mono-
    filament t.
  shear t.
  tilt t.
  tilt table t.
  two-point discrimination t.
  Watson scaphoid shift t.
  Weber two-point discrimi-
    nation t.

tester
  Accu-Measure personal
    body fat t.

testing
  epidermal t.
  hypersensitivity skin t.
  provocative dose t.

tetany
  parathyroid t.
  postoperative t.

tethered

tetrastichiasis

Tevdek suture

text
  mathetic t.

textured saline breast implant

TFCC
  triangular fibrocartilage
    complex
      TFCC meniscus tear
      TFCC tear

TGF
  transforming growth factor

TGF-β
  transforming growth factor
    beta

TG Osseotite single-stage procedure implant

thalassemia
  t. major

thecostegnosis

theleplasty

thelerethism

thenar
  t. atrophy
  t. cleft
  t. compartment
  t. eminence
  t. fascia
  t. flap
  t. muscle hypoplasia
  t. space
  t. web
  t. web space

theory
  columnar carpus t.
  markedness t.
  mendelian t.
  myoelastic t.
  myoelastic-aerodynamic t.
    of phonation

Therabite jaw motion rehabilitation system

Thera-Boot compression dressing

therapy
    adjuvant t.
    antirejection drug t.
    antiretroviral t.
    helmet t.
    immunosuppressive t.
    incremental t.
    myofunctional t.
    occlusal t.
    prophylactic antibiotic t.
    radiation t.
    roentgen t.
    vascular lesion t.
    x-ray t. (XRT)

Thermafil Plus obturator

thermal
    t. burn
    t. injury
    t. quenching

thickened
    t. bone
    t. skin

thickening
    sclerodermalike skin t.

thickness
    Breslow t.
    soft tissue t.

Thiersch
    T. canaliculi
    T. graft
    T. graft operation
    T. medium-split free graft
    T. method
    T. operation
    T. skin graft knife
    T. thin-split free graft

thigh
    cricket t.
    t. lift

thin-shaft nasal scissors

THINSite with BioFilm

third intention wound closure

Thom flap laryngeal reconstruction

Thompson
    T. line
    T. syndrome

thoracectomy

thoracic
    t. duct
    t. nerve block
    t. outlet compression
    t. outlet syndrome

thoracoacromial
    t. artery
    t. flap

thoracoceloschisis

thoracocyllosis

thoracocyrtosis

thoracodidymus

thoracodorsal
    t. artery
    t. fascia flap
    t. nerve

thoracogastroschisis

thoracoplasty

thoracoschisis

thoracostenosis

thorax *pl.* thoraces
    amazon t.
    barrel-shaped t.
    pyriform t.

THORP
    titanium hollow-screw os-
        seointegrating reconstruc-
        tion plate
            THORP system
            THORP-type mandibu-
                lar reconstruction
                plate

three
    t.-armed stellate incision

three *(continued)*
    t.-paddle tensor fasciae latae free flap
    t.-pronged retractor
    t.-step tenotomy
    t.-wall orbital decompression

three-dimensional
    t.-d. biocompatible scaffolding
    t.-d. computed tomography (3D CT)
    t.-d. computed tomography scans
    t.-d. plating system

threshold
    absolute t.

thromboangiitis obliterans

thrombophlebitis
    sinus t.

thrombosis
    inferior dental t.
    microvascular t.
    sinus t.

through-and-through
    t.-a.-t. avulsion injury
    t.-a.-t. buttonhole fashion excision
    t.-a.-t. defect
    t.-a.-t. reabsorbable suture

Thudichum nasal speculum

thumb
    bifid t.
    biphalangeal t.
    Blauth classification of hypoplasia of t. *(types I, II, IIIA, IIIB, IV, V)*
    Blauth hypoplastic t. *(Types I, II, IIIA, IIIB, IV, V)*
    clasped t.
    t. duplication
    floating t.
    t. fusion
    gamekeeper's t.
    hitchhiker's t.

thumb *(continued)*
    t. hypoplasia
    hypoplastic t.
    t.-in-palm deformity
    t. polydactyly
    t. reconstruction
    rodeo t.
    skier's t.
    tennis t.
    trigger t.
    triphalageal t.
    ulnar t.

thyremphraxis

thyroarytenoid

thyroepiglottic

thyrofissure

thyroglossal
    t. fistula

thyrohyoid
    t. fold
    t. laryngotomy
    t. ligament
    t. membrane
    t. muscle

thyroid
    aberrant t.
    accessory t.
    t. acropachy
    t. adenoma
    t. ala
    t. artery
    t. capsule
    t. carcinoma
    t. cartilage
    t. collar
    t. ima artery
    t. ima vein
    intrathoracic t.
    t. isthmus
    lingual t.
    t. lobe
    t. lobectomy
    t. nodule
    t. notch
    t. plexus
    retrosternal t.

thyroid *(continued)*
    t. storm
    t. tissue

thyroidectomy
    subtotal t.
    total t.

thyroiditis
    de Quervain granuloma-
        tous t.
    fibrous t.

thyroidotomy

thyroparathyroidectomy

thyropharyngeal muscle

thyrotomy

thyrotoxic
    t. complement-fixation fac-
        tor
    t. myopathy

tibialis
    t. anterior (anticus) flap
    t. anterior muscle
    t. posterior muscle

tibioscaphoid

tibiotarsal

tic-tac-toe classification for mu-
    tilating injuries of the hand
    (*types I–VII; subtypes A–C;
    vascular status 0–I*)

tie
    cable t.
    catgut plain t's

Tieck nasal speculum

tie-over
    t.-o. bolster
    t.-o. dressing

tightening
    eyelid t.
    plastyma muscle t.

TILT
    triquetral impingement lig-
        ament tear

tilt
    t. table test
    t. test

time
    ischemic t.

timer
    accuracy t.

TiMesh
    T. cranial mesh
    T. craniomaxillofacial plat-
        ing system
    T. emergency screw
    T. orbital mesh
    T. orthognathic strap plate
    T. patient-configured tita-
        nium craniomaxillofacial
        implant
    T. rigid fixation bone plat-
        ing system
    T. titanium mesh

T-incision

tinea
    t. amiantacea
    t. corporis
    t. dermatitis
    t. glabrosa
    t. kerion
    t. nigra
    t. tarsi
    t. unguium
    t. versicolor

Tinel sign

tip
    accelerator t.
    Becker t.
    Becker dissector t.
    Becker flat dissector t.
    Becker twist dissector t.
    t. bossing
    buccal fat extractor t.
    bulbous nasal t.
    cannula t.
    Cobra cannula t.
    Cobra K t.
    Cobra K+ cannula t.

tip *(continued)*
    Colorado electrocautery t.
    droopy nasal t.
    flap t.
    Grossan nasal irrigator t.
    Illouz modified t.
    Illouz standard t.
    Implantech SE-100 smoke
        aspiration t.
    Keel t.
    Klein cannula t.
    Klein 1-hole infiltrator t.
    Klein multihole infiltrator t.
    Leon cobra t.
    mastoid t.
    Mercedes t.
    nasal t.
    nasal t. projection
    Omni laser t.
    overprojecting nasal t.
    Pinocchio t.
    Radovan tissue expander t.
    t. rhinoplasty
    t. rotation
    soft palate t.
    suction t.
    Toledo dissector t.
    Toledo flap dissector t.
    Toledo V-dissector t.
    uvula t.
    Woolner t.

tip-plasty
    nasal t.-p.

Tisseel
    T. biologic fibrogen adhe-
        sive
    T. fibrin glue

tissue
    abdominal adipose t.
    aberrant t.
    aberrant breast t.
    t. ablation
    accessory mammary t.
    adipose t.
    adjacent t.
    areolar t.
    autogenous composite t.
    avascular t.

tissue *(continued)*
    axillary breast t.
    basement t.
    breast t.
    brown adipose t.
    calcified t.
    cancellous t.
    cartilaginous t.
    caseated t.
    cicatricial t.
    t. compression
    connective t.
    cribriform t.
    t.-cultured skin
    denuded t.
    dermoadipose t.
    devitalized soft t.
    earlobe adipose t.
    elastotic t.
    endoscopically harvested t.
    t.-engineered cartilage
    t. engineering
    ethanol-treated freeze-dried
        bone t.
    t. expander
    t. expansion
    fibroadipose t.
    fibroblastic t.
    fibrofatty t.
    fibrofatty subcutaneous t.
    fibroglandular t.
    fibromyxomatous connec-
        tive t.
    t. forceps
    friable t.
    glandular t.
    t. glue
    t.-graft engineering
    granulation t.
    granulomatous t.
    hard t.
    hemangiomatous t.
    heterologous t.
    t. hyperplasia
    incorporated t.
    interstitial t.
    keratinized t.
    mineralized t.
    t. molding

tissue *(continued)*
    nasion soft t.
    osteogenic t.
    perichondrial-periosteal t.
    radionecrotic t.
    t. reactivity
    redundant t.
    t. remodeling
    t. repair
    scar t.
    t. scissors
    SMAS (superficial muscu-
        loaponeurotic system) t.
    soft t.
    subcutaneous t.
    subcutaneous adipose t.
    subdermal nasal t.
    subjacent t.
    submucosal connective t.
    supporting t.
    thyroid t.
    vascularized t.
    weight-bearing t.

tissue expander
    AccuSpan t. e.
    Becker t. e.
    BioDIMENSIONAL t. e.
    Biospan anatomical t. e.
    Heyer-Schulte t. e.
    Heyer-Schulte subcutane-
        ous t. e.
    Integra t. e.
    Radovan t. e.
    Radovan subcutaneous t. e.
    Silastic HP t. e.
    soft t. e.
    subperiosteal t. e. (STE)
    Surgitek T-Span t. e.
    T-Span t. e.
    Versafil t. e.

titanium
    t. hollow-screw osseointe-
        grating reconstruction
        plate (THORP)
    t. hollow-screw osseointe-
        grating reconstruction
        plate (THORP) system

titanium *(continued)*
    t. hollow-screw osseointe-
        grating reconstruction
        plate (THORP)-type man-
        dibular reconstruction
        plate
    t. mandibular staple
    t. mini bur hole covering
    t. miniplate
    t. rigid fixation
    t.-sprayed IMZ implant
    t. tack

TKS laser

TLG
    tumescent liposuction gar-
        ment

TLP
    total laryngopharyngec-
        tomy

TMD
    temporomandibular dys-
        function
    temporomandibular joint
        dysfunction

TMEP
    telangiectasia macularis
        eruptiva perstans

TMI
    transmandibular implant
        TMI implant

TMJ
    temporomandibular joint
        TMJ syndrome
    temporomandibular joint
        dysfunction

TMJ-OA
    temporomandibular joint
        osteoarthritis

TMPD
    temporomandibular pain-
        dysfunction
    temporomandibular pain-
        dysfunction disorder

TNM tumor staging

Tobin
  anatomical T. malar pros-
    thetic implant

toe
  t. fillet flap
  t. fillet flap procedure
  great t.
  great t. implant
  great t. transplant
  great t. wraparound flap
  microvascular t. transfer
  t. pulp neurosensory flap
  sausage t.
  second t.
  t.-to-thumb flap
  t.-to-thumb microvascular
    transplant
  transplanted t.
  webbed t's

Toledo
  T. dissector
  T. dissector tip
  T. flap dissector tip
  T. V-dissector cannula
  T. V-dissector tip

tomography
  axial computed t. scan
  computed t. (CT)
  computed t. laser mam-
    mography
  coronal computed t. scan
  spiral computed t.
  three-dimensional compu-
    ted t. (3D CT)

tone
  cheek t.

tongue
  amyloid t.
  bald t.
  beefy t.
  bifid t.
  t. biting
  cerebriform t.
  cleft t.
  coated t.
  cobblestone t.

tongue *(continued)*
  t. depressor
  fissured t.
  forked t.
  t.-jaw-neck dissection
  lobulated t.
  magenta t.
  mappy t.
  raspberry t.
  scrotal t.
  smoker's t.
  white hairy t.
  wrinkled t.

tonsil
  Gerlach t.
  palatine t.
  pharyngeal t.

tonus
  muscle t.

tool
  Pressure Ulcer Scale for
    Healing (PUSH) T.

Toomey
  T. angled cannula
  T. G-bevel cannula
  T. standard cannula

tooth *pl.* teeth
  cheek t.
  inferior teeth
  labial teeth
  malacotic teeth
  malpositioned t.
  mandibular teeth
  maxillary teeth
  maxillary anterior t.
  maxillary posterior t.
  migrated t.
  missing t.

toothbrushing
  maxillofacial and facioprox-
    imal surface t.
  maxillopalatal and palato-
    proximal surface t.

TopiFoam gel-backed self-adhering foam pad

Topinard angle

Tornwaldt
    T. abscess
    T. cyst

Toronto
    T. two-stage mammaplasty

torque
    labial t.

torticollis
    labyrinthine t.
    muscular t.
    ocular t.

torus *pl.* tori
    t. frontalis
    t. levatorius
    mandibular t.
    t. mandibularis
    t. occipitalis
    palatine t.
    t. palatinus

total
    t. autogenous latissimus
        (TAL)
    t. body surface area (TBSA)
    t. laryngectomy
    t. laryngopharyngectomy
        (TLP)

Toti operation

Tourtual canal

tower skull

Towne projection roentgeno-
    gram

toxin
    botulinum t.
    botulinum t. type A

TPFF
    temporoparietal fascia flap
    temporoparietal fascial flap

trachea
    scabbard t.

tracheal
    t. agenesis

tracheal *(continued)*
    t. atresia
    t. fenestration
    t. stenosis
    t. web

tracing
    cephalometric t.

tract
    sinonasal t.
    sinus t.
    spinal t. of trigeminal nerve

traction
    balanced t.
    internal t.
    maxillomandibular t.

tragal
    t. border
    t. cartilage
    t. notch

tragus *pl.* tragi

Trainor-Nida operation

TRAM
    transverse rectus abdomi-
        nis musculocutaneous
        distraction TRAM
        TRAM flap
        TRAM flap breast re-
            construction
        TRAM flap hernia
        free TRAM flap
    transverse rectus abdomi-
        nis myocutaneous
        distraction TRAM
        TRAM flap
        TRAM flap breast re-
            construction
        TRAM flap hernia
        free TRAM flap

TRAMP
    transversus and rectus ab-
        dominis musculoperito-
        neal

transareolar mastectomy

transaxillary breast augmentation

transblepharoplasty
t. approach
t. forehead lift
t. procedure
t. subperiosteal midface elevation

transconjunctival
t. blepharoplasty (TCB)
t. endoscopic orbital de-
compression
t. lower lid blepharoplasty

transcoronal eyebrow lift

transcranial
t. facial bipartition
t. monobloc frontofacial advancement

Transcyte skin substitute graft

transection
platysmal t.

transfer
buried free forearm flap t.
dermal fat free tissue t.
facial paralysis reconstruction with free muscle t.
facial paralysis reconstruction with gracilis free
muscle t.
facial paralysis reconstruction with pectoralis minor
muscle t.
facial paralysis reconstruction with rectus abdomi-
nis muscle t.
free muscle t.
free omental flap t.
free tissue t. (FTT)
gracilis free muscle t.
hypoglossal-to-facial
nerve t.
ilium microvascular t.
island frontalis muscle t.
masseter muscle t.
microvascular bone t.

transfer *(continued)*
microvascular free flap t.
microvascular free gracilis t.
microvascular free tissue t.
microvascular toe t.
muscle t.
nerve t.
pectoralis minor muscle t.
rectus abdominis muscle t.
regional muscle t.
scapular flap t.
segmental microvascular
t's
staged muscle t.
temporalis muscle–fascia t.
tendon t.
toe-to-hand t.
toe-to-thumb t.
vascularized whole joint t.
Zancolli lasso tendon t.

transfixation
t. incision
t. suture

transformation
malignant t.

transforming
t. growth factor (TGF)
t. growth factor beta (TGF-
β)

transition
feather the t.

transmandibular
t. implant (TMI)
t. reconstruction

Transonic laser Doppler perfusion monitor

transosseous implant

transpalpebral approach

transplant
alloplastic t.
autogenous t.
bone marrow t. (BMT)
great toe t.

transplant *(continued)*
  homogenous t.
  laser hair t.
  toe-to-thumb microvascu-
    lar t.

transplantation
  allogeneic t.
  allograft tissue t.
  autologous fat t.
  free t. of nipple
  hair t.
  heterotopic t.
  laser hair t.
  segmental gracilis muscle t.
  tendon t.
  valve t.

transport
  mucociliary t. (MCT)

transposition
  bilateral advancement t.
    (BAT)
  bilateral gluteus maximus t.
  t. flap
  t. of graft
  muscle t.
  nipple t.
  omental t.
  parotid duct t.
  temporalis muscle t.
  valve t.
  Z-plasty t.

transseptal

transsexual
  male-to-female t.

transudate
  mucosal t.

Trans-Ver-Sal AdultPatch

transverse
  t. abdominal island flap
  t. arytenoid muscle
  t. muscle of tongue
  t. myocutaneous flap
  t. rectus abdominis muscu-
    locutaneous (TRAM)
  t. rectus abdominis myocu-
    taneous (TRAM)

transversus
  t. abdominis muscle
  t. linguae muscle
  musculus t. menti muscle
  t. perinei profundus muscle
  t. and rectus abdominis
    musculoperitoneal
    (TRAMP) composite flap
  t. thoracis muscle

trap
  Lukens t.

trapezius
  t. muscle
  t. muscle/myocutaneous
    flap

trauma
  auricular t.
  iatrogenic t.
  laryngotracheal t.
  midface t.
  occlusal t.
  occult t.
  oral t.

traumatism
  secondary occlusal t.

Trautmann
  T. angle
  T. triangular space

Treacher Collins
  T. C. deformity
  T. C. syndrome (TCS)

treatment
  Abdopatch Gel Z self-adhe-
    sive scar t.
  burn scar t.
  Mammopatch gel self-adhe-
    sive scar t.
  Obagi Blue Peel skin peel t.
  Pad Medipatch Gel Z self-
    adhesive scar t.

Treitz ligament

Trelles metal scleral shield

trench foot

trephine
  Blakesley lacrimal t.
  Boiler septal t.
  mini t.

tretinoin

triad
  Franke t.
  Kartagener t.

trial
  Multicenter Selective Lymphadenectomy t.

triangle
  Assézat t.
  Béclard t.
  Bonwill t.
  Burow t. deformity
  calibrated t. of septal cartilage
  digastric t.
  facial t.
  Kiesselbach t.
  Macewen t.
  retromandibular t.
  soft t. of the nose
  submandibular t.
  submaxillary t.
  submental t.
  suboccipital t.

triangular
  t. cartilage
  t. crest
  t. eminence
  t. fibrocartilage complex (TFCC)
  t. fibrocartilage complex (TFCC) débridement
  t. fibrocartilage complex (TFCC) meniscus tear
  t. fibrocartilage complex (TFCC) tear
  t. fibrocartilage compound
  t. fibrocartilage meniscus
  t. fold
  t. fontanelle
  t. fossa

triangular (continued)
  t. island flap
  t. muscle

trichloroacetic acid (TCA)
  t. a. peel

trichorhinophalangeal syndrome

Tricodur compression support bandage

trigger finger

trigone
  submandibular t.

trigonocephaly

trilobed
  t. cloverleaf skull
  t. skull

trim
  lateral t. of the adenoid

trimmer
  model t.

trimming
  muscle t.

Tripier operation

triquetral impingement ligament tear (TILT)

triscaphe joint

triturator
  mechanical t.

Trömner reflex

trophoneurosis
  lingual t.
  Romberg t.

trough
  infraorbital tear t.

Trousseau spot

Truc operation

Tru-Pulse
  T.-P. carbon dioxide laser

Tru-Pulse *(continued)*
  T.-P. CO$_2$ skin resurfacing laser

trusion
  mandibular t.
  maxillary t.

T-shaped
  T-s. graft
  T-s. scar

T-Span tissue expander

TSTI
  tumor-specific transplantation immunity

tube
  anesthetic t.
  aspirating t.
  Gore-Tex t.
  Guibor Silastic t.
  Hemovac suction t.
  Laryngoflex reinforced endotracheal t.
  Laser-Shield XII wrapped endotracheal t.
  Laser Trach wrapped endotracheal t.
  Lukens collecting t.
  Montgomery T t.
  Moss balloon triple-lumen gastrostomy t.
  neural t.
  salivary t.
  silicone t.
  suction t.
  tear duct t.
  Wookey skin t.

tubercle
  articular t.
  articular t. of temporal bone
  auricular t.
  auricular t. of Darwin
  corniculate t.
  darwinian t.
  genial t.
  labial t.

tubercle *(continued)*
  Lister t.
  marginal t.
  marginal t. of zygomatic bone
  mental t.
  mental t. of mandible
  Montgomery t's
  philtral t.
  Santorini t.
  scaphoid t.
  t. of upper lip
  Whitnall t. of zygoma
  Wrisberg t.
  zygomatic t.

tuberculosis
  laryngeal t.

tuberculum
  t. dentis

tuberosity
  malar t.
  maxillary t.
  pterygoid t. of mandible
  pyramidal t. of palatine bone

Tubigrip elastic support bandage

d-tubocurarine block

tubule
  mucous t.

tuck
  chin t.

Tucker mediastinoscope

Tulip cannula

tumescent liposuction garment (TLG)

tumor
  t. ablation
  acinic cell t.
  adenopapillary t.
  adnexal skin t.
  t. angiogenic factor (TAF)

tumor *(continued)*
  anterior pillar t.
  atypical carcinoid t.
  basaloid t.
  Bednar t.
  benign t.
  benign mesenchymal t.
  benign mixed t.
  Brooke t.
  calcifying epithelial odonto-
    genic t.
  carotid body t.
  central giant cell t.
  cerebellopontine angle t.
  craniopharyngeal duct t.
  deep-lobe parotid t.
  de novo t.
  dermal analogue t.
  epidermoid t.
  fatty t.
  fibrofatty t.
  fungating t.
  glomus t.
  Godwin t.
  Hürthle cell t.
  infantile vascular t.
  intracranial t.
  intraparotid mesenchy-
    mal t.
  keloid t.
  keratinizing epithelial
    odontogenic t.
  lipogenic t.
  t. lysis factor
  malignant odontogenic t.
  melanotic neuroectoder-
    mal t.
  melanotic neuroectodermal
    t. of infancy
  mesenchymal t.
  mesodermal t.
  metachronous t.
  mixed t.
  mixed t. of salivary gland
  mucoepidermoid t.
  multicentric glomus t.
  t. necrosis factor
  neural sheath t.
  neuroendocrine t.

tumor *(continued)*
  neuroendocrine t. of larynx
  neurogenic t.
  parapharyngeal t.
  parotid t.
  pilar t. of scalp
  ropy t.
  salivary gland t.
  Schwann t.
  SCM (sternocleidomastoid)
    t. of infancy
  serous t.
  skin t.
  soft tissue t.
  t.-specific transplantation
    immunity (TSTI)
  spindle cell t.
  squamous odontogenic t.
  sternocleidomastoid (SCM)
    t. of infancy
  strawberry t.
  vascular t.
  vasoformative t.
  villous t.
  Warthin t.
  Wharton t.

tunable
  argon t. dye laser
  t. dye laser
  t. dye laser with Hexascan
  t. flashlamp-excited pulsed
    dye laser
  pulsed t. dye laser
  t. tinnitus masker

tunica
  t. adventitia
  t. conjunctiva
  t. media
  t. palpebrarum
  t. vaginalis

tunnel
  double t.
  fibro-osseous t.
  stylomandibular t.

tunneled supraclavicular island
  flap for head and neck reconstruction

turbinate
    bulbous t's
    inferior t.
    middle t.
    superior t.
turgor
"turnover" flap
turricephaly
Tweed
    T. analysis
    T. method
twig
    nerve t.

twin
    conjoined t's

Twist
    T. MTX implant
    T. Ti implant

tympanomastoid fissure

type
    collagen t.

Typhoon cutter blade

Tyrrell skin hook

U
  U-flap
  reverse U-flap
  U-shaped arch
  U-shaped curve
  U-shaped incision
  U-shaped interdigitated
    muscle flap
  U-shaped scar
  U-shaped skin excision

UAL
  ultrasound-assisted lipec-
    tomy

UCLA
  unilateral cleft lip/alveolus
    isolated UCLA

U-flap
  reverse U-f.

UHMWP
  ultra-high-molecular-weight
    polyethylene

ulatrophy
  ischemic u.

ulcer
  amputating u.
  aphthous u.
  arterial u.
  atonic u.
  Barrett u.
  cold u.
  decubitus u.
  diabetic foot u.
  follicular u.
  gravitational u.
  hard u.
  herpetic u.
  hindfoot u.
  indolent u.
  inflamed u.
  ischemic u.
  Jacob u.
  Marjolin u.
  Meleney u.
  metatarsal u.
  moorean u.

ulcer *(continued)*
  necrotic u.
  oropharyngeal u.
  perambulating u.
  perforating u. of foot
  phagedenic u.
  phlegmonous u.
  plantar forefoot u.
  recalcitrant u.
  recurrent u.
  recurrent aphthous u.
  ring u.
  rodent u.
  Saemisch u.
  serpiginous u.
  sickle cell u.
  sloughing u.
  soft u.
  stasis u.
  stasis vascular u.
  steroid u.
  sublingual u.
  Sutton u.
  tarsal u.
  traumatic u.
  trophic u.
  undermining u.
  varicose u.
  vascular u.
  venous stasis u.
  venous u.
  warty u.

ulcerated granuloma

ulceration
  agranulocytic u.
  corneal u.
  superficial u.
  venous leg u.

Ulloa operation

ulnar
  u. deviation
  u. deviation deformity

ulnarward

Ultimatics
  U. demineralized cortical
    bone powder

Ultimatics *(continued)*
U. flexible laminar bone strip

ultrabrachycephalic

Ultraflex ankle dorsiflexion dynamic splint

ultra-high-molecular-weight polyethylene (UHMWP)

ultraprognathous

UltraPulse
U. carbon dioxide laser
U. carbon dioxide laserbrasion
U. CO_2 laser

ultrasonic
u. liposculpturing
u. liposuction
u. scalpel

ultrasound-assisted
u.-a. lipectomy (UAL)
u.-a. liposuction

ultrasound-guided biopsy

umbilical
u. ring
u. stalk
u. vein

umbilicoplasty

umbilicus

umbrella
u. graft
u. punctum plug

unaesthetic *(variant of* unesthetic)

unciform

uncinate process

uncinatum

undercut
soft tissue u.

underlayer cantilever bone graft

underlay fascia technique

undermine

undermining
cross-hatching u.
u. resorption
single-hatching u.
u. ulcer

undifferentiated
u. carcinoma of nasopharyngeal type
u. connective tissue disease

unesthetic *(also spelled* unaesthetic)
u. contour deformity

unfurling
u. of anthelix

unicoronal synostosis

unilambdoid synostosis

unilaminar
u. membrane
u. skin substitute

Unilase CO_2 laser

unilateral
u. abductor paralysis
u. adductor paralysis
u. cleft lip
u. cleft lip nose deformity
u. cleft lip and palate
u. coronal synostosis
u. facial hypertrophy
u. hypertrophy
u. macroglossia
u. Millard repair
u. plagiocephaly
u. vocal cord paralysis (UVCP)

UniMax 2000 laser micromanipulator

union
bony u.
fracture with cross u.

union *(continued)*
    fracture with delayed u.

unit
    Dalbo extracoronal u.
    Dalbo stud u.
    Ocoee scalp cleansing u.
    ostiomeatal u. (OMU)
    philtral u.

Universal
    U. handle with nasal-cutting tips
    U. nasal saw blade
    U. nerve hook

unmeshed
    u. split-thickness skin graft

unmyelinated
    u. nerve fiber

Unna disease

unoperated cleft

unpedicled flap

unrepositioned flap

unresectable squamous cell carcinoma

upper
    u. airway
    u. arch
    u. bound
    u. cervical nerve
    u. face rejuvenation
    u. lateral nasal cartilage
    u. lip
    u. lip length
    u. reticular dermal peel
    u. reticular dermal penetration
    u. tooth to u. lip relationship
    u. universal forceps

upturned forceps

upward
    u. bent forceps
    u. masking

uraniscochasma

uraniscoplasty

uraniscorrhaphy

uranoplastic

uranoplasty
    Wardill-Kilner four-flap u.

uranorrhaphy

uranoschisis

uranoschism

uranostaphyloplasty

uranostaphylorrhaphy

uranostaphyloschisis

uranosteoplasty

urethra
    hypoplastic u.

urethral
    u. meatus
    u. plate
    u. reconstruction
    u. stricture

urethrocutaneous fistula

urethroplasty

Uroplastique material

urticaria
    cold u.
    solar u.

U-shaped
    U-s. arch
    U-s. curve
    U-s. incision
    U-s. interdigitated muscle flap
    U-s. scar
    U-s. skin excision

uteroplasty

utility
    u. arch

utility *(continued)*
    u. glove

utricular duct

utriculosaccular duct

UVCP
    unilateral vocal cord paral-
        ysis

uveoparotid fever

uvula
    bifid u.
    cleft u.
    forked u.
    u. palatina
    palatine u.
    pendulous u.
    split u.
    u. muscle
    u. tip

uvular
    u. muscle

uvulatome

uvulectomy

uvulitis

uvulopalatopharyngoplasty
    (UPPP)

uvulopalatoplasty (UPP)
    laser-assisted u. (LAUP)
    u. procedure

uvulopharyngeal

uvuloptosis

uvulotome

uvulotomy

V

V flap
V-shaped erosion
V-shaped skin excision
V-shaped wound

VAC
vacuum-assisted closure

vaginal
v. agenesis
v. atresia
v. dimple
v. epithelialization
v. malformation
v. process of sphenoid
bone

vaginalis
tunica v.

vaginoperineal reconstruction

vaginoperineoplasty

vaginoplasty
colon interposition v.
free flap v.
intestinal v.
penile skin inversion v.
v. procedure

vagotomy

vagus nerve

Vail syndrome

Valentin
V. ganglion
V. nerve

vallate papilla

vallecula *pl.* valleculae
v. epiglottica
v. for petrosal ganglion

Valsalva
V. antrum
V. ligaments
V. maneuver
V. muscle

Valtrac anastomosis ring

valve
anterior nasal v.
BacStop check v.
Béraud v.
Bianchi v.
Bochdalek v.
breast implant v.
check v.
dysfunctional nasal v.
Foltz v.
Hasner v.
Huschke v.
incompetent v.
Krause v.
Montgomery speaking v.
nasal v.
Rosenmüller v.
Taillefer v.
v. transplantation
v. transposition
velopharyngeal v.

valvular
v. incompetence
superficial v. insufficiency

valvuloplasty

Van Beek-Zook technique

van Buchem
van B. disease
van B. syndrome

van Buren disease

van der Hoeve syndrome

Van der Woude syndrome

vanishing bone disease

Van Lint
Van L. akinesia
Van L.-Atkinson lid akinetic
block

Van Millingen
Van M. eyelid repair tech-
nique
Van M. graft
Van M. operation

Van Nes procedure

vaporization

variance
ulnar v.
ulnar-minus v.
ulnar-plus/neutral v.
ulnar-plus v.
ulnar-positive v.
zero v.

variant
dystrophic v.
Miller-Fisher v. of Guillain-
Barré syndrome
v. nerve
v. neurofibromatosis
orthokeratinized v.
parakeratinized v.

varicella
v. gangrenosa

varicella-zoster

varicelliform
v. lesion
v. rash

varicoblepharon

varicophlebitis

varicose
v. ulcer
v. vein

varicosity
spider v.
superficial v.
venous v.

varicosis

variegated lesions

varix *pl.* varices
anastomotic v.
esophageal v.
papillary varices

varnish
mastic v.

Vasconez tensor fasciae latae
flap

vascular
v. birthmark
v. bulldog
v. bundle
v. bundle implantation
v. bundle implantation into
bone
cutaneous v. anomaly
v. endothelial growth factor (VEGF)
v. endothelium
v. graft
v. hypotension
infantile v. tumor
v. lesion therapy
macular v. birthmark
v. malformation
v. mass
v. neoplasm
v. nevus
v. nidus
v. occlusive disease
v. pedicle
v. pericyte of Zimmerman
v. proliferation
v. tumor
v. ulcer

vascularis
nevus v.

vascularity
v. flap

vascularization
reverse flow v.

vascularize

vascularized
v. bone graft (VBG)
v. calvarial flap
v. fascial patch
v. island bone flap
v. tendon graft
v. tibial bone flap
v. whole joint transfer

vasculitic lesion

vasculitis
Churg-Strauss v.

vasculitis *(continued)*
    cutaneous v.
    granulomatous v.
    large vessel v.
    livedo v.
    necrotizing v.
    nodular v.
    nodular granulomatous v.
    rheumatoid v.
    segmental hyalinizing v.
    small vessel v.
    urticarial v.

vasculogenesis

vasculum *pl.* vascula

Vaseline
    V.-coated gauze
    V. petrolatum packing

vaselinized nasal tamponage

vasoconstriction

vasoconstrictive agent

vasodilating agent

vasodilation
    active v.
    local v.
    passive v.

vasoformative tumor

vasoganglion

vasomotor
    v. rhinitis

vasopressor

vasospasm

vastus
    v. lateralis flap
    v. lateralis muscle
    v. medialis
    v. medialis muscle
    v. medialis obliquus muscle

Vater
    V. corpuscles
    papilla of V.

Vater *(continued)*
    V.-Pacini corpuscles

Vaughan-Jackson lesion

vault
    cartilaginous v.
    nasal v.
    v. of pharynx

Vbeam pulsed dye laser

VBG
    vascularized bone graft

Veau
    V. classification
    V. cleft lip repair
    cleft muscle of V.
    V. elevator
    V. operation
    V. palatoplasty
    V. straight-line closure
    V.-Axhausen operation
    V.-Wardill palatal pushback
    V.-Wardill-Kilner cleft palate repair
    V.-Wardill-Kilner palatoplasty
    V.-Wardill-Kilner pushback operation
    V.-Wardill-Kilner repair

vector
    v. of aging
    lift v.
    v. of skin pull
    suspension v.

Veeneklaas syndrome

vegetans
    pemphigus v.

VEGF
    vascular endothelial growth factor

Vehe carver

veiling
    v. of the alar rim

vein
    angular v.

    angular facial v.
    anterior auricular v.
    anterior condylar v.
    anterior tibial v.
    auricular v's
    Breschet v's
    common anterior facial v.
    common facial v.
    condylar emissary v.
    deep v.
    deep inferior epigastric v.
    dorsal v.
    external jugular v.
    inferior thyroid v.
    internal jugular v.
    jugular v.
    Labbé v.
    laryngeal v.
    mastoid emissary v.
    maxillary v.
    middle thyroid v.
    palmar digital v's
    perforating v.
    peroneal v.
    posterior tibial v.
    ranine v.
    retroauricular v.
    retromandibular v.
    Santorini v.
    spider v.
    spiral v.
    sternocleidomastoid v.
    v. stripping
    stylomastoid v.
    sublingual v.
    submental v.
    superficial v.
    superficial circumflex il-
      iac v.
    superficial temporal v.
    superior laryngeal v.
    superior palpebral v.
    superior thyroid v.
    temporal v.
    temporal diploic v.
    thyroid ima v.
    umbilical v.
    varicose v.

vein *(continued)*
    vesalian v.
    Vesalius v.
    vidian v.

velar
    v. area
    v. assimilation
    v. insufficiency

vellus hair

velocardiofacial syndrome

velopharyngeal
    v. closure
    v. competence (VPC)
    v. competency
    v. function
    v. incompetence (VPI)
    v. insufficiency (VPI)
    v. isthmus
    v. portal
    v. seal
    v. valve

velopharynx

veloplasty
    functional v.
    intravelar v.

velosynthesis

velum *pl.* vela
    artificial v.
    Baker v.
    nursing v.
    v. palati
    palatine v.
    v. palatinum
    v. pendulum palati

vena comitans *pl.* venae co-
mitantes

venogram

venography
    jugular v.

venous
    ambulatory v. hypertension
    v. anomaly
    v. claudication

venous *(continued)*
  v. drainage
  v. engorgement
  v. flap
  v. flow
  v. hemodynamics
  v. hemorrhage
  v. hypertension
  v. insufficiency
  v. lake
  v. leg ulceration
  v. loop
  v. malformation
  v. pressure gradient support stockings (VPGSS)
  v. ulcer
  v. valvular competence

venous-to-venous anastomosis

vented earmold

venter
  v. frontalis musculi occipitofrontalis
  v. musculi
  v. propendens

Ventex dressing

ventricle
  Galen v.
  laryngeal v.
  Morgagni v.

ventriculocordectomy

ventriculus *pl.* ventriculi
  v. laryngis

venula *pl.* venulae
  v. nasalis retinae inferior
  v. nasalis retinae superior
  v. temporalis retinae inferior
  v. temporalis retinae superior

venule
  inferior nasal v. of retina
  inferior temporal v. of retina
  main v. (MV)

venule *(continued)*
  pericytic v's
  postcapillary v's
  superior nasal v. of retina
  superior temporal v. of retina

vera
  neuralgia facialis v.

Verdan
  V. graft
  V. tendon repair
  V. zone system

Verga lacrimal groove

verge
  nasal v.

vermilion
  v. Abbe flap
  v. border
  v. border of lip
  central v.
  dry v.
  v. enhancement
  v. margin
  v. notching
  philtral v.
  projection of v.
  v.-skin junction
  v. surface of lip
  wet v.
  v.–white line malalignment

vermilionectomy

Vernet syndrome

Verneuil
  hidradenitis axillaris of V.
  V. neuroma

Verocay bodies

verruca *pl.* verrucae
  v. digitata
  v. filiformis
  v. plana juvenilis
  v. plana senilis
  recalcitrant v.
  seborrheic v.

verruca *(continued)*
  v. senilis
  v. simplex
  v. vulgaris

verruciform
  v. xanthoma

verruciformis
  acrokeratosis v.
  epidermodysplasia v.

verrucose

verrucosis
  lymphostatic v.

verrucosus
  lichen planus v.
  lupus v.
  nevus v.

verrucous
  v. angiokeratoma
  v. carcinoma
  v. hemangioma
  v. hyperplasia
  v. nevus
  v. scrofuloderma
  v. xanthoma

Versafil tissue expander

VersaLight laser

Versi-Splint

vertex *pl.* vertices
  v. of bony cranium
  v. cranii
  v. cranii ossei

vertical
  v. angulation
  v. axis
  v. bipedicle flap
  v. bone loss
  v. bony height
  v. corrugator line
  v. dysplasia
  v. elliptical incision
  v. face-lift
  v. facial height
  v. fracture

vertical *(continued)*
  v. glabellar crease
  v. glabellar frown lines
  v. lip biopsy
  v. mammaplasty
  v. mandibular opening
  v. mattress suture
  v. maxillary excess (VME)
  v. midline approach
  v. oblique pattern fracture
  v. osteotomy
  v. osteotomy of ramus of
    mandible
  v. overbite
  v. plate of palatine
  v. ramus mandibular oste-
    otomy
  v. resorption
  v. rhomboid deepithelializ-
    ation
  v. scar

verticalis linguae muscle

verticomental

vertigo
  labyrinthine v.

Verwey eyelid operation

vesalian vein

Vesalius
  V. bone
  V. foramen
  V. vein

vesicant
  epidermolytic v.

vesicle
  matrix v's
  olfactory v.
  simple v.

vesicobullous lesion

vesicopustular eruption

vesicula *pl.* vesiculae

vesicular
  v. dermatitis

vesicular *(continued)*
    v. eruption
    v. stomatitis

vesiculated

vesiculation
    creeping v.
    intraepidermal v.
    subepidermal v.

vesiculiform

vesiculobullous
    v. lesion

vesiculopapular

vesiculopustular

vessel
    absorbent v's
    afferent v.
    anastomotic v.
    capillary v.
    choke v.
    circumflex v.
    collateral v.
    efferent v.
    fasciocutaneous v.
    feeding v's
    friable v.
    intercostal v.
    lymphatic v.
    lymphatic v's of mouth
    mucosal blood v.
    nutrient v.
    palatine v.
    perforator v.
    periosteal v.
    recipient v.
    submucosal v's
    supporting v.

vestibular
    v. abscess
    v. cyst
    v. deafferentation
    v. epithelium
    v. mucosa
    v. oral plate
    v. papilla

vestibule
    buccal v.
    v. of cheek
    labial v.
    laryngeal v.
    mandibular v.
    v. of mouth
    nasal v.
    v. of pharynx
    v. of vagina

vestibulitis
    nasal v.

vestibulo-ocular

vestibuloplasty
    Kazanjian v.

vestibulotomy
    Edlan v.
    Kazanjian v.

vestibulum *pl.* vestibula
    v. glottidis
    v. laryngis
    v. nasi
    v. oris
    v. vaginae

V flap

vibesate

vibex

Viboch iliac graft retractor

vibrissa *pl.* vibrissae

Vicryl
    braided V. suture
    coated V. Rapide suture
    V. mesh
    V. Rapide absorbable suture
    V. suture
    V. suture material

Victoreen digital densitometer

vide infra

vidian
    v. artery

vidian *(continued)*
- v. canal
- v. nerve
- v. neuralgia
- v. vein

Viegas staging for lunotriquetral instability

Vienna nasal speculum

Vienns Britetrac nasal speculum

view
- anterior v.
- bird's eye v.
- buccal v.
- bucket-handle v. of facial
  bones
- Caldwell v.
- caudocranial v.
- chin-nose v.
- frontal v.
- incisal quadrant v.
- intaglio v.
- jughandle v.
- laryngoscopic v.
- lateral oblique transcranial v.
- mandibular occlusal v.
- maxillary occlusal v.
- Mayer v.
- occipitomeatal v.
- occlusal quadrant v.
- panoramic v.
- Panorex v.
- retromammary v.
- roentgenographic v.
- submentocervical v.
- supinated oblique v. on
  x-ray
- tangential v.
- Waters v.
- worm's eye v.

Vigilon
- V. gel dressing
- V. semipermeable nonoc-
  clusive dressing
- V. synthetic occlusive
  dressing

Vilex plastic surgery instrument

villonodular
- v. synovitis

villous
- v. fold
- v. papillae of tongue
- v. tumor

villus *pl.* villi
- lingual villi
- synovial villi

villusectomy

Vincent
- V. angina
- V. disease
- V. infection
- V. stomatitis
- V. white mycetoma

viral
- v. arthritis
- v. envelope
- v. hepatitis
- v. infection
- v. sialadenitis
- v. vesicular stomatitis
- v. wart

Virchow
- V. angle
- V. cells
- V. corpuscles
- V. crystals
- V. disease
- V. law
- V. sentinel node
- V. skin graft knife
- V.-Holder angle

virginal hypertrophy

virilization

virucidal

virulence

virulent

virus
- adenosatellite v.

virus *(continued)*
  adenovirus
  attenuated v.
  bacterial v.
  Coxsackie v.
  Epstein-Barr v. (EBV)
  herpes v.
  herpes simplex v.
  herpes zoster v.
  hepatitis v.
  human mammary tumor v.
    (HMTV)
  human papilloma v.
  infectious hepatitis v.
  infectious papilloma v.
  influenza v.
  lymphadenopathy-associa-
    ted v. (LAV)
  measles v.
  mumps v.
  neurotropic v.
  oncogenic v.
  parainfluenza v.
  poliovirus
  respiratory syncytial v.
  rhinovirus
  rubella v.
  salivary gland v.
  v. shedding
  varicella-zoster v.
  West Nile v.
  western equine encephalo-
    myelitis v.

Visage Cosmetic Surgery System

VISA multi-patient monitor

viscerocranium

viscoelastic
  v. deformation
  v. property of skin

viscosity

viscous

viscus *pl.* viscera

VISI
  volar intercalated segmen-
    tal instability

Vismark skin marker

visor
  v. angle
  v. flap
  v. osteotomy

Vitallium
  V. alloy
  V. device
  V. plate
  V. screw

Vitek
  V. interpositional implant
  V.-Kent hemi TMJ replace-
    ment system
  V.-Kent total TMJ replace-
    ment system

vitiligines

vitiliginous

vitiligo
  acrofacial v.
  v. capitis
  Cazenave v.
  circumscribed v.
  localized v.
  perinevic v.
  segmental v.

Vitremer glass-ionomer restorative material

VNUS
  VNUS Closure catheter
  VNUS radiofrequency gen-
    erator
  VNUS Restore catheter

VNO
  vomeronasal organ

Vogel
  V. operation
  V. otoplasty

Vogt
  V. angle
  V. cephalodactyly

voice
  male soprano v.

voice *(continued)*
   muffled v.
   myxedema v.

volar
   v. beak ligament
   v. carpal ligament
   v. flap advancement
   v. intercalated segmental
    instability (VISI)
   v. interosseous fascia
   v. plate deficiency
   v. radiocarpal ligament
   v. tissue flap
   v. transverse incision

Volkmann
   V. bone curet
   V. bone hook
   V. canals
   V. cheilitis
   V. claw hand deformity
   V. contracture
   V. fracture
   V. ischemic contracture
   V. ischemic paralysis
   V. spoon

volume
   bony v.
   breast v.

volvulus

vomer
   v. flap
   v. mucosa

vomerine
   v. groove
   v. ridge
   v. spur

vomeronasal
   v. cartilage
   v. organ (VNO)

vomeropremaxillary crest

von Bardeleben
   prefrontal bone of von B.

von Bezold abscess

von Blaskovics-Doyen operation

von Brun flap

von Brunn membrane

von Ebner
   von E. glands
   imbrication lines of von E.
   incremental lines of von E.
   von E. line
   lines of von E.

von Ihring plane

von Koss method

von Langenbeck
   von L. bipedicle mucoperiosteal flap
   von L. method repair
   von L. palatal flap
   von L. palate closure
   von L. pedicle flap
   von L. periosteal repair
   von L. repair

von Meyenburg disease

von Recklinghausen (*see* Recklinghausen)

von Spee
   von S. curve
   curve of von S.

VPC
   velopharyngeal competence

VPGSS
   venous pressure gradient support stockings

VPI
   velopharyngeal incompetence
   velopharyngeal insufficiency

V-shaped
   V-s. erosion
   V-s. skin excision
   V-s. wound

vulgaris
    lupus v.

vulvovaginal reconstruction

vulvovaginoplasty
    Williams v.

V-Y
    V-Y advancement
    V-Y advancement for colu-
        mellar lengthening
    V-Y advancement flap
    V-Y advancement tech-
        nique
    V-Y closure
    double V-Y plasty with
        paired inverted Burow tri-
        angle excisions
    five-flap V-Y advancement
    V-Y flap
    V-Y island flap

V-Y *(continued)*
    V-Y lip roll mucosal ad-
        vancement
    V-Y mucosal flap
    V-Y muscle-plasty
    V-Y palatoplasty
    V-Y plasty
    V-Y procedure
    V-Y pushback
    V-Y pushback cleft palate
        repair
    V-Y pushback palatorrha-
        phy
    V-Y pushback procedure
    V-Y repair
    V-Y repair of cheek deficit
    V-Y retroposition cleft pal-
        ate repair
    V-Y transposition flap
    unilateral V-Y method

V-Z advancement in buccal
    sulcus

W
W-abdominoplasty
W arch
W-plasty revision
W-shaped incision

Waardenburg
W. syndrome
W.-Klein syndrome

W-abdominoplasty

Wadsworth lid clamp

Wagner
W. disease
W. operation
W. skull resection
W.-Baldwin technique
W.-Meissner corpuscle

Wakai spreader

Walden-Aufricht nasal retractor

Waldenström macroglobulinemia

Waldeyer
W. glands
W. throat ring
W. tonsillar ring

Walker retractor

walking bleach

wall
chest w.
infratemporal w.
lateral w. of sphenoid bone
medial w. of agger nasi cell
pharyngeal w.
tegmental w.

Wallace rule of nines

Wallenberg syndrome

wallerian degeneration

Wallstent expanding metallic
stent

Walsham
W. forceps

Walsham (continued)
W. straightener

Walther canals

waltzed flap

Wardill
modified W. method
W. palatoplasty
W. pharyngoplasty
W. technique
W.-Kilner four-flap urano-
plasty
W.-Kilner procedure
W.-Kilner V-Y palatal repair
W.-Kilner-Veau operation

wart
acuminate w.
filiform w.
flat w.
senile w.
telangiectatic w.
viral w.

Wartenberg
W. sign
W. symptom

Warthin
W. area
W. tumor
W.-Starry staining method

warty dyskeratoma

wash
pHisoHex facial w.

Washington regimen

Washio flap

washout
abdominal w.

Wassmund procedure

Waters
W. extraoral radiography
W. view
W. view radiograph
W. view roentgenogram

Waterson method

watertight
    w. closure
    w. skin closure

Watson
    W. duckbill forceps
    W. scaphoid shift test
    W. skin grafting knife
    W.-Williams conchotome

wattle

wavelength

wax
    bikini w.
    bone w.
    microcrystalline w.
    mineral w.
    montan w.

waxy finger

wear
    abnormal occlusal w.
    occlusal w.
    w. pattern

web
    constricted w. space
    w. creep
    esophageal w.
    first w. space
    laryngeal w.
    myringeal w.
    w. space
    w. space deepening
    w. space flap
    terminal w.
    thenar w.
    thumb-index w. space
    tracheal w.
    vestibular w.

webbed
    w. fingers
    w. toes

webbing

Weber
    W. glands
    W. two-point discrimina-
        tion test

Weber (continued)
    W.-Christian disease
    W.-Cockayne syndrome
    W.-Fergusson incision
    W.-Fergusson method
    modified W.-Fergusson inci-
        sion
    modified W.-Fergusson pro-
        cedure
    W.-Fergusson procedure

Webster
    W. cheiloplasty
    W. flap
    W. line
    W. modification of Bernard-
        Burow cheiloplasty
    W. needle holder
    W. operation
    W. skin graft knife
    four-flap W.-Bernard tech-
        nique

Wedelstaedt chisel

wedge
    w. biopsy
    w. excision
    Medpor Biomaterial w.
    w. resection

weeping
    w. dermatitis
    w. eczema
    w. lesion

Weerda distending operating la-
    ryngoscope

Wegener granulomatosis

Wei classification for mutilating
    injuries (types I, II)

weight-bearing tissue

weight loss

Weil
    W. basal layer
    W. basal zone
    W.-Blakesley conchotome

Weimert epistaxis packing

Weine technique

Weir
W. excision
W. pattern skin flap
W. pattern skin flap technique
W. resection of the alar base
W. technique

Weisbach angle

Weitlaner retractor

Welch Allyn LumiView portable binocular microscope

Welcker angle

well-differentiated carcinoma

well-epithelialized

well-healed scar

Werb rhinostomy scissors

Werdnig-Hoffmann disease

Werner syndrome

Werther
W. disease
W. nevus

Wescott stitch scissors

West
W. lacuna skull
W. nasal-dressing forceps
W.-Engstler skull

West Nile virus

wet
w. leather sign
w. strength
w. technique
w. vermilion

wet-to-dry dressing

Weyers
W. syndrome
W.-Fülling syndrome
W.-Thier syndrome

Wharton
W. duct
W. tumor

wheal
w. and flare
skin w.

Wheeler operation

Whip-Mix articulator

whistling
w. deformity
w. face syndrome

Whitaker malar sizer

White tenaculum

white
w. dural fold
w. fibrocartilage
w. graft rejection
w. hairy tongue
w. roll border
w. sponge nevus
w.-spot lesion

Whiting rongeur

whitlow
herpetic w.
melanotic w.
thecal w.

Whitlow and Constable alar cartilage correction

Whitnall
W. ligament
W. tubercle of zygoma

Wicherkiewicz operation

wick

Wickham striae

wide
w. decompression
w. excision
w.-field total laryngectomy
w. resection biopsy

widening
>   transverse w. of cribriform
>   plate

width
>   mesiodistal w.

Wiener
>   W. breast reduction
>   W. eyelid repair
>   W. nasal rasp

Wies operation

Wilde
>   W. ethmoid forceps
>   W. septal forceps

Wildermuth ear

Wildervanck
>   W. syndrome
>   W.-Smith syndrome

Wild operating microscope

Wilkes stage I–V

Williams vulvovaginoplasty

Willis
>   circle of W.

Wills retractor

Wilmer conjunctival and utility
>   scissors

Wilson
>   curve of W.

Winchester syndrome

windblown hand

window
>   bone w.
>   epineural w.
>   nasoantral w.
>   soft tissue w.

windowed balloon

wing
>   great w. of sphenoid bone
>   greater w. of sphenoid
>   greater w. of sphenoid
>   bone

wing (continued)
>   lesser w. of sphenoid bone
>   maxillary surface of
>   great w.
>   nasal w.
>   w. plate
>   sphenoidal w.
>   temporal surface of
>   great w.

Winkler disease

Winter facial fracture appliance

wire
>   arch w.
>   bone fixation w.
>   braided w.
>   Coffin transpalatal w.
>   Coffin-type transpalatal w.
>   w. fixation
>   w.-Gelfoam prosthesis
>   interdental w.
>   interosseous w.
>   Ivy w.
>   K-w.
>   Kirschner w.
>   labial w.
>   lingual w.
>   measuring w.
>   w. osteosynthesis
>   Quadcat w.
>   Risdon w.
>   subcuticular w.

wiring
>   circumferential w.
>   circummandibular w.
>   circumzygomatic w.
>   continuous loop w.
>   craniofacial suspension w.
>   Gilmer w.
>   interfragmentary w.
>   interosseous w.
>   mandibular w.
>   multiple loop w.
>   perialveolar w.
>   pyriform aperture w.
>   Stout continuous w.

Wise
>   W. breast incision

Wise *(continued)*
 W. pattern
 W. pattern in breast reduc-
  tion
 W. pattern mastopexy

witch
 w's chin
 w's chin deformity

Witkop-von Sallman syndrome

Wizard microdebrider

Wohlfart-Kugelberg-Welander
 disease

Wolfe
 W. breast dysplasia
 W. cheiloplasty
 W. classification of breast
  dysplasia
 W. eye forceps
 W. graft
 W. mammographic paren-
  chymal patterns
 W. method
 W. operation
 W. ptosis operation
 W.-Krause graft

Wolf-Hirschhorn syndrome

Wolff
 W. dermal curet
 W. operation

Wölfler gland

Wolfring glands

Wolman xanthomatosis

Wood
 W. light
 W. light examination

Wookey
 W. flap
 W. neck flap
 W. pharyngoesophageal re-
  construction
 W. radical neck dissection
 W. skin tube

Woolner tip

woolly-hair nevus

Woringer-Kolopp disease

working
 w. bite relation
 w. occlusal surface
 w. occlusion
 w. radiograph

worm-eaten appearance

wormian bones

Worth operation

wound
 w. approximation
 aseptic w.
 avulsed w.
 w. bed
 w. botulism
 burn w.
 w. care
 w. cavity
 chronic w.
 w. contraction
 w. covering
 w. débridement
 w. dehiscence
 delayed w. healing
 w. discharge
 w. drainage
 w. entrance
 w. excision
 w. fibroblast
 w. fever
 first intention w. closure
 full-jacketed bullet w.
 fungating w.
 gaping w.
 w. healing
 w. incision and suction
 w. infection
 w. irrigation
 w. ischemia
 lacerated w.
 w. margins
 w. matrix contraction
 missile-caused w.
 Mohs w.
 w. necrosis

wound *(continued)*
    nonhealing w.
    open w.
    penetrating w.
    perforating w.
    pressure w.
    primary w. closure
    problematic w.
    puncture w.
    radiation w.
    sacral w.
    secondary w. closure
    second intention w. closure
    septic w.
    w. seroma
    silicone-treated w.
    sternotomy w.
    superficial w.
    surgical w.
    w. tensile strength
    w. tension
    tertiary w. closure
    third intention w. closure
    traumatic w.
    V-shaped w.

Woun'Dres hydrogel dressing

Wound-Span Bridge II dressing

woven bone

W-plasty revision

wrap
    Ace w.
    Coban w.

wraparound flap

wreath
    hippocratic w.

wrench
    tightening w.
    torque w.
    torque ratchet w.

Wright
    W. needle
    W. operation

Wrightington wrist radiograph

wrinkle
    dynamic w.
    frontoglabellar w.
    glabellar w.
    w. lines
    periorbital w.
    radial w.

wrinkled tongue

wrinkling
    forehead w.
    implant shell w.
    perioral w.

Wrisberg
    W. cartilage
    cuneiform cartilage of W.
    W. tubercle

wrist
    w. block
    center of rotation of w.
    coronal MRI of w.
    degenerative joint disease
      of w.
    dorsal w. syndrome (DWS)
    dorsal w. syndrome test
    w. drop
    dynamic instability of w.
    w. extension
    extra-articular causes of w.
      pain
    w. flexion
    four-bone SLAC (scapholu-
      nate advanced collapse)
      w. reconstruction
    w. ganglion
    w. ganglionectomy
    w. mechanics
    w. radial deviation
    radial w. examination
    range of motion of the w.
    SLAC (scapholunate ad-
      vanced collapse) w.
    SLAC (scapholunate ad-
      vanced collapse) w. re-
      construction
    spaghetti w.

wrist *(continued)*
    static instability of w.
    w. ulnar deviation
    ulnar w. pain

Wristaleve

wristlet

W-shaped incision

Wucher atrophy

Würzburg
    W. fracture system
    W. maxillofacial plating system
    W. plating system
    W. reconstruction system

Würzburg *(continued)*
    revised W. mandibular reconstruction system

W-Y
    W-Y operation
    W-Y palatal repositioning
    W-Y palatoplasty

Wyburn-Mason syndrome

Wynn
    W. cleft lip operation
    W. cleft lip repair

Wyse
    W. pattern for reduction mammaplasty
    W. reduction mammaplasty

X

X
X paralysis

X-act cutaneous x-ray marker

X-Acto
X-A. blade
X-A. gouge

xanthelasma
generalized x.
x. palpebrarum

xanthelasmatosis

xanthochromia

xanthoderma

xanthoerythrodermia perstans

xanthofibroma thecocellulare

xanthogranuloma
juvenile x.
necrobiotic x.

xanthogranulomatous

xanthoma
x. diabeticorum
x. disseminatum
eruptive x.
fibrous x.
x. of joint
x. multiplex
x. palpebrarum
x. striata palmaris
x. tendinosum
tendinous x.
tuberous x.
verruciform x.
verrucous x.

xanthomatosis
x. of bone
Wolman x.

xanthomatous

xanthopsydracia

xanthosarcoma

xanthosis

Xantopren impression material

XenoDerm graft

xenogeneic
x. bone
x. graft

xenogenous

xenograft
porcine x.
x. wound covering

xenotransplantation

xeransis

xerocheilia

xeroderma
x. pigmentosum

Xeroform
X. dressing
X. gauze

xerogram

xerography

xeroma

xeromammography

xeromycteria

xerophthalmia

xeroradiography

xerosis
x. parenchymatosa
x. vulgaris

xerostomia
postradiation x.

xerostomic mucositis

xerotic
x. keratitis

xiphisternum

xiphicostal

xiphoid
x. to os pubis incision

xiphoid *(continued)*
    x. process
    x. to umbilicus incision

Xomed Doyle nasal airway
   splint

Xpanderm

X paralysis

XPS Sculpture system

x-ray
    x-r. absorption

x-ray *(continued)*
    x-r. beam
    x-r. burn
    x-r. calipers
    x-r. dermatitis
    x-r. image
    serial cephalometric x-r's
    x-r. therapy (XRT)

XRT
    x-ray therapy

Y
Y bone plate
Y configuration closure
Y flap
Y graft
Y incision
Y-plasty
Y-port connector
Y-shaped fracture
Y-shaped incision
Y-shaped scar
Y-shaped skin paddle

YAG
yttrium-aluminum-garnet
diode pumped Nd:YAG
laser
holmium:YAG laser
KTP/YAG laser
LaseAway ruby and
Q-switched Nd:YAG
laser
YAG laser
MedLite Q-Switched
YAG laser
NaturaLase Er:YAG la-
ser
QS Nd:YAG laser
Q-switched neodym-
ium:YAG laser
Q-switched ruby/YAG
laser
SharpLase Nd:YAG la-
ser
Skinlight YAG laser

YagLazr system

Yangtze edema

Yankauer
Y. ethmoid-cutting forceps
Y. nasopharyngeal specu-
lum

yaw
mother y.

yaws
Bosch y.
crab y.
foot y.

Y bone plate

Y configuration closure

yellow cartilage

Yersinia arthritis

Y flap

Y graft

Y incision

yoke
alveolar y's of mandible
alveolar y's of maxilla
cerebral y's of bone of cranium
y. of mandible
y. of maxilla
sphenoidal y.

Young
Y. frame
Y. rubber dam holder

Y-plasty

Y-port connector

Y-shaped
Y-s. fracture
Y-s. incision
Y-s. scar
Y-s. skin paddle

yttrium-aluminum-garnet (YAG)

Yunas-Varon syndrome

yuppie flu

Z
Z angle
double opposing Z-plasty
four-flap Z-plasty
Furlow double Z-plasty
Furlow double-opposing Z-plasty
Furlow double-reversing Z-plasty
Z-mammaplasty
Z-plasty
Z-plasty revision
Z-plasty technique
Z-plasty transposition
Straith Z-plasty
Tennison Z-plasty

Zancolli lasso tendon transfer

Z angle

Zeiss
Z. glands
Z. microscope
Z. operating camera
Z. operating microscope
Z./Jena surgical microscope

zero variance of articular surfaces

Zest
Z. implant
Z. implant anchor

ZF
zygomaticofrontal
bone step-off at ZF suture
ZF region
ZF suture

Zimany flap

Zimmer clip

Zimmerman
vascular pericyte of Z.

Zinn
Z. artery

Zinn (continued)
Z. ligament
Z. tendon

zipper
abdominal z.

zippered mesh

Zisser-Madden method of upper lip reconstruction

Zitelli bilobed nasal flap

Z-mammaplasty

ZMC
zygomatic malar complex
zygomatic maxillary complex

Zocchi ultrasound-assisted lipoplasty technique

zona
z. arcuata
z. corona
z. facialis
z. ophthalmica
z. serpiginosa
z. vasculosa

zone
abdominal z's
abdominal wall z's (1–4)
barrier z.
basement tissue z.
calcification z.
cell-free z.
degenerative z.
dentofacial z.
facial danger z's
grenz z.
inflammatory z.
z. of injury
intermediate z.
interpalpebral z.
Looser z's
Marchant z.
marginal z.
middle z.
necrotic z.
occlusal z.

zone *(continued)*
    red z. of lip
    three z's of a burn wound
    vermilion z.
    vermilion transitional z.
    Weil basal z.

zoograft

zoografting

zooplasty

zoster
    herpes z.

zosteriform

Zovickian flap

Z-plasty
    double opposing Z-p.
    four-flap Z-p.
    Furlow double Z-p.
    Furlow double-opposing Z-p.
    Furlow double-reversing Z-p.
    Z-p. revision
    Straith Z-p.
    Z-p. technique
    Tennison Z-p.
    Z-p. transposition

Z-stent
    Gianturco-Rösch Z-s.

Zuckerkandl's dehiscence

Zyderm
    Z. I collagen
    Z. II collagen
    Z. collagen implant
    Z. collagen injection

zygal

zygion *pl.* zygia

zygodactyly

zygoma
    depressed fracture of z.
    z. elevator
    z. hook
    malunion of z.
    Whitnall tubercle of z.

zygomatic
    z. arch
    z. arch fracture
    z. bone
    z. branch
    z. breadth
    z. buttress
    z. buttress of maxilla
    z. complex fracture
    z. crest
    displaced z. fracture
    z. eminence
    z. fissure
    z. foramen
    z. frontal nerve
    z. ligament
    z. malar complex (ZMC)
    z. margin
    z. maxillary complex (ZMC)
    z. maxillary complex fracture
    z. muscle
    z. osteocutaneous ligament
    z. osteomyelitis
    z. process
    z. process of frontal bone
    z. process of maxilla
    z. process of temporal bone
    z. recess
    z. reflex
    z. retaining ligaments
    z. suture line
    z. tubercle
    unstable z. complex fracture

zygomatic-coronoid ankylosis

zygomaticoauricular

zygomaticoauricularis

zygomaticofacial
    z. canal
    z. foramen
    z. nerve

zygomaticofrontal (ZF)
    bone step-off at z. suture
    z. region
    z. suture

zygomaticomandibular muscle

zygomaticomaxillary
    z. buttress
    z. complex
    z. fracture
    z. hypoplasia
    z. osteotomy
    z. suture

zygomatico-orbital
    z. artery
    z. foramen
    z. fracture

zygomaticosphenoid
    z. fissure

zygomaticosphenoidal suture

zygomaticotemporal
    z. canal

zygomaticotemporal *(continued)*
    z. foramen
    z. nerve
    z. suture

zygomaticus
    arcus z.
    z. major muscle
    z. minor muscle

zygomaxillare

zygomaxillary

zygon

Zylik-Joseph hook

Zyplast
    Z. collagen
    Z. implant
    Z. injectable collagen

Drugs Used in Plastic Surgery

Below are the names of generic and ℞ brand name drugs used in plastic surgery, as shown in the *Saunders Pharmaceutical Xref Book*. The drugs are categorized by their "indications"—also called "designated use," "approved use," or "therapeutic action"—which group together drugs used for a similar purpose. The indications shown below are broad categories of therapeutic action. Individual drugs may be placed in subcategories or have specifically targeted diseases beyond the scope of this listing. For complete information about the drugs listed below, including each drug's availability, specific indications, forms of administration, and dosages, please consult the current edition of *Saunders Pharmaceutical Word Book*.

Burns [*see: Wound Treatment*]
Debriding Agents [*see: Wound Treatment, Debriding Agents*]
Dressings [*see: Hemostatics; Wound Treatment, Medicated Dressings*]

Hemostatics
[*see also: Wound Treatment, Medicated Dressings*]
acetylhydrolase
Alphanate
AlphaNine
AlphaNine SD
Amicar
aminocaproic acid
anti-inhibitor coagulant complex
antihemophilic factor (AHF)
Antihemophilic Factor (Porcine) Hyate:C
aprotinin
AquaMEPHYTON
argatroban
Autoplex T
Avitene Hemostat
Benefix
Bioclate
calcium alginate fiber
cellulose, oxidized
collagen sponge, absorbable
Cyklokapron
DDAVP

Hemostatics (continued)
desmopressin acetate
Ethamolin
ethanolamine oleate
factor IX complex
factor VIIa, recombinant
factor VIII SQ, recombinant
factor XIII, plasma-derived
Feiba VH Immuno
Fibrogammin P
gelatin film, absorbable
gelatin powder, absorbable
gelatin sponge, absorbable
Gelfilm; Gelfilm Ophthalmic
Gelfoam
Helistat
Helixate
Hemaseel HMN
Hemofil M
Hemonyne
Hemopad
Hemotene
Humate-P
Koāte-DVI
Koāte-HP
KoGENate
KoGENate SF
Konakion
Konyne 80
Mephyton
microfibrillar collagen hemostat (MCH)

Hemostatics (continued)
Monoclate
Monoclate P
Mononine
nonacog alfa
Novastan
NovoSeven
Oxycel
Pafase
phytonadione (vitamin K_1)
Profilate HP
Profilate OSD
Profilnine SD
Proplex T
Recombinate
ReFacto
Sorbsan
Stimate
Surgicel
thrombin
Thrombin-JMI
Thrombinar
Thrombogen
Thrombostat
tranexamic acid
Trasylol

Wound Treatment
Wound Treatment, Debriding Agents
Accuzyme
ananain
collagenase
comosain
Debrisan
Dermuspray

Wound Treatment, Debriding Agents (continued)
desoxyribonuclease
dextranomer
Elase
Elase-Chloromycetin
fibrinolysin, human
Granulderm
Granulex
GranuMed
Panafil
Panafil White
papain
Santyl
sutilains
Travase
trypsin, crystallized
Vianain
Wound Treatment, Medicated Dressings
[see also: Hemostatics]
Adcon-L
Adcon-P
Apligraf
cadexomer iodine
carbohydrate polymer gel
DuraGen
Furacin Soluble Dressing
Iamin
mafenide
mafenide acetate
nitrofurazone
povidone-iodine
prezatide copper acetate
scarlet red
Scarlet Red Ointment Dressings
Sulfamylon

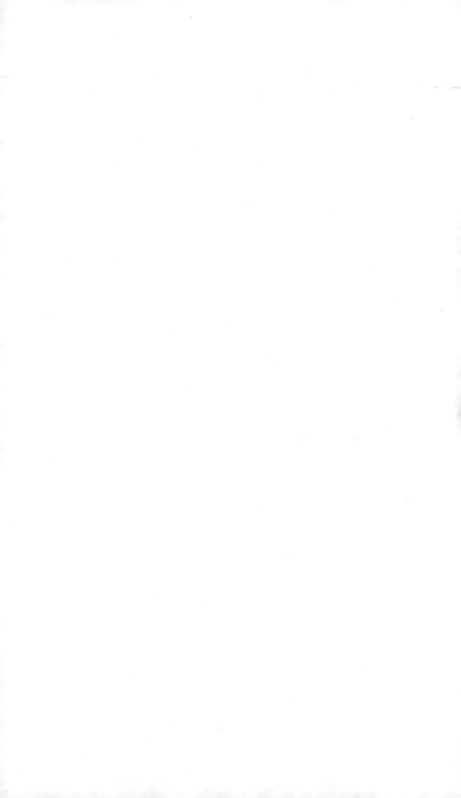